Ovarian Cancers

Eric Pujade-Lauraine
Isabelle Ray-Coquard • Fabrice Lécuru
Editors

Ovarian Cancers

Advances through International Research Cooperation (GINECO, ENGOT, GCIG)

Springer

Editors
Eric Pujade-Lauraine
AP-HP
Hôtel-Dieu
Paris
France

Fabrice Lécuru
Chirurgie cancérologique
HEGP
Paris
France

Isabelle Ray-Coquard
Centre Léon Bérard
Université Claude Bernard
Lyon
France

ISBN 978-3-319-32108-0 ISBN 978-3-319-32110-3 (eBook)
DOI 10.1007/978-3-319-32110-3

Library of Congress Control Number: 2016953670

Printed on acid-free paper

This Springer imprint is published by Springer Nature
The registered company is Springer International Publishing AG Switzerland

Preface

Ovarian cancer is the leading cause of death from gynecological cancers in western countries. A huge effort in clinical research has been conducted during the last 20 years thanks to a unique organization of national networks dedicated to gynecology oncology. National networks, such as GINECO (Groupe des Investigateurs Nationaux pour l'Etude des Cancers de l'Ovaire et du sein) in France, have grouped together and joined forces at the European level through the ENGOT (European Network of Gynecology Oncology Trials). This European network has been integrated at a global level within GCIG (Gynecologic Cancer InterGroup) with twice a year meetings, offering to Europe, America, Asia, and Australia a platform for scientific exchange and debates.

Treatment of advanced ovarian cancer (FIGO stages III and IV) until recently consisted of cytoreductive surgery and paclitaxel/carboplatin chemotherapy. However, a great debate has risen when two consecutive trials have suggested that three cycles of neoadjuvant chemotherapy could decrease the toxicity of extensive debulking surgery. In this debate presented by F Lecuru, the most important is the selection of patients likely to benefit from neoadjuvant chemotherapy, a topic extensively covered by A Fagotti. The role of lymphadenectomy during debulking surgery with its potential side effects will be discussed by P Harter, while JM Classe will introduce hyperthermic intraperitoneal chemotherapy (HIPEC) as an experimental procedure complementary to extensive debulking surgery.

Standard intravenous paclitaxel/carboplatin chemotherapy delivered every 3 weeks is no more the only option for primary systemic treatment. Dose-dense weekly administration of paclitaxel and intraperitoneal therapy will be discussed by S Pignata. His paper will introduce the first biological therapy used in ovarian cancer (OC), namely, bevacizumab, first in class among the antiangiogenic agents.

The poly (ADP-ribose) polymerase *(*PARP*)* inhibitor olaparib is also first in class and has been recently approved in OC for patients in late relapse with a breast cancer (BRCA) gene mutation as shown by J Ledermann. This BRCA predictive value for olaparib has highlighted the increasing importance of BRCA testing in OC and the role of oncogenetics, and these are extensively outlined by D Stoppa-Lyonnet. PARP inhibitor has augmented the armamentarium of active drugs used in patients in relapse as described by J Pfisterer. However, the increasing number of lines of therapy administered to the patients with recurrent disease has raised the question of balancing benefit with quality of life, and F Joly is documenting this increasingly important topic.

New areas of extensive clinical research have appeared these last years. It has been recognized that epithelial ovarian cancer is not a unique disease, but a constellation of at least four separate diseases in addition to the predominant high-grade serous OC. D Gershenson, K Fujiwara, JE Kurtz, and J Brown are introducing you to the borderline/low-grade, clear cell, endometrioid, and mucinous carcinomas. Each of these entities has a unique molecular profile and will deserve specific therapy in the future. D Berton-Rigaud is giving an update on carcinosarcoma which is currently considered as a form of poor prognosis in high-grade serous OC. The domain of rare malignant tumors is, however, extending beyond the infrequent epithelial OC. M Seckl, N Colombo, and P Pautier are discussing the issues of germ cell, sex cord, and other very rare malignant tumors such as small cell carcinomas where tremendous advances in their knowledge have been made recently.

These rare ovarian malignant tumors are mainly diagnosed in young women for whom fertility issue is critical, pointing out the importance of this topic addressed by P Morice. On the other side of the age scale, elderly/frail patients are a growing population of OC patients, and the question of how to handle their management is addressed by C Falandry.

Finally, in this era of overflowing progress, A Makkouk is making us dream with the new perspectives in OC, including immunotherapy.

Paris, France — Eric Pujade-Lauraine
Lyon, France — Isabelle Ray-Coquard
Paris, France — Fabrice Lécuru

Holbrook Kohrt in Memoriam

Holbrook was a great personality. All who encounter him have been impressed by his brightness and his smile and charm. His great knowledge and optimism together with his eagerness to help were unique and led to his natural leadership. He was an outstanding man with a creative and strategic intelligence dedicated to cure cancer. His novel preclinical work in immunotherapy has opened the path to new hopes in fighting cancer. Holbrook gave us an impressive lecture on immunotherapy in March 2015 as Special Invited International Guest during our ARCAGY-GINECO Annual Scientific Meeting in France which generated a lot of enthusiasm. We worked together on different clinical projects, including the recent OvaCure program which he was cofounder, a not-for-profit scientific innovation incubator, accelerating curative cancer treatments particularly in immunotherapy in the fight against ovarian cancer. In this book, he is a coauthor of the chapter on immunotherapy, and this is one of the last witness of his sharp brain and ability of innovation.

On the 24th of February, we lost too young not only a dear friend but also a great figure in tumor immunology. He will be greatly missed.

Contents

Part I

Ovarian Cancer Management

Clinical Research in France, Europe, and in the World Dedicated to Ovarian Cancers

1

Eric Pujade-Lauraine, Florence Joly, Anne-Claire Hardy-Bessard, Isabelle Ray-Coquard, Fabrice Lecuru, and Jean-Emmanuel Kurtz

Abstract

During these last 20 years has been woven a worldwide spider web of cooperative groups dedicated to running Gynecology clinical trials. In Europe, the longest standing national groups are GINECO in France, AGO in Germany and NSGO in Nordic Countries. They have been the core groups of the very active ENGOT (European Network of Gynecology Oncology Trials) gathering 20 groups in West and East Europe and Middle East. Many of these European groups are also members of the international GCIG (Gynecological Cancer InterGroup) including also networks from North/Central America, Asia and Australia. The regular meetings twice a year of these organizations has allowed

E. Pujade-Lauraine (✉)
AP-HP, Hôtel-Dieu, Centre des cancers de la femme,
Place du Parvis Notre-Dame 1, Paris 75004, France
e-mail: epujade@arcagy.org

F. Joly
Centre François Baclesse, Avenue du Général Harris, 14000 CAEN, France
e-mail: f.joly@baclesse.fr

A.-C. Hardy-Bessard
Centre CARIO - HPCA, 10 Rue François Jacob, 22190 PLERIN-SUR-MER, France
e-mail: ac.hardy@cario-sante.fr

I. Ray-Coquard
Centre Léon Bérard, Université Claude Bernard, Lyon, France
e-mail: isabelle.ray-coquard@lyon.unicancer.fr

F. Lecuru
Chirurgie cancérologique, HEGP, Paris, France
e-mail: fabrice.lecuru@aphp.fr

J.-E. Kurtz
Département Hémato-Oncologie, Hôpitaux Universitaires de Strasbourg, 1 Place de l'Hôpital, 67000 STRASBOURG, France
e-mail: jemkurtz@yahoo.fr

E. Pujade-Lauraine et al. (eds.), *Ovarian Cancers*,
DOI 10.1007/978-3-319-32110-3_1

to complete numerous large phase III trials in complementary ways. In addition, brainstorming meetings and Consensus Conferences alternate over time and are opportunities to build the future together at an international level

The French ARCAGY-GINECO Group

This was the first cooperative group in France for clinical research organized by medical oncologists. At that time, in 1993, medical oncology was a new specialty recognized as such since only 5 years. Cooperative groups were already functioning in the field of cancer but either in hematology or in digestive cancer organized by gastroenterologists.

To overcome the potential struggles for power by competitive structures, a triumvirate was put at the head of this new ARCAGY-GINECO group representing the main different medical French structures treating GYN cancers: academic hospital (Pujade-Lauraine Eric), comprehensive cancer center (Guastalla Jean-Paul), and private center (Vincent Pascal).

Twenty-three years after its birth, ARCAGY-GINECO is the only French GYN network and is among the 12 cooperative groups labeled by the French National Cancer Institute (INCA) and is supported by the Ligue Nationale du Cancer as a clinical platform for GYN clinical research.

ARCAGY (Association de Recherche sur les CAncers dont GYnécologiques) is the legal structure as a nonprofit organization, and GINECO (Groupe des Investigateurs Nationaux pour l'Etude des Cancers de l'Ovaire) is the scientific part organized as a scientific society.

ARCAGY is responsible for the operational management of trials. Under the umbrella of Bénédicte Votan, the manager, 23 employees, mainly project managers, are working to make the trials launched and run in time with the best quality.

GINECO is led by a board including the current chair elected for 1 year, the vice-chair and the past-chairs, which meet every month either by teleconference or face-to-face meetings. Account of the board decisions is done to the Scientific Committee comprising 30 regional leaders meeting every 4 months. Globally, 150 centers are active in ARCAGY-GINECO trials with around a 1000 investigators. A total of 7000 patients have been included in the database. Currently 25 trials are ongoing.

Nine working groups are responsible for proposing new trial ideas to the Board and the Scientific Committee and for commenting trial designs. Some working groups are devoted to particular tumor location such as ovarian cancer-first line, ovarian cancer-relapse, endometrial cancer, or cervix cancer. Others are transversal working groups such as Cancer in the Elderly, Rare Tumors, Surgery, Early Phase and translational (GINEGEPS or GINEco Group for Early Phase Study) or Statistical Committee.

Integrated into ENGOT and GCIG, ARCAGY-GINECO has participated or led the great majority of the trials which have changed the landscape of GYN cancer patient management. The combination of carboplatin-paclitaxel which is still the standard regimen for initial chemotherapy in ovarian cancer was developed by GINECO in patients in relapse [1]. The French group participated to several large phase III first-line trials, including the European phase III ICON7 trial whose results supported the EMA approval of first-line bevacizumab in ovarian cancer [2]. In first line, GINECO is leading the international PAOLA trial evaluating the role of the anti-PARP olaparib in maintenance. In ovarian cancer relapse, GINECO has led the large international CALYPSO phase III trial, allowing carboplatin-pegylated liposomal doxorubicin to be a standard chemotherapy in late relapse (platinum-free interval over 6 months) [3]. GINECO has also led the AURELIA trial in early relapse allowing bevacizumab to be approved in this setting both in Europe and in the USA [4]. Among other major international phase III trials, GINECO is leading the olaparib phase III trial in BRCA-mutated patients with late relapse (SOLO2) and two phase III trials with the immune checkpoint inhibitor anti-PDL1 in early and late relapse.

Cancer in the Elderly and Rare Tumor are the oldest transversal working groups being settled nearly 15 years ago. Their success can't be denied. The Cancer in the Elderly working group has been the first to introduce geriatric assessment in ovarian cancer and has completed three consecutive prospective phase II trials for over 70-year-old patients. Currently, this group is running a unique international randomized phase III trial assessing the best chemotherapy regimen for frail elderly patients selected through a GVS score (Geriatric Vulnerability Score) described by Claire Falandry [5]. The Rare Tumor working group has developed a French network of 20 expert centers including selected expert oncologists and expert pathologists brought together in regular multidisciplinary meetings for cases reported on a specific website (www.ovaire-rare). This network called TMRG (Tumeurs Malignes Rares Gynecologiques), initially focused on rare ovarian tumors, and labeled by the French INCA, is including more than 1200 cases of rare malignant ovarian cancer patients each year. Isabelle Ray-Coquard, TMRG network coordinator, is running with success the sole international phase III ever done in recurring granulosa tumors (ALIENOR). The surgery group, with Fabrice Lecuru as coordinator, is more recent but has also shown its great potential for accrual in being a major contributor to the German AGO-led DESTOP trial evaluating surgery in late relapse. In addition, this group is leading with Gwenaël Ferron the first randomized phase III in the neoadjuvant setting (CHIVA) in the first line of ovarian cancer whose accrual is completed.

Translational research and statistics are two fields of great interest for ARCAGY-GINECO. A lot of work has been initiated in collaboration with biological platforms and laboratories particularly in genetics through the BRCA and HRD (homologous recombination deficiency) issues and in immunology where a network of lab are working together since 3 years through an INCA program. The GINEGEPS working group which gather the "young" investigators with translational experience are doing the bridge between the clinical and the translational research. The Statistical Committee includes a mix of experienced and young academic statisticians. Their area of expertise includes international trial design, quality of life and PRO (patient-reported outcome) design and analyses, megadatabase, and innovative statistic methodology.

The European ENGOT Network

As soon as 1997, ARCAGY-GINECO and the German cooperative group AGO decided to cooperate tightly for all phase III trials in ovarian cancer, particularly in first-line therapy. A few years later, the Nordic countries (NSGO group) joined this French-German axis. Further on, Italian MITO and Spanish GEICO came on and formed with the NCRI-MRC from UK the core of what will be in 2007 the European Network of Gynecological Oncological Trial Groups (ENGOT) under the umbrella of ESGO (European Society for Gynecology Oncology).

Currently, the ENGOT is a research network of 20 European academic gynecological cancer trial groups from Western Europe (almost all the Western European countries), Eastern Europe (Czech Republic, Slovakia, and Poland), and Middle East (Israel and Turkey).

Gynecological cancer trial groups represented in European Network of Gynecological Oncological Trial Groups

Study group (country)
AGO – Austria, *Arbeitsgemeinschaft Gynäkologische Onkologie Austria*
AGO Study Group, *Arbeitsgemeinschaft Gynäkologische Onkologie Studiengruppe, Germany*
BGOG, *Belgian Gynaecological Oncology Group*
CEEGOG, *Central and Eastern Gynaecological Oncology Group, Czech Republic, Slovakia, Poland*
DGOG, *The Dutch Gynecological Oncology Group, The Netherlands*
EORTC-GCG, *European Organisation for Research and Treatment of Cancer-Gynaecological Cancer Group*
GEICO, *Grupo Español de Investigación en Cáncer de Ovario, Spain*
GINECO, *Groupe d'Investigateurs Nationaux pour l'Etude des Cancers Ovariens, France*
GROINS, *GROningen INternational Study on Sentinel nodes in vulvar cancer, The Netherlands*
HeCOG, *Hellenic Cooperative Oncology Group, Greece*
ICORG, *The All Ireland Cooperative Oncology Research Group*
ISGO, *Israeli Society of Gynecologic Oncology*
MaNGO, *Mario Negri Gynecologic Oncology group, Italy*
MITO, *Multicenter Italian Trials in Ovarian Cancer, Italy*
NCRI-MRC, *National Cancer Research Institute-Medical Research Council, UK*
NOGGO, *North-Eastern German Society of Gynaecologic Oncology*
NSGO, *Nordic Society of Gynecologic Oncology*
SAKK, *Switzerland Group for Clinical Research*
SGCTGC, *Scottish Gynaecologic Cancer Trials Group, Scotland*
TRSGO, *Turkish Society of Gynecologic Oncology*

ENGOT coordinates and promotes clinical trials within Europe in patients with gynecological cancer trial groups. This coordination is particularly relevant for academic trials, translational research, research on rare diseases, and for clinical trials sponsored by the industry to perform multinational studies in Europe. ENGOT also stimulates young investigators to be involved in clinical trials and promotes the creation of new clinical study groups in parts of Europe where ENGOT is not yet represented.

The ENGOT Mission statement is the following:

ENGOT is a platform that guarantees that the European spirit and culture is incorporated into the medical progress in gynecological oncology and that all European patients and countries can participate in an active way in clinical research and progress.

The ultimate goal is to bring the best treatment to gynecological cancer patients through the best science and enabling every patient in every European country to access a clinical trial.

In 2010, ENGOT published the requirements for trials between the academic ENGOT and pharmaceutical companies [6], and this paper has been recently updated in 2015 [7]. In this paper, ENGOT defined the following items: development of the protocol, statistical analysis, the ownership of the database, the development of case report forms, sponsorship of the trial, monitoring of the trial, publication rules, participation of investigators from non-European countries, appointment of the independent data monitoring committee, and the standard operating procedures for trials between ENGOT and the industry. The three possible models for cooperation between the ENGOT lead group of the trial and industry are shown in the table below.

Models of cooperation between ENGOT groups (lead group) and industry according to option chosen for handling the database and statistical and publications rules
Database (DB) could be organized as
Option A: DB itself at the academic lead group (1st choice)
Audits by company or company assigned auditors
Transfer of database for registration issues and analysis to the company
Option B: DB at CRO and CRO is contracted by the academic lead group (2nd choice)
Audits by company and by lead study group
Installation of SOPs for the respective protocol and information system for any violation to the sponsor
Transfer of the complete database to lead study group for scientific analysis and to company for registration purposes
Option C: DB at CRO and CRO is contracted by industry (3rd choice)
Quality assurance and certified database software with 100% tracing of any access or changes made
Audits by study group or study group assigned auditors

Models of cooperation between ENGOT groups (lead group) and industry according to option chosen for handling the database and statistical and publications rules
Installation of SOPs for the respective protocol and information system for any violation to the lead study group
Transfer of the complete database for further scientific evaluations to the lead study group after final analysis of predefined endpoints
Statistical and publications rules
Lead Study group performs independent analysis of the complete DB for primary and secondary endpoints
The DB may be used later for further meta-analyses or subgroup analyses of the study group or within an intergroup consortium
The publication is the sole responsibility of the lead study group
The company may comment within a predefined period but cannot prohibit any publication

ENGOT has also published a roadmap and a charter for GYN trials performed in Europe [8, 9]. The aim of this roadmap is to facilitate cooperation between the different ENGOT groups, to clarify the role of the leading group, to determine the publication rules, to provide templates for intergroup contracts and contracts between academic groups and the pharmaceutical industry, and to determine the communication flow during ENGOT trials. This roadmap and charter will facilitate the performance of ENGOT studies and also improve the speed of starting ENGOT trials.

ENGOT has been quite successful in developing new trials in Europe and is certainly the most powerful consortium to run GYN trials worldwide. Although ENGOT has only existed for 8 years, the network has already been able to set up more than 20 trials in the field of gynecological cancer, and as of today, more than 4000 patients were included in ENGOT trials. A number of other new trials are in development in ovarian, endometrial, and cervical cancer and will be initiated in 2016 and 2017.

Further goals for ENGOT are to increase translational research in ENGOT trials and to develop more trials in cervical cancer, endometrial cancer, and rare gynecological cancers. Discussion of how to create an ENGOT multicenter European BioBank is ongoing. Challenges include investigator motivation, financial support, sample quality, data quality, sense of equity, storage logistics, governance, and oversight. Teaching and motoring has been delineated as one of the major ENGOT goals. This aim has been nicely fulfilled thanks to two initiatives: the Gynaecological Cancer Academy (GCA) and the e-learning program. GCA consists in mentoring future leaders of ENGOT cooperative groups through 2-day courses every 6 months during 2 years. The key goal of the GCA is to maintain the high quality of clinical trials in gynecological oncology within ENGOT into the future.

Nurturing and developing the next generation of leaders in gynecological oncology is of critical importance to ensure continuity and transfer of knowledge and experience within the clinical trial community.

The main objectives of the GCA are to provide an international networking, strategic partnership, and development opportunity for senior investigators within

ENGOT, to enable them to achieve their potential as future leaders of gynecological oncology study groups, and to develop their experience and knowledge of effective clinical trial development and conduct.

This program started in 2013 which brings together future and current leaders around working groups, and presentations is very successful. Similarly, the e-learning portal accessible from the ESGO website has encountered a sustainable interest.

In conclusion, ENGOT has succeeded in its goal to improve the collaboration between European gynecological cancer trial groups and to initiate trials. These trials have been accruing rapidly with good quality of data.

The Worldwide GCIG Network

The mission of the Gynecologic Cancer InterGroup (GCIG) has been to enhance the global impact of clinical trials in gynecologic cancer [10, 11]. The GCIG formalized in 1997 through a collaboration of European and Canadian cooperative groups that recognized the need for large-scale trials sufficiently powered to answer important clinical questions in a timely and efficient manner. The InterGroup is now comprised of 27 international member organizations and 11 industry partners. The primary focus has been the conduct of high-quality phase III clinical trials in populations of women affected by ovarian, endometrial, and cervical cancer. Recently, there has been a focus on rare tumors, translational research, and patient-reported outcomes. The GCIG has conducted and published the results in the peer-reviewed literature of multiple phase III international trials. Additionally the GCIG has convened Ovarian Cancer Consensus Conferences [12] and State-of-the-Science meetings [13] and published on methodology and endpoints [14] on the conduct of clinical trials. The GCIG, incorporated in 2011, has a governance structure with an Executive Board of Directors and has adopted a formal set of bylaws and statutes to guide operational activity. The group meets at least twice per year. Recently, a Cervical Cancer Research Network (CCRN) has been formally created by the GCIG to engage countries with developing capacity for the conduct of high-quality phase III trials.

Each cooperative clinical trial group sends six representatives to attend meetings of the GCIG, which are held biannually, always at the American Society of Clinical Oncology Meeting each year and alternating between the biannual meetings of the International Gynecologic Cancer Society or another meeting.

The GCIG is managed by an executive board consisting of a chair (Eric Pujade-Lauraine was Chair until end of 2014), a past chair, and chair-elect together with representatives from each of the groups; this executive board oversees the work of the various committees, including harmonization, translational research, ovarian cancer, cervix cancer, and endometrial cancer. The rare tumors group is currently chaired by Isabelle Ray-Coquard from GINECO [15]. Florence Joly, who was the GINECO chair in 2015, is also a very active Chair of the "Symptom Benefit Working Group" [16].

The committees and working groups come together to develop new concepts which, in turn, have been brought forward by the various member groups; once these concepts have been matured and are ready for adoption, they are passed to the executive board for support. Publication guidelines are determined prior to any study commencement.

Any international or national research cooperative group that performs clinical trials in gynecological cancer can become a member, but such cooperative groups have to consist of several centers and must be able to show that they have been part of at least one randomized multicenter phase III trial in gynecological cancer. All groups are required to follow GCP, to follow the guidelines of the declaration of Helsinki, and to ensure as good quality assurance as possible.

The graphs below show how GCIG has succeeded to increase cooperation and exchange during the last 20 years in GYN oncology. A steep increase with time in the number of ties between the groups within GCIG has been observed, allowing to validate a posteriori the GCIG initiative.

In conclusion, GCIG has been intensively productive in collaborative trials, intellectual exchanges and learning, brainstorming, and consensus conferences. A lot remains to do, including translational science applied to clinical trials collaboration and rare tumors collaboration.

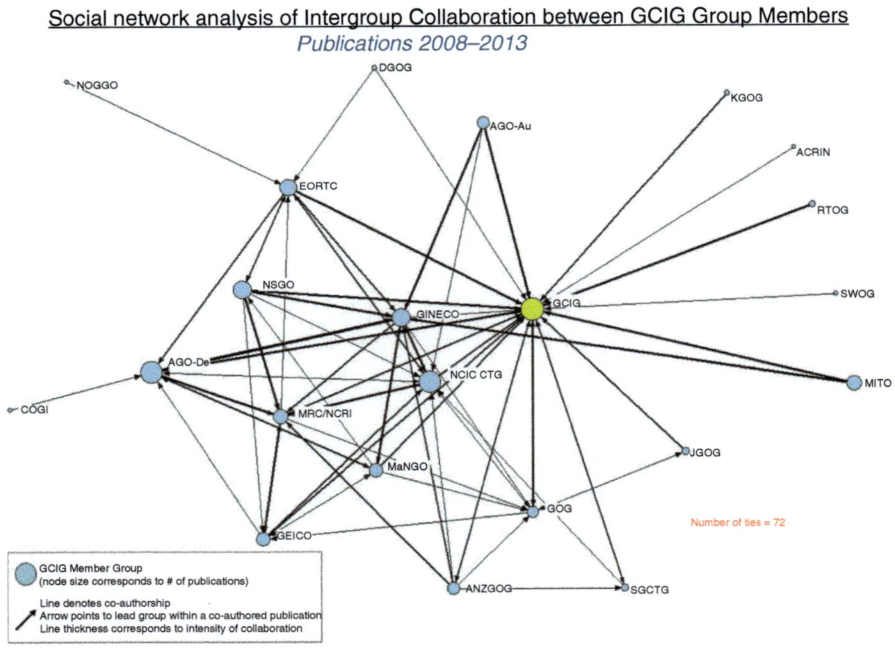

By courtesy of Stuart Gavin

References

1. Pujade-Lauraine E, Guastalla JP, Weber B, Curé H, Orfeuvre H, Mousseau M, Vincent P, Diéras V, Tubiana-Mathieu N, Jacquin JP, Mignot L, Leduc B, Paraïso D, Viens P. Efficacy and safety of the combination paclitaxel/carboplatin in patients with previously treated advanced ovarian carcinoma: a multicenter French Groupe des Investigateurs Nationaux pour l'Etude des Cancers Ovariens phase II study. Semin Oncol. 1997;24(5 Suppl 15):S15-30–5.
2. Perren TJ, Swart AM, Pfisterer J, Ledermann JA, Pujade-Lauraine E, Kristensen G, Carey MS, Beale P, Cervantes A, Kurzeder C, du Bois A, Sehouli J, Kimmig R, Stähle A, Collinson F, Essapen S, Gourley C, Lortholary A, Selle F, Mirza MR, Leminen A, Plante M, Stark D, Qian W, Parmar MK, Oza AM, ICON7 Investigators. A phase 3 trial of bevacizumab in ovarian cancer. N Engl J Med. 2011;365(26):2484–96.
3. Pujade-Lauraine E, Wagner U, Aavall-Lundqvist E, Gebski V, Heywood M, Vasey PA, Volgger B, Vergote I, Pignata S, Ferrero A, Sehouli J, Lortholary A, Kristensen G, Jackisch C, Joly F, Brown C, Le Fur N, du Bois A. Pegylated liposomal Doxorubicin and Carboplatin compared with Paclitaxel and Carboplatin for patients with platinum-sensitive ovarian cancer in late relapse. J Clin Oncol. 2010;28(20):3323–9.
4. Pujade-Lauraine E, Hilpert F, Weber B, Reuss A, Poveda A, Kristensen G, Sorio R, Vergote I, Witteveen P, Bamias A, Pereira D, Wimberger P, Oaknin A, Mirza MR, Follana P, Bollag D, Ray-Coquard I. Bevacizumab combined with chemotherapy for platinum-resistant recurrent ovarian cancer: the AURELIA open-label randomized phase III trial. J Clin Oncol. 2014;32(13):1302–8.
5. Falandry C, Weber B, Savoye AM, Tinquaut F, Tredan O, Sevin E, Stefani L, Savinelli F, Atlassi M, Salvat J, Pujade-Lauraine E, Freyer G. Development of a geriatric vulnerability score in elderly patients with advanced ovarian cancer treated with first-line carboplatin: a GINECO prospective trial. Ann Oncol. 2013;24(11):2808–13.
6. Vergote I, Pujade-Lauraine E, Pignata S, Kristensen GB, Ledermann J, Casado A, Sehouli J, Mirza M, Fossati R, Marth C, Creutzberg C, Del Campo J, Siddiqui N, Calvert P, Bamias A, Tulunay G, van der Zee AG, du Bois A, European Network of Gynaecological Oncological Trial Groups. European network of gynaecological oncological trial groups' requirements for trials between academic groups and pharmaceutical companies. Int J Gynecol Cancer. 2010;20(3):476–8.
7. du Bois A, Reuss A, Pujade-Lauraine E, Pignata S, Ledermann J, Casado A, Sehouli J, Mirza M, Colombo N, Marth C, Witteveen E, Del Campo J, Calvert P, Aravantinos G, Vardar MA, van der Zee AG, Korach J, Taskiran C, Fehr M, Glasspool R, Pfisterer J, Cibula D, Vergote I, Member trial groups of the European Network of Gynaecological Oncological Trial Groups (ENGOT). European network of gynaecological oncological trial groups' requirements for trials between academic groups and industry partners--first update 2015. Int J Gynecol Cancer. 2015;25(7):1328–30.
8. Vergote I, Elser G, Votan B, Farrelly L, De Roover J, Bryce J, du Bois A, member trial groups of the European Network of Gynaecological Trial groups (ENGOT). Roadmap for the European network of gynaecological trial groups (ENGOT) trials. Int J Gynecol Cancer. 2013;23(7):1339–43.
9. Marth C, du Bois A, Schauer C, du Bois A, Casado A, Vergote I, del Campo JM, Goudopoulou A, Pujade-Lauraine E, Bruchim I, Colombo N, Pignata S, Ledermann J, Chekerov R, Raza Mirza M, Westermann A, Glasspool R, Taskiran C, Fehr M, Cibula D. The European network for gynaecological oncological trial groups Charta for privileged partnership. Int J Gynecol Cancer. 2015;25(6):1094–5.
10. Quinn M. Developing an international network for clinical research: the gynecological cancer intergroup experience. Clinical Investigation. 2012;2(1):29–33.
11. Bacon M, Kitchener H, Stuart GC, Vermorken JB, Gynecologic Cancer InterGroup and participants of 4th Ovarian Cancer Consensus Conference. The global impact of the gynecologic

cancer InterGroup in enhancing clinical trials in ovarian cancer. Int J Gynecol Cancer. 2011;21(4):746–9.

12. Stuart GC, Kitchener H, Bacon M, du Bois A, Friedlander M, Ledermann J, Marth C, Thigpen T, Trimble E, participants of 4th Ovarian Cancer Consensus Conference (OCCC); Gynecologic Cancer Intergroup. 2010 gynecologic cancer InterGroup (GCIG) consensus statement on clinical trials in ovarian cancer: report from the fourth ovarian cancer consensus conference. Int J Gynecol Cancer. 2011;21(4):750–5.
13. Sagae S, Monk BJ, Pujade-Lauraine E, Gaffney DK, Narayan K, Ryu SY, McCormack M, Plante M, Casado A, Reuss A, Chávez-Blanco A, Kitchener H, Nam BH, Jhingran A, Temkin S, Mileshkin L, Berns E, Scholl S, Doll C, Abu-Rustum NR, Lecuru F, Small Jr W, participants of the Gynecologic Cancer InterGroup Cervix Cancer brainstorming day. Advances and concepts in cervical cancer trials: a road Map for the future. Int J Gynecol Cancer. 2016;26(1): 199–207.
14. Rustin GJ, Vergote I, Eisenhauer E, Pujade-Lauraine E, Quinn M, Thigpen T, du Bois A, Kristensen G, Jakobsen A, Sagae S, Greven K, Parmar M, Friedlander M, Cervantes A, Vermorken J, Gynecological Cancer Intergroup. Definitions for response and progression in ovarian cancer clinical trials incorporating RECIST 1.1 and CA 125 agreed by the gynecological cancer intergroup (GCIG). Int J Gynecol Cancer. 2011;21(2):419–23.
15. Ray-Coquard I, Brown J, Harter P, Provencher DM, Fong PC, Maenpaa J, Ledermann JA, Emons G, Rigaud DB, Glasspool RM, Mezzanzanica D, Colombo N. Gynecologic cancer InterGroup (GCIG) consensus review for ovarian sex cord stromal tumors. Int J Gynecol Cancer. 2014;24(9 Suppl 3):S42–7.
16. McAlpine JN, Greimel E, Brotto LA, Nout RA, Shash E, Avall-Lundqvist E, Friedlander ML, Joly F, Gynecologic Cancer InterGroup (GCIG). Quality of life research in endometrial cancer: what is needed to advance progress in this disease site? Methodological considerations from the gynecologic cancer InterGroup symptom benefit working group brainstorming session, Leiden 2012. Int J Gynecol Cancer. 2014;24(9):1686–92.

Genetics of Ovarian Carcinomas

2

Claire Sénéchal, Bruno Buecher, Antoine de Pauw, Claude Houdayer, Etienne Rouleau, Catherine Nogués, and Dominique Stoppa-Lyonnet

Abstract

It is estimated that 15–20 % of ovarian carcinomas arise in women carrying a monoallelic germline cancer-predisposing gene mutation. The two main known hereditary forms of ovarian carcinoma are hereditary breast/ovarian cancer (HBOC) linked to *BRCA1* or *BRCA2* mutations, genes involved in DNA double-strand break repair by homologous recombination (HR), and Lynch syndrome linked to mutations in genes involved in DNA mismatch repair (MMR): *MLH1, MSH2, MSH6* or *PMS2*. The contribution of *BRCA1/ BRCA2* mutations is at least tenfold higher than that of MMR genes. Identification of a cancer-predisposing mutation is useful for the prevention of breast, ovarian or colon cancers in affected women and their relatives and

C. Sénéchal
Department of Tumour Biology, Institut Curie, Paris, France

B. Buecher • A. de Pauw • E. Rouleau
Department of Tumour Biology, Institut Curie, Paris, France

C. Houdayer • D. Stoppa-Lyonnet (✉)
Department of Tumour Biology, Institut Curie, Paris, France

Institut Curie, INSERM U830, Paris, France

Université Paris Descartes, Sorbonne Paris-Cité, Paris, France
e-mail: dominique.stoppa-lyonnet@curie.fr

C. Noguès
Department of Tumour Biology, Institut Curie, Saint-Cloud, France

E. Pujade-Lauraine et al. (eds.), *Ovarian Cancers*,
DOI 10.1007/978-3-319-32110-3_2

is now becoming a major part of the treatment of women with ovarian carcinoma, as poly-ADP-ribose-polymerase (PARP) inhibitors have been demonstrated to be useful in HBOC syndrome. New perspectives are opening up in Lynch syndrome with immunotherapy targeting Lynch syndrome-related cancers, characterised by their immunogenicity. Other genes involved in the HR pathway (*PALB2*, *RAD51*, *ATM*) are good candidates to be associated with an increased risk of ovarian and breast cancers that would be expected to be also sensitive to PARP inhibitors. As the identification of women harbouring germline or tumour inactivation of HR genes and probably, in the near future, MMR gene mutations is now becoming essential for their treatment, increasing test demands and the need for rapid and complete analyses are going to modify current genetic counselling and testing practices.

Introduction

Up until now, the aim of genetic testing in a woman with ovarian carcinoma was to allow identification of a predisposing factor and therefore the prevention of other cancers as well as testing of her relatives in order to adapt their management. Ovarian cancer prevention of relatives has been and remains a major goal of cancer genetics, particularly because of the absence of reliable ovarian cancer screening. The scope of genetic testing has now been widened, especially in women carrying a germline *BRCA1* or *BRCA2* mutation: identification of such a mutation may change the treatment of the disease and may therefore have a major impact on the patient's medical management.

Two main ovarian carcinoma (OC) genetic predisposition syndromes have been identified to date. Hereditary breast and ovarian cancer (HBOC) syndrome is linked to germline *BRCA1* or *BRCA2* gene mutations. Mutations in other genes also involved in DNA damage repair and especially in homologous recombination (HR), like *BRCA1* and *BRCA2* genes, may also be associated with an increased risk of breast and ovarian cancers. Lynch syndrome is mainly characterised by a high risk of colorectal, endometrial and ovarian cancers and is linked to germline *MLH1*, *MSH2*, *MSH6* or *PMS2* gene mutations.

These two cancer predisposition syndromes are estimated to be involved in 15–20 % of all OCs, with the contribution of HBOC at least tenfold greater than that of Lynch syndrome. These two syndromes are transmitted according to an autosomal dominant mode. At-risk women carry a monoallelic germline loss of function mutation of a responsible gene. However, the tumour presents somatic inactivation of the wild-type allele via a partial chromosomal defect (deduced from the observation of loss of heterozygosity at the gene locus) or via a point mutation or promoter methylation. Thus, according to Knudson's "two-hit" theory, although the predisposition is transmitted according to a dominant mode, its effect on the tumour is recessive.

Hereditary Breast and Ovarian Cancers

Identification of *BRCA1* and *BRCA2* Genes and Their Molecular Pathology

The *BRCA1* and *BRCA2* genes were identified in 1994 and 1995, respectively, after preliminary genetic linkage studies performed in breast cancer families [1–3] that allowed their chromosomal location. *BRCA1* is located in chromosome 17 (17q21) and *BRCA2* is located in chromosome 13 (13q12). Soon after localisation of these genes, it was observed that families including at least one case of OC were more frequently linked to the *BRCA1* locus than families with breast cancer cases only [4], thus highlighting that *BRCA1* and subsequently *BRCA2* genes are also OC-predisposing genes.

The *BRCA1* gene has a coding sequence of 5589 nucleotides distributed over 23 exons, and the *BRCA2* gene has a coding sequence of 10,254 nucleotides distributed over 26 exons. More than one thousand different loss of function mutations spread over large coding sequences has been reported to date in the various mutation databases. Most mutations are point or small mutations introducing a stop codon. Large gene rearrangements also account for 8.5 % of *BRCA1* mutations and 2 % of *BRCA2* mutations [5].

In addition to deleterious mutations, variants of uncertain significance (VUS) are detected in about 8 % of *BRCA1* or *BRCA2* analyses currently performed in breast and breast/ovarian cancer families. Considerable efforts, combining complementary approaches (epidemiological, genetic, functional studies), have been performed to characterise the significance of these variants [6]. These efforts are coordinated by the international ENIGMA consortium [7], which, in 2014, fused with the *BRCA* Challenge, the Global Alliance for Genomics and Health (GA4GH) designed to characterise VUS of all genes involved in genetic diseases. It is difficult to provide patients with suitable information regarding VUS because the geneticist must inform them that a VUS has been identified, that it cannot be currently used for genetic testing of his or her relatives, but that it could be used in the future.

Due to the complexity of *BRCA1/BRCA2* molecular pathology in terms of analyses and interpretation and the low yield of positive tests in many severe breast and ovarian cancer families, suggesting that other genes may also be involved, sequential genetic testing of the family needs to be performed, as, whenever possible, full screening of the *BRCA1/BRCA2* genes is performed in the individual most likely to be predisposed: a woman with a history of breast or ovarian cancer. When a deleterious mutation has been identified, a mutation-targeted test can be performed in the patient's relatives. Thus, in *BRCA1/BRCA2*-positive families, a negative result in a relative is reassuring.

Functions of BRCA1 and BRCA2 Proteins, the Homologous Recombination Pathway

The observation of the nucleus colocalisation of the BRCA1 and RAD51 proteins during the cell cycle S phase was a breakthrough in the knowledge of BRCA1 function [8], as the amino-acid sequence of BRCA1 did not provide any clues to a specific cellular pathway. BRCA1 and BRCA2 proteins are involved in the repair of DNA double-strand breaks (DSB) by HR, a critical function for the survival of normal cells [9, 10], and Fig. 2.1. In the absence of functional HR, unrepaired or incorrectly repaired DSBs lead to a massive loss of genetic information, genomic

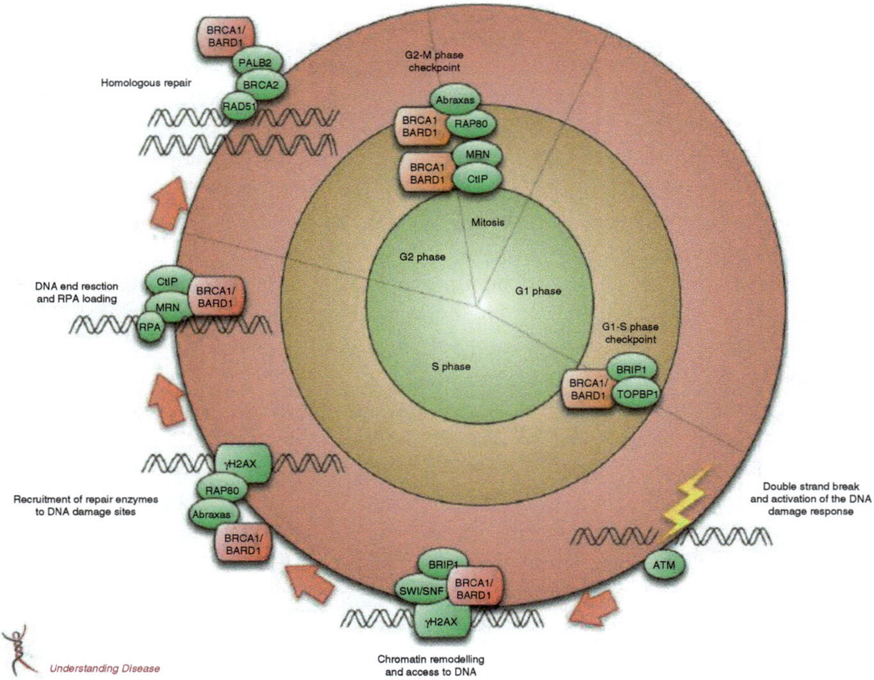

Fig. 2.1 BRCA, DNA repair and the cell cycle (Foulkes and Shuen [9]). In response to DNA damage, BRCA1 mediates HR (depicted in the outer ring) and cell cycle regulation (depicted in the inner ring) when bound to different various macrocomplexes. Following a double-strand break, ATM (ataxia telangiectasia mutated) and *ATR* (ataxia telangiectasia and Rad3-related) phosphorylate a number of downstream effectors, including H2AX, MRN (MRE11-RAD50-NBN), BRCA1 and its binding partner BARD1 (BRCA1-associated RING domain protein 1), initiating the DNA damage response (*DDR*). BRCA1 binds to BRIP1 (BRCA1-interacting protein 1), and SWI/SNF regulates histone deacetylases to open up the chromatin, perhaps allowing access of repair enzymes to the site of DNA damage. Following complex enzymatic modifications by ubiquitin and *SUMO* (small ubiquitin-like modifier), *RAP80* (receptor-associated protein 80) and FAM175A (Abraxas) recruit BRCA1 and other downstream repair enzymes to the site of DNA damage. BRCA1, coupled with MRN and *CtIP* (C-terminal binding protein interacting protein), is involved in resecting the DNA ends to create single-stranded DNA (ssDNA), which is protected by *RPA* (replication protein A). The BRCA1/PALB2/BRCA2 macrocomplex is then required for RPA displacement and RAD51 loading onto ssDNA. Finally, RAD51 mediates sister chromatid strand invasion and homologous repair. Acting in parallel with the DNA damage response are BRCA1 complexes that regulate the cell cycle. BRCA1 coupled with BRIP1 and TOPBP1 regulates G1 – S and intra-S phase checkpoints, while BRCA1/MRN/CtIP and BRCA1/RAP80/FAM175A (Abraxas) regulate the G2 – M phase checkpoint

rearrangements or cell death. BRCA1 appears to have an early and broad role in the HR process via a ubiquitin ligase function: BRCA1 is involved in genome surveillance by the transmission and amplification of the signal induced by DSB; in addition, BRCA1 promotes HR via a modulatory role in the PALB2-dependent loading of BRCA2-RAD51 repair machinery. Moreover, BRCA1 exerts negative control on the cell cycle, thereby allowing the cell to repair its DNA damages especially during S phase. Inversely, BRCA2 is directly involved in the HR process via the sequestration and release of small RAD51 recombinase molecules at the site of the DSB (Fig. 2.1). Bi-allelic germline *BRCA2* mutations are responsible for Fanconi disease, a recessive disease with strong genetic heterogeneity, as 15 genes have been identified to date.

The involvement of BRCA1 and BRCA2 in DNA damage response (DDR) has led to the hypothesis that cells with a BRCA1 or BRCA2 defect could be more sensitive to alkylating agents that considerably increase DSBs and to molecules inhibiting DNA repair pathways other than HR, such as base excision repair (BER) [11]. Poly-ADP-ribose-polymerase inhibitors are an emerging family of DDR inhibitors (see Chap. 13 J Ledermann).

As mentioned above, *BRCA1* and *BRCA2* mutations cannot account for all severe breast/ovarian cancer families, suggesting that other predisposing genes have yet to be identified. Consequently, partner genes of *BRCA1* and *BRCA2,* especially those involved in the HR pathway, are good candidates to be associated with high cancer risks and higher tumour sensitivity to alkylating agents or DDR inhibitors in case of gene inactivation. Numerous genes have been tested in association studies, for example, *CHEK2* and *CHEK1* involved in cell cycle control; *ATM*, *MRE11A* and *NBN* involved in the detection of DNA damage; and *PALB2* and *BRIP1* which are also Fanconi disease genes. Of note, no monoallelic deleterious mutation of *RAD51* has yet been reported, probably because such mutations would be lethal. In contrast, mutations of *RAD51* paralogs (duplicated genes during species evolution that have slightly diverged but still have very similar functions to those of the original gene) have been reported and are associated with an increased risk of ovarian cancer (see below). Most of these genes are currently at the stage of research, and genetic testing has not been proposed to date.

Histology of Ovarian Carcinoma in *BRCA1/BRCA2* Mutation Carriers

Lakhani et al. compared the pathological characteristics of 178 *BRCA1* and 29 *BRCA2* OCs to those of 235 age-matched controls [12]. Both *BRCA1* and *BRCA2* tumours were of higher grade than control tumours ($p < 0.0001$ and $p = 0.028$, respectively). Well-differentiated and grade 1 tumours do exist in *BRCA1/BRCA2* mutation carriers but tend to be rare. Similarly to sporadic cases, papillary serous OC is the most prevalent type, observed in 44 and 48 % of *BRCA1* and *BRCA2* mutation carriers, respectively, followed by the endometrioid type, 36 and 38 % in *BRCA1* and *BRCA2* mutation carriers, respectively. The frequency of serous tumours is reported to be significantly higher among *BRCA1* mutation carriers (OR 1.84, 95 %CI 1.21–2.79), while the frequency of mucinous tumours is much lower (OR 0.13, 95 % CI 0.05–0.34, p <0.0001). The distribution of histological types in *BRCA2* tumours is similar to that in *BRCA1* tumours but not significantly different from the control distribution. The frequency of borderline tumours does not appear to be increased in *BRCA1/BRCA2* mutation carriers. In the study by Zhang et al., no *BRCA1/BRCA2* mutation was identified in a series of 112 cases of unselected mucinous carcinomas [13]. As in the general population, clear cell forms and carcinosarcomas are rare. In summary, *BRCA1/BRCA2* OCs are classically poorly differentiated and of high grade, corresponding to the "type 2" pathway of ovarian carcinogenesis [14]. OCs in *BRCA1/BRCA2* mutation carriers are thought to arise from serous intraepithelial tubal carcinoma (STIC) in the fallopian tubes, associated with *TP53* somatic mutations [15].

Prevalence of *BRCA1/BRCA2* and Other HR Pathway Gene Germline Mutations Among Ovarian Cancer Cases

Before reporting the prevalence of *BRCA1/BRCA2* germline mutations in women with OC, it is useful to recall the prevalence of these mutations in the general population (males and females). According to the Anglian Breast Cancer Study, and taking into account the Hardy and Weinberg law, the allelic frequency for *BRCA1* mutations in the general population was estimated to be 0.051 % (95 % CI: 0.021 – 0.125 %), and the allelic frequency for *BRCA2* mutations was estimated to be 0.068 % (95 % CI: 0.033 – 0.141 %). The frequencies of *BRCA1* and *BRCA2* mutation carriers were therefore estimated to be 1/974 and 1/734, respectively. In other words, the frequency of *BRCA1/BRCA2* mutation carriers in the general population is about 1/400 [16]. In the study by Song et al. described below, the observed frequency of *BRCA1/BRCA2* mutation carriers among the 1528 cancer-free controls was 0.37 % (one *BRCA1* mutation, 4 *BRCA2* mutations), corresponding to 1/270 *BRCA1/BRCA2* carriers in the general population, with 1/1428 *BRCA1* mutation carrier and 1/333 *BRCA2* mutation carrier [17].

Numerous studies have examined the prevalence of *BRCA1/BRCA2* germline deleterious mutations in women with OC. The most recent studies performed in the largest series were based on a molecular testing approach that was as complete as possible [17, 18].

Song et al. performed germline analyses of *BRCA1, BRCA2, MLH1, MSH2, MSH6* and *PMS2* genes in a series of 2222 women with invasive OC unselected for breast or ovarian cancer and in 1528 controls. Proportions of histological subtypes, serous (57 %), endometrioid (14 %), clear cell (8.6 %), mucinous (7.1 %) and high grade (66 %), were consistent with unselected OCs. Among the 2222 OCs, 178 (8 %) *BRCA1/BRCA2* mutation carriers were identified: 84 *BRCA1* mutation carriers (3.8 %) and 94 *BRCA2* mutation carriers (4.2 %). The proportion of *BRCA1/BRCA2* carriers was higher in the high-grade subgroup, with 11 % of carriers.

Alsop's study, conducted in a series of 1001 consecutive cases of non-mucinous, non-borderline OC, identified 141 *BRCA1/BRCA2* mutation carriers: 14.1 % (95 % CI: 11.9–16.3). About 2/3 of these cases were *BRCA1* mutation carriers (88 cases), and 1/3 were *BRCA2* mutation carriers (53 cases). In the serous and high-grade subgroups, 16.6 % and 16.8 % of cases were associated with a *BRCA1 or BRCA2* germline mutation, respectively, and 17.1 % of cases harboured combined characteristics. Notably, 45 % of mutation carriers did not present a positive family history for breast and/or ovarian cancers, highlighting the fact that family history is not a sensitive marker for *BRCA1/BRCA2* detection [18]. The indications for *BRCA1/BRCA2* germline mutation testing in a patient with ovarian cancer are summarised in Table 2.3.

Walsh et al. used a high-throughput sequencing method to screen 21 *BRCA1/BRCA2* partner genes that are candidates to be associated with an increased risk of breast or ovarian cancers in a series of 360 women with ovarian, peritoneal or fallopian tube carcinoma. Mucinous carcinomas were excluded, and a selection bias towards high-grade cases was observed, as 91 % of tumours were high grade. Among the 360 women tested, 24 % carried a deleterious mutation: 18 % in *BRCA1* or *BRCA2* (a figure similar to Alsop's study) and 6 % in *BARD1*, *BRIP1*, *CHEK2*, *MRE11A*, *MSH6, NBN, PALB2, RAD50, RAD51C* or *TP53* [19].

BRCA1, BRCA2 and HR-Associated Genes: Breast and Ovarian Cancer Risks

Two meta-analyses examined the risk of breast and ovarian cancers in *BRCA1* and *BRCA2* carriers [20, 21]. Note that the meta-analysis by Antoniou, performed without selection for family history, was included in the meta-analysis by Chen and Parmigiani, which combined both family and population-based studies and which mainly concerned the risks of breast and ovarian cancers (Table 2.1). Cumulative risks of ovarian cancer at ages 40, 50, 60 and 70 are reported in Table 2.2 [21]. The mean age at onset for both breast and ovarian cancers was younger in *BRCA1* and *BRCA2* carriers compared to the general population. In

Table 2.1 70-year cumulative risk of breast and ovarian cancer in *BRCA1* and *BRCA2* mutation carriers

Cumulative cancer risk at age 70	*BRCA1* (95 %CI)	*BRCA2* (95 %CI)
Breast cancer		
Antoniou et al. (2003)	65 % (44–78)	45 % (31–56)
Chen and Parmigiani (2007)	57 % (47–66)	49 % (40–57)
Ovarian cancer		
Antoniou et al. (2003)	39 % (18–54)	11 % (2.4–19)
Chen and Parmigiani (2007)	40 % (35–46)	18 % (13–23)

Table 2.2 Predicted ovarian cancer risk of a 30-year-old woman carrying a *BRCA1* or *BRCA2* germline mutation

Risk (%) of developing ovarian cancer by age				
30-year-old woman with a *BRCA1/BRCA2* mutation	Risk at age 40 Mean (95 %CI)	Risk at age 50 Mean (95 %CI)	Risk at age 60 Mean (95 %CI)	Risk at age 70 Mean (95 %CI)
BRCA1	2.2 (1.6–3.4)	8.7 (6.7–12)	22 (18–27)	39 (34–43)
BRCA2	0.52 (0.28–1)	2.4 (1.5–4.2)	7.4 (5.1–11)	16 (12–20)

From Chen and Parmigiani [21]

addition, according to the recent study by Alsop performed in a large series of OC women, the mean age at onset in sporadic cancer patients was 60.5 years versus 53.4 years and 59.8 years in patients with *BRCA1* and *BRCA2* mutations, respectively [18].

These figures correspond to mean cancer risks. Shortly after the identification of *BRCA1* and *BRCA2,* it was observed that cancer risks may differ from one family to another (defined by close relatives) and among relatives of the same family. These differences were not chance differences but were underpinned by modifying factors that can be either genetic or non-genetic or by the nature/location of the causative mutation. Two international consortia have been established in order to identify such modifying factors: HBCCS and CIMBA. A recent study performed by CIMBA in a very large number of women (19,581 *BRCA1* and 11,900 *BRCA2* mutation carriers) identified regions of the coding sequence in both genes in which the relative risk of ovarian cancer may be higher than the relative risk of breast cancer [22]. A genome-wide association study conducted on a series of 11,403,952 SNPs disseminated throughout the genome on 15,437 sporadic cases, 15,252 *BRCA1* carriers, 8211 *BRCA2* mutation carriers and 30,845 controls has also identified 6 SNPs associated with a slight increase of the relative risk of ovarian cancer. However, only two of these SNPs increase the risk of ovarian cancer in *BRCA1* mutation carriers, and only one increases the risk of ovarian cancer in *BRCA2* mutation carriers [23]. The results of these extensive studies are disappointing at the present time, as they do not lead to any modification of the management of at-risk women, but they need to be pursued by combining factors of various origins.

Few data are available concerning ovarian cancer risk associated with germline mutation of genes involved in HR. At the present time, estimated cancer risks are only available for two *RAD51* paralogs, *RAD51D* and *RAD51C* [24, 25]. The relative risk of ovarian cancer was estimated to be 6.30 (95 % CI: 2.86–13.85) in *RAD51D* mutation carriers and 5.88 (95 % CI: 2.91–11.88) for *RAD51C* mutation carriers, which constitutes a >9 % cumulative risk by age 80 [25, 26]. The lack of precise estimates of cancer risk associated with these newly identified genes is a major limitation to their use for genetic counselling in clinical practice. However, genes involved in HR could be used to guide treatment.

Prevalence of Somatic Inactivation of *BRCA1/BRCA2* and HR Genes in Ovarian Cancer and Related Diseases

Although it has been clearly demonstrated that, in the presence of a germline *BRCA1/ BRCA2* mutation, the second allele is somatically inactivated, identification of the *BRCA1* gene immediately raised the question of its possible bi-allelic somatic inactivation. The article reporting the identification of *BRCA1* in the October 1994 issue of *Science* was accompanied by another article reporting a study based on a series of 32 breast carcinomas selected for a deletion of the 17q arm, in which *BRCA1* is located. Although three *BRCA1* mutations were detected in the tumour, they all corresponded to germline mutations [27]. Consequently, up until recently, tumour inactivation of *BRCA1/BRCA2* genes was considered to be mainly associated with germline mutations. However, recent studies, based on high-throughput sequencing techniques in large series of ovarian cancers, have thrown new light on this issue, which is of critical importance with the recent development of DDR inhibitors, to which strictly somatically *BRCA1/BRCA2* inactivated tumours are expected to also be sensitive.

The Cancer Genome Atlas (TCGA) project selected 316 high-grade serous ovarian carcinomas. Exome, promoter methylation, transcriptome, microRNA expression and DNA copy number were studied for each tumour [28]. Germline DNA was matched. Tumour analyses identified 73 *BRCA1/BRCA2* mutations (23 %), which were of germline origin in 52 cases (17 %). Conversely, in 21 (6 %) tumours, *BRCA1/BRCA2* inactivation was strictly somatic. In summary, 25 % (21/73) of *BRCA1/BRCA2* inactivations may be somatic. The *BRCA1* promoter has also been shown to be methylated in about 10 % of tumours, suggesting loss of expression. Genes of the HR pathway (*EMSY, FANC, RAD51C, PALB2, CHEK2, BRIP1*) have also been found to be mutated in the absence of *BRCA1/BRCA2* inactivation.

In the study by Pennington et al., providing an update to the study by Walsh et al., 30 genes, including *BRCA1, BRCA2* and 13 genes involved in the HR pathway and cell cycle control (*BRCA1, BRCA2, ATM, BARD1, BRIP1, CHEK1, CHEK2, FAM175A, MRE11A, NBN, PALB2, RAD51C, RAD51D*), were sequenced in a series of 390 cases of high-grade OC at both germline and tumour levels [19, 29]. A deleterious *BRCA1/ BRCA2* mutation was identified in 24 % of tumours (18 % germline and 6 % strictly somatic). Deleterious mutations of other genes were also identified in 8.6 % of cases (6 % germline and 2.6 % strictly somatic). The somatic/germline inactivation ratio was 25 %, similar to that observed in the TCGA study (Fig. 2.2). It is noteworthy that although germline HR pathway gene mutations do exist in low-grade serous carcinoma (11 % of cases), no strictly somatic gene inactivation has been observed.

The Pennington study also reported that tumours demonstrating inactivation of the *BRCA1/BRCA2* or HR pathway genes, regardless of its origin, are more sensitive to platinum-based therapy than non-mutated tumours [29]. Due to the complexity of genetic testing, especially on formalin-fixed, paraffin-embedded tissues, the availability of a tumour BRCAness or HRness signature would be highly desirable to select patients for clinical trials and specific treatments. Such signatures, which

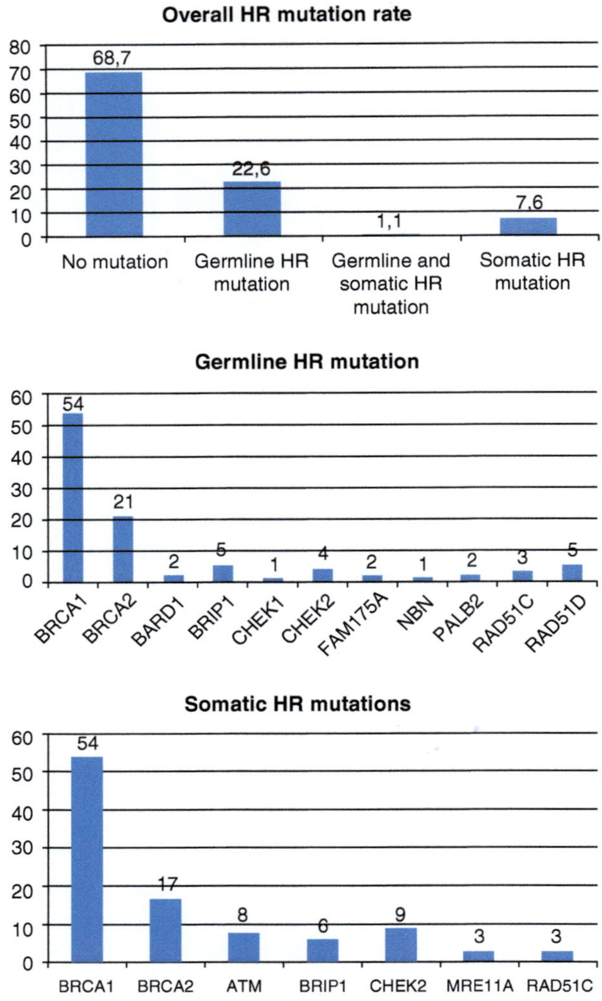

Fig. 2.2 Mutation rates in homologous recombination (HR) genes (From Pennington et al. [29]). (**a**) According to Pennington's study in 367 subjects, 115 (31.3 %) had deleterious mutations in one of 13 HR genes tested: 83 (22.6 %) with germline mutations, 28 (7.6 %) with somatic mutations and 4 (1.1 %) with both germline and somatic mutations. (**b**) According to Pennington's study in 367 subjects, 87 subjects (24 %) had *germline mutations* in 11 HR genes: 49 (13.4 %) in *BRCA1*, 17 (4.6 %) in *BRCA2* and 22 (6 %) in other homologous recombination genes, including *BARD1, BRIP1, CHEK1, CHEK2, FAM175A, NBN, PALB2, RAD51C* and *RAD51D*. (**c**) According to Pennington's study in 367 subjects, 32 carcinomas (8.7 %) had a total of 35 *somatic mutations* in 7 HR genes: 19 (5.2 %) in *BRCA1*, 6 (1.6 %) in *BRCA2* and 10 (2.7 %) in other homologous recombination genes, including *ATM, BRIP1, CHEK2, MRE11A and RAD51C*

correspond to genomic scars of the HR defect, are currently under development [30–32] and are starting to be used in clinical trials [33].

Lynch Syndrome

Definition

Lynch syndrome, also known as hereditary non-polyposis colorectal cancer (HNPCC), was first described by Henry Lynch, who reported rare familial aggregations of colorectal, gastric, endometrium, small bowel, biliary tract, urothelium tract and ovarian cancer with early onset and whose distribution in one side of the family suggested a predisposing gene transmitted according to an autosomal dominant mode [34]. The Amsterdam clinical criteria, initially defined arbitrarily in order to select families for identifying responsible genes, should now be abandoned. The current definition of Lynch syndrome is molecular, based on identification of an inactivating monoallelic germline mutation in a gene involved in the DNA mismatch repair pathway (MMR): *MLH1*, *MSH2, MSH6* or exceptionally *PMS2* [35]. As indicated for *BRCA1* and *BRCA2*, Lynch syndrome is associated with a marked heterogeneity of deleterious mutations. In addition, there are also a large number of variants of unknown significance that require complementary classification studies.

Function of the Mismatch Repair Pathway

The function of the MMR pathway is to correct DNA polymerase nucleotide misincorporations that may occur during DNA replication. Seven proteins compose the human MMR system with three MutS-homologs (MSH2, MSH3 and MSH6) and four MutL homologs (MLH1, MLH3, PMS1 and PMS2). MutS proteins recognise a mismatch and recruit the ATP-bound MutL protein and then correct the mismatch. The MutS homodimer is formed by either MSH2/MSH6 (the MutSα complex) for single-base mismatches and short insertion–deletion loops or MSH2/MSH3 (the MutSβ complex) for larger loops. The endonuclease function in the PMS2 subunit of MutLα (formed by MLH1 and PMS2) excises the DNA strand containing the wrong nucleotide and resynthesises the excision gap via the replicative DNA polymerase.

In MMR pathway-deficient cells, short tandem repeat sequences, i.e. microsatellites, appear particularly prone to nucleotide misincorporations. The resulting microsatellite instability (MSI) is a hallmark for MMR defects (for review, see [36]). Lynch syndrome with genome-wide microsatellite instability therefore presents a signature of MMR dysfunction. This signature is applied in routine diagnosis. This signature is sensitive – the absence of MSI can almost formally exclude the diagnosis of Lynch syndrome (sensitivity of about 90 %, but less reliable with *MSH6*) – and nonspecific, as MSI may result from *MLH1* promoter methylation in late-onset

Table 2.3 Indications for molecular testing in women with OC

Indications for *BRCA1/BRCA2* germline testing
Individual criteria: **woman with ovarian cancer**
Diagnosed **before age 71 years** (except for mucinous OC, borderline tumour and non-epithelial OC) irrespective of family history or with **high-grade serous ovarian cancer,** regardless of age at diagnosis if a targeted therapy is available
Or associated with a **personal history of breast cancer**, regardless of age at diagnosis
Family criteria
Woman with ovarian cancer with (at least) one first-degree relative (or second degree if the link is a man) with breast or ovarian cancer, regardless of age at diagnosis
Indications for screening for MMR gene germline mutations
Woman with ovarian cancer diagnosed before 61 years
Woman diagnosed with ovarian cancer and a Lynch syndrome spectrum cancer (colon, rectum, endometrium, ovary, stomach, urinary tract, biliary tract, small bowel) regardless of age at diagnosis
Woman with ovarian cancer and a first-degree relative with a Lynch syndrome spectrum cancer (see above)
AND with MSI tumour (Lynch syndrome-associated ovarian or tumour)
OR in the absence of a somatic study with clinical features highly suggestive of Lynch syndrome and familial aggregation of Lynch syndrome spectrum cancers concerning at least two generations and with at least one case diagnosed before the age of 50 years

colorectal cancers [37, 38]. Techniques and interpretation are now well standardised. Immunohistochemistry (IHC) analyses of MMR protein expression should also be performed, as the mutated gene is expected to lead to loss of expression of the corresponding protein in tumour tissue, which may guide genetic screening [38].

Any case of Lynch syndrome spectrum cancer (see below) occurring before the age of 60 or even 70 years should be tested somatically for MMR system deficiency (deficient MMR phenotype (dMMR) defined by microsatellite instability (MSI) and/or loss of expression of MMR protein) (Table 2.3), as OCs can be considered to be like endometrial cancer, for which the combination of MMR protein expression followed by evaluation of *MLH1* promoter region methylation in cases demonstrating MLH1/PMS2 IHC loss provided the highest positive predictive value for identification of mutation carriers in women younger than 60 years of age at diagnosis [39]. However, the current development of high-throughput sequencing techniques will radically change this stepwise diagnostic strategy by combining somatic prescreening analyses followed by germline MMR testing in selected patients. Nevertheless, these somatic analyses will still be useful, particularly for interpretation of the results and especially in the case of identification of VUS, rather than to define the indications for MMR gene screening.

Histology of Ovarian Carcinoma in Lynch Syndrome Carriers

Chui et al. performed a review of the published literature [40]. Among 168 ovarian carcinomas observed in Lynch syndrome patients, 54 (32.1 %) were serous, 43

(25.6 %) were endometrioid, 24 (14.3 %) were clear cell, 14 (8.3 %) were mucinous and 33 (19.6 %) were not otherwise specified, i.e. an overrepresentation of non-serous ovarian cancers, such as endometrioid, clear cell and mucinous carcinomas. Chui et al. then performed a centralised pathology review on 20 ovarian cancers from patients carrying a confirmed germline MMR mutation [41]. Surprisingly, this review revealed that all carcinomas were either pure endometrioid (14 cases, grade 1 or grade 2, no grade 3), mixed with an endometrioid component (4 cases) or clear cell (2 cases). No serous or mucinous carcinomas were identified in this small series. All tumours presented MSI. It should be noted that 19 of the 20 OCs were diagnosed at stage pT1 or pT2, consistent with low or intermediate grade, as Lynch syndrome-associated OCs result from type 1 carcinogenesis (*TP53*-negative, low-grade [42]), but associated with a particular molecular profile, *KRAS/BRAF* non-mutated, and with a frequency of 30 %, *PIK3CA* mutations, comparable to type 1 sporadic tumours [43].

Prevalence of Lynch Syndrome Among Ovarian Cancer Cases

To our knowledge, few studies have examined the frequency of Lynch syndrome in the general population. Based on the results of MMR gene screening performed in two series of colorectal cancer cases combined with 1044 Finnish cases, 2.7 % of patients were MMR mutation carriers. Figures were extrapolated to estimates in the general population. The frequency of Lynch syndrome was estimated to be 1/740 in the general population [44]. In the above-mentioned study by Song, germline MMR mutations were identified in 5 out of 1528 cancer-free controls tested for *MLH1*, *MSH2*, *MSH6* and *PMS2* germline mutations; extrapolation to the general population results in a prevalence of one carrier for 306 individuals [17].

Also in the study by Song, germline analysis of the MMR genes in a series of 2222 patients with invasive OC identified a pathogenic mutation in 17 cases (0.76 %), namely, 10 *MSH6* mutations, 4 *MSH2* mutations, 2 *MLH1* mutations and one *PMS2* mutation.

Pal et al. screened *MLH1*, *MSH2* and *MSH6* genes in a population-based series of 1893 women with ovarian tumours, including borderline tumours (13.5 % of the series) [45]. Nine deleterious mutations were identified in nine individuals [0.5 %; 95 % CI: 0.2–0.8)], including 5 *MSH6* mutations, 2 *MLH1* mutations and 2 *MSH2* mutations.

Walsh et al. screened 21 tumour suppressor genes, including *MLH1*, *MSH2*, *MSH6* and *PMS2*, in a series of 360 women with primary ovarian, peritoneal or fallopian tube carcinoma [18]. Cases of mucinous ovarian cancer were excluded. Most tumours (91 %) were high-grade tumours. Only two deleterious germline *MSH6* mutations were identified (0.5 %), with no *MLH1*, *MSH2* or *PMS2* mutations. It is noteworthy that the only MMR gene found mutated in this series of cases selected for type 2 OC, while Lynch syndrome-associated OCs tend to be type 1, was *MSH6*. These results are consistent with those reported in the two previously cited studies, indicating that most patients with Lynch syndrome-associated OC were *MSH6* mutation carriers.

In summary, Lynch syndrome patients represent a small proportion of ovarian cancer cases. Carrier frequency may be only about 1 %, and mutations involve the

MSH6 gene in the majority of cases. However, Lynch syndrome should be suspected in any patient diagnosed with ovarian cancer before the age of 61 years and/or with a personal or family history of Lynch syndrome spectrum cancers (Table 2.3).

Cancer Risks in Lynch Syndrome

The "narrow cancer spectrum" of Lynch syndrome, defined by a relative risk higher than 8, includes colorectal, endometrial, urinary tract and small bowel cancers. The "broad cancer spectrum", defined by a relative risk between 5 and 8, includes ovarian, stomach and biliary tract cancers. Good estimates of cancer risks were provided by the ERISCAM study that was designed to avoid ascertainment bias in cases with a positive family history [46]. This study examined 537 individuals and their relatives with a germline mutation in one of the MMR genes [*MLH1* ($n=248$), *MSH2* ($n=256$) and *MSH6* ($n=33$)]. Table 2.4 reports cancer risks according to the gene identified. The specific ovarian cancer cumulative risk at the age of 70 years was estimated to be 8 % (95%CI: 2–37 %) in the entire study population. This risk was estimated to be 20 % (95%CI: 1–65 %) in patients with *MLH1* mutation, 24 % (95%CI: 3–52 %) in patients with *MSH2* mutation and 1 % (95%CI: 0–3 %) in patients with *MSH6* mutation (Table 2.5). Globally, the

Table 2.4 Cumulative risks of cancers in Lynch syndrome for all genes

Cumulative risks of cancer at the age of 70 years	% (95 %CI)
Colorectal cancer	35 (25–49)
Endometrial cancer	34 (16–58)
Ovarian cancer	8 (2–37)
Stomach	0.7 (0.08–4.4)
Urothelium	1.9 (0.3–5.3)
Small bowel	0.6 (0.1–1.3)
Biliary tract	0.6 (0.07–2.5)

From Bonadona et al. [46]

Table 2.5 Age-specific cumulative risks of ovarian cancer according to genes for MMR mutation carriers

	Cumulative ovarian cancer risks			
Age (year)	All % (95 %CI)	*MLH1* % (95 %CI)	*MSH2* % (95 %CI)	*MSH6* % (95 %CI)
30	0	0	0 (0–1)	0
40	1 (0–1)	0 (0–2)	1 (0–3)	0
50	3 (1–5)	4 (0–11)	4 (1–9)	0 (0–1)
60	7 (2–21)	15 (1–45)	11 (2–28)	1 (0–2)
70	8 (2–37)	20 (1–65)	24 (3–52)	1 (0–3)

From Bonadona et al. [46]

ovarian cancer cumulative risk at age 40 years was less than 1 %. However, assessment of ovarian cancer risks is subject to caution in view of the small number of families, especially those with *MSH6* germline mutations.

Impact of Tumour Microsatellite Instability in the Clinical Management of Patients

Survival with MMR deficiency has been extensively investigated in patients with colorectal cancer, but much less extensively in patients with ovarian cancer. The prognosis is definitely better with MMR deficiency, which can be explained by reactive immunity [47]. The microsatellite instable subset in colorectal cancer seems to be a good immunotherapy checkpoint candidate [48]. Anti-PD-1 and anti-PD-L1 are new emerging therapeutic agents responsible for blockade of the programmed death (PD-1) pathway, a negative feedback system that represses the Th1 cytotoxic immune response. This pathway is upregulated in many tumours, and blockade of this pathway by antibodies targeting either PD-1 or its ligands (PD-L1, PD-L2) has resulted in remarkable clinical responses. Some experimental and clinical data suggest that tumours with deficient MMR (dMMR) phenotype may be more responsive to PD-1 blockade than proficient MMR tumours (pMMR), as dMMR tumours have 10 to 100 times as many somatic mutations that have the potential to encode "non-self" immunogenic antigens, compared to pMMR tumours. dMMR tumours may therefore be more immunogenic and consequently more sensitive to these new immunotherapeutic approaches, as suggested by the results of the recently published phase II study by Le et al. evaluating the activity of pembrolizumab, an anti-PD 1 immune checkpoint inhibitor, in a small number of pMMR colorectal cancers, dMMR colorectal cancers and in other dMMR cancer types (cholangiocarcinoma, endometrial, small bowel and gastric) [49]. If these results are further confirmed and extended to ovarian cancers, patients with sporadic or Lynch-associated dMMR ovarian cancers may benefit from the administration of these new agents.

Cancer Genetic Testing Issues: Adding to Prevention Management and Specific Treatment Choices

As mentioned in the introduction, the aim of genetic testing for "a cancer-predisposing gene" up until now has been cancer prevention in the tested individual and his/her relatives. A new era is opening with the advent of PARP inhibitors for the treatment of women with OC with *BRCA1* or *BRCA2* gene inactivation and, in the near future, for genes involved in HR. As up to 25 % of *BRCA1/BRCA2* inactivation may have occurred only in the tumour and may therefore be strictly somatic, it would be useful to start by testing the *BRCA1/BRCA2* genes in the tumour. This new genetic testing issue and new testing strategies raise a number of challenges for molecular and clinical geneticists, oncologists as well as patients. The resolution of these challenges may lead to a modification of current genetic testing practices.

Genetic testing is expected to increase in the future, as most women with ovarian cancer, including women with high-grade OC after 70 years of age, and their oncologists will systematically require *BRCA1/BRCA2* genetic tests. Result delivery time will need to be shortened. Technical difficulties of *BRCA1/BRCA2* full gene screening, including screening for large gene rearrangements on formalin-fixed, paraffin-embedded tissues, must not be underestimated. To avoid loss of opportunity, *BRCA1/BRCA2* tests will probably need to be performed at both the germline and tumour levels.

Patients will be asked to consent to a test comprising multiple issues that are often difficult to understand. They will be required to give their consent at the time of diagnosis, associated with a high level of stress. Will patients really be able to provide their free and informed consent? Genetic testing starting with the tumour could be considered to dissociate genetic predisposition from therapeutic issues. However, even if the technical difficulties of tumour genetic testing are resolved in the near future, allowing tumour testing to be performed first, a positive result, corresponding to the presence of a germline mutation in 75 % of cases, will still constitute a cancer-predisposing genetic test. Patient information concerning genetic testing issues, support to help them communicate a positive result to their relatives, and their own personal psychological support will still be required.

Improvement of the interpretation of *BRCA1/BRCA2* sequencing will remain of utmost importance, especially in terms of VUS. It is essential to enter VUS into specialised databases in order to contribute to their classification so that the patient can subsequently be informed once the significance of a VUS has been determined. As mentioned above, the international ENIGMA consortium and the BRCA Challenge of the Global Alliance for Genomics and Health are actively involved in this field. Maintenance of the participation of patients, oncologists and geneticists in these initiatives constitutes a real challenge. Similarly, although new ovarian cancer genes have recently been identified as a result of high-throughput sequencing, precise estimates of cancer risk are impossible and screening tests cannot be performed in relatives in a diagnostic setting. Further epidemiological studies in patients and their relatives are required.

In summary, two principles must be taken into account for the definition of new cancer genetic testing guidelines: (1) patient information and support and (2) improvement of test quality, especially concerning interpretation of the results. More genetic counsellors specialised in cancer genetics are needed, oncologists must be educated about genetic testing issues and the difficulties of interpretation of the results and new information media (phone, web, booklets) must be developed [50]. Epidemiological studies must be conducted and variant databases must be established. Networks between oncologists and clinical and molecular geneticists therefore need to be set up and will be a central component of these new guidelines.

References

1. Miki Y, Swensen J, Shattuck-Eidens D, Futreal PA, Harshman K, Tavtigian S, Liu Q, Cochran C, Bennett LM, Ding W, et al. A strong candidate for the breast and ovarian cancer susceptibility gene BRCA1. Science. 1994;266:66–71.
2. Wooster R, Bignell G, Lancaster J, Swift S, et al. Identification of the breast cancer susceptibility gene BRCA2. Nature. 1995;378(6559):789–92.
3. Tavtigian SV, Simard J, Rommens J, Couch F, Shattuck-Eidens D, Neuhausen S, Merajver S, Thorlacius S, Offit K, Stoppa-Lyonnet D, et al. The complete BRCA2 gene and mutations in chromosome 13q-linked kindreds. Nat Genet. 1996;12:333–7.
4. Narod SA, Feunteun J, Lynch HT, Watson P, Conway T, Lynch J, Lenoir GM. Familial breast-ovarian cancer locus on chromosome 17q12-q23. Lancet. 1991;338(8759):82–3.
5. INCa annual activity report 2013. http://www.e-cancer.fr/publications/59-recherche/811-synthese-de-lactivite-doncogenetique-2013-consultations-et-laboratoires
6. Caputo S, Benboudjema L, Sinilnikova O, Rouleau E, Béroud C, Lidereau R, French BRCA GGC Consortium. Description and analysis of genetic variants in french hereditary breast and ovarian cancer families recorded in the UMD-BRCA1/BRCA2 databases. Nucleic Acids Res. 2012;40(Database issue):D992–1002.
7. Spurdle AB, Healey S, Devereau A, Hogervorst FB, Monteiro AN, Nathanson KL, Radice P, Stoppa-Lyonnet D, Tavtigian S, Wappenschmidt B, Couch FJ, Goldgar DE. ENIGMA--evidence-based network for the interpretation of germline mutant alleles: an international initiative to evaluate risk and clinical significance associated with sequence variation in BRCA1 and BRCA2 genes. Hum Mutat. 2012;33(1):2–7.
8. Scully R, Chen J, Plug A, Xiao Y, Weaver D, Feunteun J, Ashley T, Livingston DM. Association of BRCA1 with Rad51 in mitotic and meiotic cells. Cell. 1997;88(2):265–75.
9. Foulkes WD, Shuen AY. In brief: BRCA1 and BRCA2. J Pathol. 2013;230(4):347–9.
10. Prakash R, Zhang Y, Feng W, Jasin M. Homologous recombination and human health: the roles of BRCA1, BRCA2, and associated proteins. Cold Spring Harb Perspect Biol. 2015;7(4):a016600.
11. Lee JM, Ledermann JA, Kohn EC. PARP inhibitors for BRCA1/2 mutation-associated and BRCA-like malignancies. Ann Oncol. 2014;25(1):32–40.
12. Lakhani SR, Manek S, Penault-Llorca F, Flanagan A, Arnout L, Merrett S, et al. Pathology of ovarian cancers in BRCA1 and BRCA2 carriers. Clin Cancer Res. 2004;10(7):2473–81.
13. Zhang S, Royer R, Li S, et al. Frequencies of *BRCA1* and *BRCA2* mutations among 1,342 unselected patients with invasive ovarian cancer. Gynecol Oncol. 2011;121:353–7.
14. Levanon K, Crum C, Drapkin R. New insights into the pathogenesis of serous ovarian cancer and its clinical impact. J Clin Oncol. 2008;26(32):5284–93.
15. Kindelberger DW, Lee Y, Miron A, Hirsch MS, Feltmate C, Medeiros F, Callahan MJ, Garner EO, Gordon RW, Birch C, Berkowitz RS, Muto MG, Crum CP. Intraepithelial carcinoma of the fimbria and pelvic serous carcinoma: evidence for a causal relationship. Am J Surg Pathol. 2007;31(2):161–9.
16. Antoniou AC, Pharoah PD, McMullan G, Day NE, Stratton MR, Peto J, et al. A comprehensive model for familial breast cancer incorporating BRCA1, BRCA2 and other genes. Br J Cancer. 2002;86(1):76–83.
17. Song H, Cicek MS, Dicks E, Harrington P, Ramus SJ, Cunningham JM, Fridley BL, Tyrer JP, Alsop J, Jimenez-Linan M, Gayther SA, Goode EL, Pharoah PD. The contribution of deleterious germline mutations in BRCA1, BRCA2 and the mismatch repair genes to ovarian cancer in the population. Hum Mol Genet. 2014;23(17):4703–9.
18. Alsop K, Fereday S, Meldrum C, De Fazio A, Emmanuel C, George J, et al. BRCA mutation frequency and patterns of treatment response in BRCA mutation-positive women with ovarian cancer: a report from the Australian Ovarian Cancer Study Group. J Clin Oncol. 2012;30(21):2654–63. Erratum in J Clin Oncol. 2012; 30(33):4180.

19. Walsh T, Casadei S, Lee MK, Pennil CC, Nord AS, Thornton AM, Roeb W, Agnew KJ, Stray SM, et al. Mutations in 12 genes for inherited ovarian, fallopian tube, and peritoneal carcinoma identified by massively parallel sequencing. Proc Natl Acad Sci U S A. 2011;108(44): 18032–7.
20. Antoniou A, Pharoah PDP, Narod S, Risch A, et al. Average risks of breast and ovarian cancer associated with BRCA1 or BRCA2 mutations detected in cases series unselected for family history: a combined analysis of 22 studies. Am J Hum Genet. 2003;72(5):1117–30.
21. Chen S, Parmigiani G. Meta-analysis of BRCA1 and BRCA2 penetrance. J Clin Oncol. 2007;25:1329–33.
22. Rebbeck TR, Mitra N, Wan F, Sinilnikova OM, Healey S, et al. Association of type and location of BRCA1 and BRCA2 mutations with risk of breast and ovarian cancer. JAMA. 2015;313(13):1347–61.
23. Kuchenbaecker KB, Ramus SJ, Tyrer J, Lee A, Shen HC, Beesley J, Lawrenson K, et al. Identification of six new susceptibility loci for invasive epithelial ovarian cancer. Nat Genet. 2015;47(2):164–71.
24. Meindl A, Hellebrand H, Wiek C, Erven V, Wappenschmidt B, Niederacher D, Freund M, Lichtner P, et al. Germline mutations in breast and ovarian cancer pedigrees establish RAD51C as a human cancer susceptibility gene. Nat Genet. 2010;42(5):410–4.
25. Loveday C, Turnbull C, Ramsay E, Hughes D, et al. Germline mutations in RAD51D confer susceptibility to ovarian cancer. Nat Genet. 2011;43(9):879–82.
26. Loveday C, Turnbull C, Ruark E, Xicola RM, Ramsay E, Hughes D, Warren-Perry M, Snape K, Breast Cancer Susceptibility Collaboration (UK). Germline RAD51C mutations confer susceptibility to ovarian cancer. Nat Genet. 2012;44(5):475–6.
27. Futreal PA, Liu Q, Shattuck-Eidens D, Cochran C, Harshman K, Tavtigian S, Bennett LM, Haugen-Strano A, Swensen J, Miki Y, et al. BRCA1 mutations in primary breast and ovarian carcinomas. Science. 1994;266(5182):120–2.
28. Cancer Genome Atlas Research Network. Integrated genomic analyses of ovarian carcinoma. Nature. 2011;474(7353):609–15.
29. Pennington KP, Walsh T, Harrell MI, Lee MK, Pennil CC, Rendi MH, et al. Germline and somatic mutations in homologous recombination genes predict platinum response and survival in ovarian, fallopian tube, and peritoneal carcinomas. Clin Cancer Res. 2014;20(3):764–75.
30. Popova T, Manié E, Rieunier G, Caux-Moncoutier V, Tirapo C, Dubois T, Delattre O, et al. Ploidy and large-scale genomic instability consistently identify basal-like breast carcinomas with BRCA1/2 inactivation. Cancer Res. 2012;72(21):5454–62.
31. Abkevich V, Timms KM, Hennessy BT, Potter J, Carey MS, Meyer LA, Smith-McCune K, Broaddus R, Lu KH, Chen J, et al. Patterns of genomic loss of heterozygosity predict homologous recombination repair defects in epithelial ovarian cancer. Br J Cancer. 2012;107(10):1776–82.
32. Birkbak NJ, Wang ZC, Kim JY, Eklund AC, Li Q, Tian R, Bowman-Colin C, Li Y, Greene-Colozzi A, Iglehart JD, Tung N, Ryan PD, Garber JE, Silver DP, Szallasi Z, Richardson AL. Telomeric allelic imbalance indicates defective DNA repair and sensitivity to DNA-damaging agents. Cancer Discov. 2012;2(4):366–75.
33. Isakoff SJ, Mayer EL, He L, Traina TA, Carey LA, Krag KJ, Rugo HS, Liu MC, Stearns V, et al. TBCRC009: a multicenter phase II clinical trial of platinum monotherapy with biomarker assessment in metastatic triple-negative breast cancer. J Clin Oncol 2015;33(17):1902–9.
34. Lynch HT, Shaw MW, Magnuson CW, et al. Hereditary factors in cancer: study of two large Midwestern kindreds. Arch Intern Med. 1966;117:206–12.
35. Piñol V, Castells A, Andreu M, Castellví-Bel S, Alenda C, Llor X, Xicola RM, Rodríguez-Moranta F, Payá A, Jover R, Bessa X, Gastrointestinal Oncology Group of the Spanish Gastroenterological Association. Accuracy of revised Bethesda guidelines, microsatellite instability, and immunohistochemistry for the identification of patients with hereditary nonpolyposis colorectal cancer. JAMA. 2005;293(16):1986–94.

36. Martín-López JV, Fishel R. The mechanism of mismatch repair and the functional analysis of mismatch repair defects in Lynch syndrome. Fam Cancer. 2013;12(2):159–68.
37. de la Chapelle A, Hampel A. Clinical relevance of microsatellite instability in colorectal cancer. J Clin Oncol. 2010;28(20):3380–7.
38. Giardiello FM, Allen JI, Axilbund JE, Boland CR, Burke CA, Burt RW, Church JM, Dominitz JA, Johnson DA, et al. Guidelines on genetic evaluation and management of Lynch syndrome: a consensus statement by the US multi-society task force on colorectal cancer. Am J Gastroenterol. 2014;109(8):1159–79.
39. Buchanan DD, Tan YY, Walsh MD, Clendenning M, Metcalf AM, Ferguson K, Arnold ST, Thompson BA, Lose FA, et al. Tumor mismatch repair immunohistochemistry and DNA MLH1 methylation testing of patients with endometrial cancer diagnosed at age younger than 60 years optimizes triage for population-level germline mismatch repair gene mutation testing. J Clin Oncol. 2014;32(2):90–100.
40. Chui MH, Gilks CB, Cooper K, et al. Identifying Lynch syndrome in patients with ovarian carcinoma: the significance of tumor subtype. Adv Anat Pathol. 2013;20:378–86.
41. Chui MH, Ryan P, Ferguson SE, Pollett A, Aronson M, Semotiuk K, et al. The histomorphology of Lynch syndrome-associated ovarian carcinomas: toward a subtype-specific screening strategy. Am J Surg Pathol. 2014;38(9):1173–81.
42. Kurman RJ, Shih IM. The origin and pathogenesis of epithelial ovarian cancer: a proposed unifying theory. Am J Surg Pathol. 2010;34(3):433–43.
43. Niskakoski A, Kaur S, Renkonen-Sinisalo L, Lassus H, Järvinen HJ, Mecklin JP, Bützow R, Peltomäki P. Distinct molecular profiles in Lynch syndrome-associated and sporadic ovarian carcinomas. Int J Cancer. 2013;133(11):2596–608.
44. Salovaara R, Loukola A, Kristo P, Kääriäinen H, Ahtola H, Eskelinen M, Härkönen N, Julkunen R, Kangas E, Ojala S, Tulikoura J, Valkamo E, Järvinen H, Mecklin JP, Aaltonen LA, de la Chapelle A. Population-based molecular detection of hereditary nonpolyposis colorectal cancer. J Clin Oncol. 2000;18(11):2193–200.
45. Pal T, Akbari MR, Sun P, Lee JH, Fulp J, Thompson Z, Coppola D, et al. Frequency of mutations in mismatch repair genes in a population-based study of women with ovarian cancer. Br J Cancer. 2012;107(10):1783–90.
46. Bonadona V, Bonaïti B, Olschwang S, Grandjouan S, Huiart L, Longy M, Guimbaud R, Buecher B, French Cancer Genetics Network, et al. Cancer risks associated with germline mutations in MLH1, MSH2, and MSH6 genes in Lynch syndrome. JAMA. 2011; 305(22):2304–10.
47. Radman M, Wagner R. Carcinogenesis. Missing mismatch repair. Nature. 1993;366(6457):722.
48. Xiao Y, Freeman GJ. The microsatellite instable subset of colorectal cancer is a particularly good candidate for checkpoint blockade immunotherapy. Cancer Discov. 2015;5(1):16–8.
49. Le DT, Uram JN, Wang H, Bartlett BR, Kemberling H, Eyring AD, et al. PD-1 blockade in tumors with mismatch-repair deficiency. N Engl J Med. 2015;372(26):2509–20.
50. Schwart MD, Valdimarsdottir HB, Peshkin BN, Mandelblatt J, Nusbaum R, Huang AT, Chang Y, Graves K, et al. Randomized noninferiority trial of telephone versus in-person genetic counseling for hereditary breast and ovarian cancer. J Clin Oncol. 2014;32(7):618–26.

Debulking Surgery: Interval Debulking Surgery Versus Primary: Pros and Cons on How to Evaluate Quality

3

Fabrice Lécuru, Charlotte Ngo, Anne Sophie Bats, Chérazade Bensaid, Pierre Combe, Eric Pujade-Lauraine, Marie Aude le Frère Belda, and Laure Fournier

Abstract

Surgery for advanced ovarian cancer should now take into account the modern data on the pathophysiology of these diseases and the results of randomized trials.

Initial management of chemosensitive diseases such as high-grade serous carcinoma, grade 3 endometrioïd cancer, and carcinosarcomas relies on surgery and chemotherapy. The goal of surgery is the complete resection of macroscopic lesions. The remaining question is the timing of surgery, primary or interval. Owing to results of four randomized trials, we can state that patients with operable disease and good general status should receive surgery first. Patients in poor general

F. Lécuru (✉) • C. Ngo • A.S. Bats • C. Bensaid
Surgery, Centre Expert Oncologie Gynécologique Paris Descartes- Hôpital Européen Georges Pompidou, APHP, Paris, France

Faculté de Médecine, Université Paris Descartes, Paris, France

Faculté de Médecine, Université Paris Descartes, UMR S 747, Paris, France
e-mail: fabrice.lecuru@egp.aphp.fr

P. Combe • E. Pujade-Lauraine
Medical Oncology, Centre Expert Oncologie Gynécologique Paris Descartes- Hôpital Européen Georges Pompidou, APHP, Paris, France

Faculté de Médecine, Université Paris Descartes, Paris, France

M.A. le F. Belda
Pathology, Centre Expert Oncologie Gynécologique Paris Descartes- Hôpital Européen Georges Pompidou, APHP, Paris, France

L. Fournier
Radiology, Centre Expert Oncologie Gynécologique Paris Descartes- Hôpital Européen Georges Pompidou, APHP, Paris, France

Faculté de Médecine, Université Paris Descartes, Paris, France

E. Pujade-Lauraine et al. (eds.), *Ovarian Cancers*,
DOI 10.1007/978-3-319-32110-3_3

condition or with large or disseminated metastases should receive chemotherapy first. For other patients, surgery or neoadjuvant chemotherapy can be proposed.

Integration of biological data in the decision making process seems relevant, but few data are now available and of clinical interest.

Role, objective, and time of surgery of carcinomatosis from adnexal origin has been in debate for the past 30 years.

Griffith was the first to establish a clear relation between residual disease and survival [1]. Since then, all the studies that addressed this issue found the same result: residual disease is the most important prognostic factor in these patients, i.e., survival is correlated to the surgical output.

Conversely, some authors argued that extensive surgery was frequently responsible of severe intra- and postoperative morbidity and had a detrimental impact on initiation of chemotherapy (and prognosis?), as well as on quality of life [2, 3]. The concept of interval debulking surgery after some cycles of chemotherapy has emerged in order to decrease morbidity, improve quality of life, and even improve survival [4].

During the same period, the understanding of "ovarian cancer" as a disease improved. Several diseases were identified according to histological but also molecular characteristics [5].

All the ideas that will be developed in this chapter are mainly applicable to chemosensitive diseases such as high-grade serous carcinoma, grade 3 endometrioïd tumors, and carcinosarcomas. Other types, like low-grade serous cancers and mucinous and clear cell carcinomas, should probably follow different concepts.

Goals and Results of Cytoreduction

Bristow et al. published a meta-analysis including only cohorts of patients with stage III/IV ovarian cancer who received a "modern" platinum-based chemotherapy [6]. He reported that "maximal cytoreductive surgery" (largest residual ≤3 cm) was obtained in 41.9 % of patients (0 – 100 %) and that survival of each cohort was significantly correlated to the rate of patients having a maximal cytoreductive surgery. Clearly, a cohort with less than 25 % of maximal cytoreductive surgery had a median survival of 23.0 months. On the other hand, cohorts with more than 75 % of maximal cytoreductive surgery reached a median survival time of 36.8 months. Increasing the rate of maximal cytoreductive surgery by 10 % led to an increased median survival of 5.5 %. In other words, the simple respect of surgical standard of care provides survival benefits similar to that obtained by addition of new drugs. Finally, multiple linear regression analysis showed that rate of maximal cytoreductive surgery was the strongest prognostic factor of the cohort [6].

Subsequently numerous authors established that "optimal" surgery provided better results in terms of progression-free survival (PFS) as well as overall survival (OS), when compared to patients with larger residual disease. However, one limitation was the flexible definition of "optimal" according to authors and its lack of reproducibility [7].

Chi et al. introduced the concept of "complete macroscopic resection" [8]. He reported a series of IIIc patients and observed that OS was significantly better in patients without macroscopic residuals when compared to <1 cm and >1 cm residuals (median OS of 106 months for stage IIIc patients) [8]. Du Bois et al. confirmed this notion. He reported on survival of patients included in three drug trials, according to completeness of surgery: complete resection vs. 1–10 mm residuals vs. >10 mm residuals. 3126 patients were analyzed and complete resection was obtained in 33.5 %, whereas 1–10 mm residuals were observed in 37.8 % and >10 mm residuals in 24.7 %. Significantly longer PFS and OS were observed in patients after complete resection (up to 99.1 months OS). The same effect was observed for the overall population and also after stratification according to stage (IIb-IIIb, IIIc, or IV) or histological types [9]. On the other hand, the initial tumor burden had also an effect, since the survival improvement was lower in stage IV than in stage IIIc [9].

However, the impact of increasing the surgical effort could not be assessed by these data. Was complete resection due to the disease (limited extension, intrinsic biology) or to the surgeon (surgical aggressiveness)? Chi et al. reported two cohorts of patients, operated on in two different time periods. During the first period, surgery was mainly limited to the pelvis and nodal areas, whereas a more aggressive surgery, including procedures in the upper abdomen, was performed in the second period. Optimal surgery rate and complete resection rate were significantly higher in the second time period [10]. At last, survival (PFS and OS) was significantly improved in the second group of patients, indicating that increasing the surgical aggressiveness and increasing the rate of optimal/complete resection had an impact on survival (with the limitation that other factors could also improve survival). Major complications were also significantly more frequent in the second group of patients [11].

Morbidity of primary surgery constitutes its main limitation. A recent multicenter study showed that postoperative complications occurred in 33 % of patients with major complications in 11 % [3]. Primary surgery, extent of surgery, performing any bowel resection (especially recto-sigmoïdectomy), and high Peritoneal Cancer Index (PCI) associated with bowel resection were significant predictors of morbidity. The impact of complications on initiation of chemotherapy is an issue. Delaying the medical treatment has been proved to be detrimental in colonic cancers. Data are scarce in ovarian cancer. However, it appears that delay has no prognostic impact under the cutoff of 35 days [12].

How to Achieve Complete Surgical Resection?

The rate of optimal or complete cytoreduction is widely variable among teams. Explanations and discussions have mainly focused on surgery. However, the notion of "team" appears more and more important. Preoperative evaluation of the patient, in terms of extension of the disease, and also of the patient herself is a critical stage. Assessment of the disease extension requires a close collaboration between radiologists, pathologist, and surgeon. Logically the result is correlated to the training and level of expertise of all members of the team. Assessment of the patients "operability" is also of main importance. Age, comorbidity, nutritional status, ASA (American

Society of Anesthesiology) score, etc., will require the intervention of specialists (onco-geriatrician, cardiologists, metabolism disorder specialist, anesthesiologists, etc.). Here again, the level of expertise of all of them and their coordination is crucial. Intraoperative management of the patient requires anesthesiologists trained for long surgery, diaphragm opening, bowel resection, bleeding, fluid loss, etc. Stay in intensive care unit for the initial postoperative period and experience of trained nurses in the surgical department are also important. A quick and reliable pathological diagnosis and a quick initiation of chemotherapy will finalize the primary management of the patient.

Globally, the correct management of ovarian cancer patients requires a trained team, with a comprehensive "patient pathway" rather than only an experienced surgeon.

In terms of surgery, many people have focused on extirpation of larges masses or bowel resection. However, the way the surgeon performs (and describes in the operative report) the initial exploration with assessment of the disease burden is representative of his level of expertise: how to claim a "complete macroscopic resection" if a full and comprehensive exploration has not been performed, including liver mobilization, section of adhesions in patients with prior history of surgery, etc.? The operative record is a surrogate indicator of the surgical quality. Lack of a full description of the initial carcinomatosis with at best a score of peritoneal extension, and even more the specification of the amount of residual disease with if possible a validated score, generally indicates a less thorough operation.

A literature review shows that surgeon qualification, surgeon volume, hospital qualification, and volume have an impact with respect to standards of care, surgical output, appropriate use of chemotherapy, and even survival [13]. Participation in clinical trials could also be discriminant [14].

The results of Bristow et al.'s meta-analysis can also be interpreted according to the volume of the surgeon/hospital [6]. Nonspecialized centers generally have the lowest rate of maximal cytoreductive surgery, whereas specialized hospitals provide rates up to75%. The impact on survival of these differences in expertise offers a strong argument for centralization of ovarian cancer patient management.

Results of Neoadjuvant Chemotherapy and Interval Surgery

Neoadjuvant chemotherapy associated with interval surgery has been proposed as an alternative to primary surgery. The aims were to increase the rate of complete/optimal resection, to decrease intraoperative morbidity, to improve quality of life, and finally to improve PFS and OS [4].

Four main randomized controlled trials have been published on this topic.

The first EORTC trial reported by van der Burg et al. included patients having residual disease measuring 1 cm or more after biopsy or primary surgery [15]. Patients with a clinical response or stable disease after neoadjuvant chemotherapy were randomized between interval surgery (after three cycles of chemotherapy) or no surgery. A "second-look" surgery was performed in patients with complete clinical response at the end of the treatment. Interval surgery significantly increased the rate of clinical response and complete clinical response, but the rate of pathological response was similar in patients having second-look surgery. PFS (+5 months) and OS (+6 months) were significantly improved by interval surgery, but patients with nonoptimal surgery (residuals >1 cm) have a similar PFS than patients without surgery. In the multivariate analysis, surgery was the most important prognostic factor.

The GOG trial reported by Rose et al. had the same design but showed no significant improvement in PFS and OS [16]. The main difference between the two trials was the primary surgery, done in 95 % of cases by gynecologic oncologists with the intent of maximal cytoreduction in the American trial and mainly by nonspecialists in the European study. These two studies indicate that "interval" surgery can be considered if a surgical effort had not been made initially and if residual disease is supposed to be small or absent after interval surgery.

Two subsequent trials compared primary debulking and interval surgery. The EORTC trial published by Vergote et al. as well as the CHORUS trial reported by Kehoe et al. included patients with stage III/IV disease [17, 18]. Their design was similar and the results too. The main result was a similar PFS and OS after primary debulking or interval surgery, interpreted as "interval debulking was not inferior to primary debulking." The second result was a significant decrease in morbidity. The third result was that complete resection was confirmed to be the most significant prognostic factor. However, numerous criticisms have been addressed to these studies. Survival was lower than expected; surgical output was questionable since a complete resection was obtained in a minority of patients after primary surgery. Interestingly, the correlation between survival and residual disease was similar to that described by Bristow R. The second intriguing result was that complete/optimal resection was significantly more common after interval surgery, but this did not translate into improvement of survival. Size of the disease was also a concern, since size of the largest metastasis was 10 cm or more in 40 % of patients of the EORTC trial, indicating that the worse patients had been included in these studies.

However, despite "surgical" limitations, these trials showed that survival was similar after neoadjuvant chemotherapy and primary surgery, but obviously was not improved; that morbidity of surgery was decreased with interval surgery; and that the increase in resection rate obtained by neoadjuvant chemotherapy did not translate into improved survival.

In the future, the use of anti-angiogenic agents in the neoadjuvant setting could be an option to improve neoadjuvant chemotherapy efficiency and change our vision of this option.

Tumor Extent, Surgery, and Prognosis

The relation between the initial extension of the carcinomatosis, the surgical output, and survival is now the most interesting question. In other words, is the observed survival after complete resection the result of the limited extension of the carcinomatosis or the result of the surgical aggressiveness?

Aletti et al. reported a series of IIIc patients (FIGO 2008) with carcinomatosis [19]. He compared survival between patients having "optimal cytoreduction" (less than 1 cm) according to the aggressiveness of surgery. He observed that residual disease was the strongest prognostic factor. However, the use of radical surgery increased the rate of "optimal cytoreduction" as well as 5-year OS. Radical surgery, residual disease, age, ASA score, and operative time were significant variables in the univariate analysis. In the multivariate model, residual disease and radical surgery were independent prognostic factors. However, the performance status could be one explanation since there was a significant correlation between the ASA score and the rate of radical surgery. Other authors observed similar results [20, 21].

Conversely, Hamilton et al. reported that patients with upper abdominal disease had a worse prognosis, even with a complete resection when compared to patients with carcinomatosis limited to the pelvis [22]. More recently, Horowitz et al. reported recently on the correlation between initial extent of the carcinomatosis, aggressiveness of surgery, and survival [23]. Complete resection was once more associated to longer survival, whatever the initial disease burden. But among patients without residual disease, prognosis significantly varied with the initial extent of the disease. In patient with disease high score, the use of complex surgery increased the rate of complete resection and provided similar survival to that of patients with disease high score and without residual obtained by less aggressive surgery. In terms of survival, there was a benefit of 3 months for PFS and 6 months for OS, in patients with initial disease high score and without residuals after complex surgery when compared to patients with macroscopic residuals after the same kind of procedures. However, complexity score of surgery was not an independent prognostic factor in the multivariate analysis. The interpretation of these results should be cautious since the definition of the disease score is questionable in this paper (high score represents a large and heterogeneous population; low score represents previous nodal IIIc patients with the best prognosis of "advanced" disease), and only 12 % of patients with high disease score underwent complete resection.

In summary, there are many arguments to think that the use of radical surgery for patients with carcinomatosis in which optimal or complete resection can be obtained will have a positive impact on survival. However, the extent of this benefit could be moderate and should be compared to morbidity and mortality of such operations.

Primary Debulking or Neoadjuvant Chemotherapy?

This issue has been raised as a systematic strategy for the management of advanced carcinomatosis of adnexal or peritoneal origin. However, a majority of physicians now consider that this alternative could constitute a personalized approach taking into account the disease characteristics and the patient history.

Detailed analysis of the EORTC trial provides some leads for future guidelines. In this study, subgroup analyses have been performed according to the extent of the initial disease (published as appendix). Tables clearly show a direct relation between

Table 3.1 Neoadjuvant trials. Impact of surgeon qualification on results

Study	*n*	% optimal primary surgery	% optimal interval surgery	PFS primary	PFS interval	OS primary	OS interval
EORTC [15]	319	0	45 %	13 months	18 months	20 months	26 months
GOG [16]	550	0	?	10.7 months	10.5 months	35.7 months	36.2 months

Table 3.2 Neoadjuvant trials. Results in patients with advanced disease

Study	*n*	% optimal primary surgery	% optimal interval surgery	PFS primary surgery	PFS interval surgery	OS primary surgery	OS interval surgery
EORTC [17]	670	41.6 %	80.2 %	12 months	12 months	29 months	30 months
Chorus [18]	552	41 %	73 %	10.7 months	12 months	22.6 months	24.1 months

the initial extent of the disease, expressed as 1988 FIGO stage or largest metastatic tumor and overall survival [17]. The same material has been subsequently used for an exploratory analysis, aiming to identify biomarkers [24]. The Kaplan-Meier estimates for a 5-year survival for each biomarker were computed according to primary surgery or neoadjuvant chemotherapy. Five-year survival was similar with both strategies according to age, WHO performance status, tumor grade, tumor histology, pleural effusion, CA125 at baseline, presence of a pelvic mass, or an omental cake. On the other hand, largest metastatic tumor size and clinical stage were significant predictors of survival according to treatment group. Combining these two biomarkers provides four groups of patients. Primary surgery provided longer survival in patients with stage IIIc and largest metastasis <45 mm (20 % of patients), whereas neoadjuvant chemotherapy provided better results in patients with stage IV disease and large metastatic deposits (16 % of patients) [24]. For intermediate patients (stage IIIc and large metastasis or stage IV with small metastasis) (64 % of patients), both strategies were similar in terms of 5-year survival. One of the limitations was the absence of information on patients with poor performance status since they could not be included in this trial (Tables 3.1 and 3.2).

A consensus exists to recommend primary surgery in patients with good performance status and limited disease (stage IIIa, IIIIb, and IIIc with largest metastasis <50 mm of the 1988 FIGO classification) [25]. This population accounts for 37 % of the overall population.

On the other hand, a minority of patients require a neoadjuvant chemotherapy due to poor general status and/or stage IV disease or large abdominal metastases.

The "grey zone" is now the most challenging population. Patients with good performance status and stage III disease associated with metastases ≥50 mm can be managed by primary surgery (with a real risk of incomplete resection and morbidity) or neoadjuvant chemotherapy and interval surgery. This accounts for 8–25 % of patients. The attitude greatly varies between centers and is mostly a question of philosophy rather than the result of scientific data. The TRUST trial which will compare OS after primary vs. interval debulking surgery in trained centers will address this issue [26]. Overall, the rate of neoadjuvant chemotherapy should not be superior to 30 % of patients.

A different way of thinking has to be used for histology types other than high-grade serous ovarian cancer, especially in types where a low response to chemotherapy is expected. The prevailing strategy may be primary surgery, even in case of expected residual disease.

Selection of patients is today mostly performed using imaging, laparoscopy (see specific chapter), and surgeon's opinion. However, in the near future, molecular data could be used to help in the decision-making process [27]. It appears logical to propose surgery when the expected rate of complete resection is high and to have an adapted approach in patients with predictable chemoresistance. Today, BRCA mutation and homologous recombination deficiency signature, as well as tumor infiltrating lymphocytes CD8+ expression, should be helpful to predict chemotherapy response and will be more and more taken into account for primary or interval surgery decision. Complex molecular signatures associated to survival have also been published, with better accuracy than classical prognostic factors, to select high- and low-risk patients [27]. The same train of thought has been applied to select patients with the goal of "optimal surgery." Interestingly, hyperactivation of the TGF-β/Smad pathway and of the RTK/Ras/MAPK/Egr-1 (+ AMPK/Egr-1, Hedgehog/Gli) pathway are associated with tumor dissemination, migration, invasion, angiogenesis, metastatic colonization, and activation of tumor-associated fibroblasts [27].

Conclusion

Several randomized trials have allowed to accumulate data on the surgical management of advanced epithelial ovarian. Complete resection of the peritoneal disease should be the goal of primary or interval debulking surgery. The choice between these two strategies should be done by trained and structured teams. Patients with good general status and low to intermediate extent of disease should be proposed for primary surgery. Patients with poor general status or very extensive disease should be candidates to neoadjuvant chemotherapy. For other patients, the choice between these two options is today mainly a question of opinion. Tomorrow, the TRUST trial will hopefully help to answer this question. We should keep in mind the survival benefit obtained by management of patients by experienced teams and the respect of guidelines.

Personalized approach taking into account molecular characteristics of the tumor will probably help the decision in the future.

References

1. Griffiths CT. Surgical resection of tumor bulk in the primary treatment of ovarian carcinoma. Natl Cancer Inst Monogr. 1975;42:101–4.
2. Chéreau E, Rouzier R, Gouy S, Ferron G, Narducci F, Bergzoll C, Huchon C, Lécuru F, Pomel C, Daraï E, Leblanc E, Querleu D, Morice P. Morbidity of diaphragmatic surgery for advanced ovarian cancer: retrospective study of 148 cases. Eur J Surg Oncol. 2011;37:175–80.
3. Rafii A, Stoeckle E, Jean-Laurent M, Ferron G, Morice P, Houvenaeghael G, Lecuru F, Leblanc E, Querleu D. Multi-center evaluation of post-operative morbidity and mortality after optimal cytoreductive surgery for advanced ovarian cancer. PLoS One. 2012;7:e39415. doi:10.1371/journal.pone.0039415.
4. Vergote I, van Gorp T, Amant F, Leunen K, Neven P, Berteloot P. Timing of debulking surgery in advanced ovarian cancer. Int J Gynecol Cancer. 2008;18 Suppl 1:11–9.
5. Prat J. Staging classification for cancer of the ovary, fallopian tube, and peritoneum. Int J Gynecol Obstet. 2014;124:1–5.
6. Bristow RE, Tomacruz RS, Armstrong DK, Trimble EL, Montz FJ. Survival effect of maximal cytoreductive surgery for advanced ovarian carcinoma during the platinum era: a meta-analysis. J Clin Oncol. 2002;20:1248–59.
7. Eisenkop SM, Spirtos NM, Friedman RL, Lin WC, Pisani AL, Perticucci S. Relative influences of tumor volume before surgery and the cytoreductive outcome on survival for patients with advanced ovarian cancer: a prospective study. Gynecol Oncol. 2003;90:390–6.
8. Chi DS, Eisenhauer EL, Lang J, Huh J, Haddad L, Abu-Rustum NR, Sonoda Y, Levine DA, Hensley M, Barakat RR. What is the optimal goal of primary cytoreductive surgery for bulky stage IIIC epithelial ovarian carcinoma (EOC)? Gynecol Oncol. 2006;103:559–64.
9. du Bois A, Reuss A, Pujade Lauraine E, Harter P, Ray-Coquard I, Pfisterer J. Role of surgical outcome as prognostic factor in advanced epithelial ovarian cancer: a combined exploratory analysis of 3 prospectively randomized phase 3 multicenter trials. Cancer. 2009;115:1234–44.
10. Chi DS, Franklin CC, Levine DA, Akselrod F, Sabbatini P, Jarnagin WR, DeMatteo R, Poynor EA, Abu-Rustum NR, Barakat RR. Improved optimal cytoreduction rates for stages IIIC and IV epithelial ovarian, fallopian tube, and primary peritoneal cancer: a change in surgical approach. Gynecol Oncol. 2004;94:650–4.
11. Chi D, Eisenhauer E, Zivanovic O, Sonoda Y, Abu-Rustum N, Levine D, Guile M, Bristow R, Aghajanian C, Barakat R. Improved progression-free and overall survival in advanced ovarian cancer as a result of a change in surgical paradigm. Gynecol Oncol. 2009;114:26–31.
12. Fournier M, Huchon C, Bats AS, Ngo C, Bensaid C, Douay Hauser N, Seror J, Dessapt AL, Poupon C, Lecuru F. Prognostic impact of chemotherapy delay after primary surgery in advanced ovarian cancer. Melbourne: Poster. IGCS; 2014.
13. Vernooij F, Heintz P, Witteveen E, van der Graaf Y. The outcomes of ovarian cancer are better when provided by gynecologic oncologist in specialized hospitals. Gynecol Oncol. 2007;105:801–12.
14. Rochon J, Pfisterer J, Hoskins W, du Bois A. Variations in institutional infrastructure, physician specialization and experience, and outcome in ovarian cancer: a systematic review. Gynecologic Oncology. 2009;112:422–36.
15. van der Burg MEL, van Lent M, Buyse M, Kobierska A, Colombo N, Favalli G, Lacave A, Nardi M, Renard J, Pecorelli S. The effect of debulking surgery after induction chemotherapy on the prognosis in advanced epithelial ovarian cancer. N Engl J Med. 1995;332:629–34.
16. Rose Rose PG, Nerenstone S, Brady MF, Clarke-Pearson D, Olt G, Rubin S, Moore D, Small J. Secondary surgical cytoreduction for advanced ovarian carcinoma. N Engl J Med. 2004;351:2489–97.
17. Vergote I, Tropé C, Amant F, Kristensen G, Ehlen T, Jonhson N, Verheijen R, van der Burg M, Lacave A, Benedetti Panici PL, Kenter G, Casado A, Mendiola C, Coens C, Verleye L, Stuart

G, Pecorelli S, Reed N, for the European Organization for Research and Treatment of Cancer–Gynaecological Cancer Group and the NCIC Clinical Trials Group — a Gynecologic Cancer Intergroup Collaboration. Neoadjuvant chemotherapy or primary surgery in stage IIIC or IV ovarian cancer. N Engl J Med. 2010;363:943–53.
18. Kehoe S, Hook J, Nankivell M, Jayson G, Kitchener H, Lopes T, Luesley D, Perren T, Bannoo S, Mascarenhas M, Dobbs S, Essapen S, Twigg J, Herod J, McCluggage G, Parmar M, Swart AM. Primary chemotherapy versus primary surgery for newly diagnosed advanced ovarian cancer (CHORUS): an open-label, randomised, controlled, non-inferiority trial. Lancet. 2015;386(9990):249–57.
19. Aletti GD, Podratz KC, Jones MB, Cliby WA. Role of rectosigmoidectomy and stripping of pelvic peritoneum in outcomes of patients with advanced ovarian cancer. J Am Coll Surg. 2006;203:521–6.
20. Eisenhauer E, Abu Rustum N, Sonoda Y, Aghajanian C, Barakat R, Chi D. The effect of maximal surgical cytoreduction on sensitivity to platinum-taxane chemotherapy and subsequent survival in patients with advanced ovarian cancer. Gynecol Oncol. 2008;108:276–81.
21. Eisenkop SM, Spirtos NM. Procedures required to accomplish complete cytoreduction of ovarian cancer: is there a correlation with "biological aggressiveness" and survival? Gynecol Oncol. 2001;82:435–41.
22. Hamilton CA, Miller A, Miller C, Krivak TC, Farley JH, Chernofsky MR, Stany MP, Rose GS, Markman M, Ozols RF, Armstrong DK, Maxwell GL. The impact of disease distribution on survival in patients with stage III epithelial ovarian cancer cytoreduced to microscopic residual: a gynecologic oncology group study. Gynecol Oncol. 2011;122:521–6.
23. Horowitz N, Miller A, Rungruang B, Richard S, Rodriguez N, Bookman M, Hamilton C, Krivak T, Maxwell L. Does aggressive surgery improve outcomes? Interaction between preoperative disease burden and complex surgery in patients with advanced-stage ovarian cancer: an analysis of GOG 182. J Clin Oncol. 2015;33(8):937–43.
24. van Meurs H, Tajik P, Hof M, Vergote I, Kenter G, Mol B, Buist M, Bossuyt P. Which patients benefit most from primary surgery or neoadjuvant chemotherapy in stage IIIc or IV ovarian cancer? An exploratory analysis of the European Organisation for research and treatment of cancer 55971 randomised trial. Eur J Cancer. 2013;49:3191–201.
25. Vergote I, Amant F, Leunen K, du Bois A, Heitz F, Harter P. Neoadjuvant chemotherapy in advanced ovarian cancer: on what do we agree and disagree? Gynecol Oncol. 2013;128:6–11.
26. TRUST. https://clinicaltrials.gov/ct2/results?term=NCT02828618.
27. Riester M, Wei W, Waldron L, Cuhlane A, Trippa L, Oliva E, Kim S, Michor F, Huttenhower C, Parmigiani G, Birrer M. Risk prediction for late stage ovarian cancer by meta-analysis of 1525 patients samples. J Natl Cancer Inst. 2014;106(5):1–12. doi:10.1093/jnci/dju048.

How to Evaluate Tumor Burden Before Therapeutic Decision

4

Anna Fagotti, Luigi Pedone Anchora, Mara Pacciani, and Giovanni Scambia

Abstract

Absent residual tumor after primary debulking surgery is one of the main prognostic factors in advanced ovarian cancer. However, complete resection is very difficult to obtain, due to the wide spread diffusion of the disease both within the abdominal cavity on peritoneal surfaces, and to the liver/spleen, or far to the lung, brain and lymphnodes. Predicting successful surgical outcome depends on many variables including patients' characteristics, serum markers, and disease extension. Here we describe more advanced techniques to assess pre-operative tumor burden, ongoing clinical trials and integrated clinical models to individualize therapeutic decision.

Introduction

Ovarian cancer mainly spreads within the peritoneum, due to anatomical and biological reasons. The low thickness of tubal epithelium favors the detachment of high-grade serous cancer cells arising from the fallopian tube into the pouch of Douglas [1]. The same mechanism is described for tumors primarily originating from the surface of the ovary, such as endometrioid and clear cell cancer.

The peristaltic movements from the gastrointestinal tract and the negative pressure exerted by the diaphragm favor a clockwise circulation of the fluids and isolated cancer cells within the abdomen. In case specific molecular changes occur, cancer cells can adhere, infiltrate, and metastasize according to a characteristic pattern of peritoneal carcinosis. Therefore, each intraperitoneal mesothelial covered surface is at risk of metastasis and needs to be evaluated preoperatively.

A. Fagotti (✉) • L.P. Anchora • M. Pacciani • G. Scambia
Gynecologic Oncology, Department Obstetrics and Gynecology,
Catholic University of Sacred Heart, Rome, Italy
e-mail: anna.fagotti@rm.unicatt.it

E. Pujade-Lauraine et al. (eds.), *Ovarian Cancers*,
DOI 10.1007/978-3-319-32110-3_4

Pleural effusion occurs in 70 % of Advanced Epithelial Ovarian Cancer (AEOC) patients and origins from cancer cell translymphatic circulation through subperitoneal lymphatic spaces [2]. Other mechanisms of metastasis are rare in ovarian cancer, but still possible: hematogenous way to the liver, spleen, lung, and brain and lymphatic route to aortic, thoracic, and paracardiac nodes [3]. Their presence can critically change the therapeutic strategy.

The ideal preoperative staging technique of AEOC should be an "all in one" technique, able to detect any size of intraperitoneal disease at any location, as well as to assess lymphonodal status and distant parenchymatous metastases. However, specific information seems crucial for the clinical management, such as the involvement of precise anatomical sites or specific patterns of disease that make a complete cytoreduction impossible to achieve. A hypothetical reliable method should provide these kinds of data.

Clinical Evaluation

Advanced ovarian cancer clinical presentation is vague and varies widely, including bloating, diffuse abdominal pain, fatigue, nausea/vomiting, and dyspnea. Clinical examination is able to assess the presence of a solid pelvic/abdominal mass with possible rectal involvement and ascites. However, the typical spread of ovarian cancer into the abdominal cavity makes the usefulness of the clinical evaluation in predicting disease diffusion and chances of cytoreduction very restricted. Nevertheless, the role of clinical evaluation in AEOC patients is crucial to achieve a correct therapeutic decision, besides imaging or intraoperative results on tumor burden. In fact, complete cytoreduction often requires extensive surgical procedures, and it is inevitably associated with high rates of postoperative morbidity and mortality. Assessment of tumor burden should be always related to the patient's clinical features in order to have an adequate balance between risk and benefits of debulking surgery, thus achieving the best therapeutic decision.

Age and nutritional status are simple data to evaluate. No study demonstrates they are clearly related to tumor burden, but with increased postoperative morbidity and mortality in surgical patients. More recently, decreased *serum albumin levels* <3.5 g/dl have been strongly correlated with postoperative morbidity and mortality [4, 5].

The *Eastern Cooperative Oncology Group (ECOG)* score [6], also called the WHO score, and American Society of Anesthesiologists physical status classification system score (ASA) are simple and commonly used in clinical practice. Aletti et al. demonstrated that an *ASA score* ≥3 is an independent prognostic factor influencing 30-day morbidity and it is the only preoperative variable correlating with patient's ability to receive planned chemotherapy [4]. Barlin et al. [5] included ASA score in their nomogram as a predictor of mortality after primary surgery.

Serum Markers

CA-125 is a membrane-associated glycoprotein expressed by ovarian surface epithelium. Elevated CA-125 serum levels can be found in benign and inflammatory conditions of the female reproductive system and in the abdominal area (i.e., endometriosis), as well in ovarian cancer. This justifies the limited specificity of CA-125 testing. Moreover, not every patient with ovarian cancer will have elevated levels of CA-125 in the blood. Rosen DG et al. detected a rate of 79 % of all ovarian cancers positive for CA-125, whereas remainders did not express this antigen at all [7]. Different CA-125 serum levels have been related to the histological types, with the highest in serous and lowest in mucinous epithelial cancers; clear cell and endometrioid ovarian cancer often have lower CA-125 values too.

In the 2000s, high preoperative CA-125 values were associated with poor chance of optimal cytoreduction at primary surgery [8, 9]. However, in the last two decades, surgical approach has changed, including procedures able to achieve higher rates of optimal cytoreduction. Consequently, a more recent study has demonstrated that preoperative CA-125 levels >500 U/mL lack the ability to predict optimal cytoreduction, accurately [9]. In a subsequent meta-analysis, Kang et al. [10] analyzed 14 studies with 2192 patients to assess the performance of CA-125 at various cutoff levels as a predictor of the outcome of cytoreductive surgery. Preoperative serum CA-125 level had a low positive and a high negative likelihood ratio in predicting cytoreductive outcome in advanced ovarian carcinoma. In other words, a preoperative serum CA-125 level >500 U/mL was strongly associated with suboptimal cytoreduction (odds ratio, 3.69; 95 % CI, 2.02–6.73) [11, 12].

Although a novel biomarker, called HE4, has been shown to be a better predictor of complete cytoreduction than CA-125 in naïve patients, CA-125 remains the principal marker used in clinical practice so far [13].

During the last years, some predictive models of optimal cytoreduction based on radiological and clinical criteria, including CA-125 ≥500 U/mL [14, 15], have been created with a high accuracy rate. Suidan et al. [14] published a prospective, nonrandomized, multicenter trial of preoperative CT of the abdomen and pelvis in combination with serum CA-125 level to predict suboptimal primary cytoreduction (≥1 cm residual disease) in 350 patients with stage III–IV disease. The results showed that the following criteria were associated with suboptimal cytoreduction: age ≥60 years, CA-125 level ≥500 U/mL, American Society of Anesthesiologists physical status 3 or 4, retroperitoneal lymph nodes above the renal hilum (including supradiaphragmatic) >1 cm, diffuse small bowel adhesions/thickening, perisplenic lesion >1 cm, small bowel mesentery lesion >1 cm, lesion in the root of the superior mesenteric artery >1 cm, and lesser sac lesion >1 cm. Based on these findings, the authors developed a predictive model in which the rate of suboptimal cytoreduction was directly proportional to a predictive value score.

However, in the last few years, patients' characterization has improved thanks to molecular biology. It has been hypothesized that surgical outcomes, i.e., residual disease at primary surgery, may be predictable based on biomarkers assessment from tumor tissue, besides the large variability between disease presentation and surgeon experience. Recently, a group of researchers from the MD Anderson Cancer Center has shown that high FABP4 and ADH1B expression is associated with significantly higher risk of residual disease in high-grade serous ovarian cancer. Therefore, women with high tumoral levels of these genes may be candidates for neoadjuvant chemotherapy [16]. Unfortunately, serous and biological markers do not have an independent role in evaluation of tumor burden to date.

Imaging Techniques

Several imaging techniques are available to provide an assessment of tumor burden in order to plan the correct therapeutic strategy and complex surgery in AEOC women (Table 4.1).

Table 4.1 Ongoing clinical trials on imaging techniques in advanced ovarian cancer

NCT#	Name	Type – site	Objective
MRI			
NCT02243059	MILO	Maastricht University Medical Center	Magnetic resonance imaging for lymph node staging in ovarian cancer
NCT02334371		Maastricht University Medical Center	MR-PET for staging and assessment of operability in ovarian cancer: a feasibility study
NCT01657747	S53580	Universitaire Ziekenhuizen Leuven	Whole-body diffusion MRI for staging, response prediction, and detecting tumor recurrence in patients with ovarian cancer
NCT01505829	DISCOVAR	Institute of Cancer Research, United Kingdom	Diffusion-weighted imaging study in cancer of the ovary
CT scan			
NCT00587093		Multicentric (MSKCC, John Hopkins University, MD Anderson CC)	A multicenter trial on the utility and impact of computed tomography and serum CA-125 in the management of newly diagnosed ovarian cancer
FDG-PET/CT scan			
NCT02258165	IMAGE	Queensland Centre for Gynaecological Cancer	Impact of gated PET/CT in the diagnosis of advanced ovarian cancer
Laparoscopy			
NCT01461850	SCORPION	Monocentric, Catholic University of the Sacred Heart	Surgical complications related to primary or interval debulking in ovarian neoplasm
NTR 2644	LapOvCa-trial	Multicentric, Gyn Onc, Netherlands	Laparoscopy to predict the result of primary cytoreductive surgery in advanced ovarian cancer patients: a multicenter randomized controlled study

Ultrasonography

Transvaginal ultrasonography is a well-established imaging modality for the assessment of pelvic masses, and usually it is the first-line imaging technique for detecting and characterizing adnexal masses. Most experienced ultrasound examiners have shown to be able to reliably discriminate between benign and malignant extrauterine pelvic masses, based on gray scale and color Doppler ultrasound findings [17]. Recently, some researchers have evaluated the abdominal disease extension by TV/TA US with promising results. Presence of ascites is often associated with peritoneal carcinosis [18]. Peritoneal involvement can be diagnosed by the presence of solid, hypoechogen nodules, which grow on the peritoneal surfaces or by bands of thickened tissue that catch intestinal loops and may cause a retraction toward mesenteric root. The peritoneal involvement includes the gastrohepatic, hepatoduodenal, gastrosplenic, and splenocolic ligaments; supra- and infracolic omentum; parietal peritoneum on the diaphragm, paracolic gutters, and anterior abdominal wall; and visceral and mesenterial peritoneum. Lymph nodes are also visible: the peripheral (inguinal or supraclavicular and axillary lymph nodes), retroperitoneal (also called parietal lymph nodes), and visceral abdominal lymph nodes (around the celiac trunk up to the splenic and hepatic hilum and around the superior and inferior mesenteric artery).

Testa et al. [19] demonstrated that ultrasound examination is highly accurate in detecting metastatic omental involvement in cases with suspicious pelvic masses, with NPV, PPV, and accuracy rates of 91.9 %, 94.6 %, and 93.8 %, respectively. Among 173 patients enrolled, sonographic detection of metastatic omentum was achieved in 104 (60.1 %), appearing as either solid aperistaltic tissue (80.8 % of cases) or as solid discrete nodules (19.2 %).

Ultrasound may also allow the targeted biopsy of advanced tumors or metastatic lesions, obtaining fast histological diagnosis, as shown by Zikan et al. [20] in 190 patients, with a complication rate of 1.0 %.

Therefore, a new interesting role is arising for completely transabdominal and pelvic US, in the hands of experienced examiners [21]. It consists of describing intraperitoneal, retroperitoneal, and parenchymal diffusion of advanced ovarian cancer and to assess the chances of optimal cytoreduction. With this purpose, a multicentric international prospective study within the IOTA group is going to be started, to compare ultrasound and CT scan evaluation in terms of prediction of residual disease in naïve advanced epithelial ovarian cancer patients.

Magnetic Resonance Imaging (MRI)

MRI may be used to define the origin and tissue characteristics of an adnexal mass. It may discriminate between benign and malignant pelvic tumors [22]. Generally, after gadolinium administration, ovarian cancer enhances earlier, more rapidly, and more avidly than benign lesions. Moreover, delayed images help in abdominal staging of ovarian cancer, increasing the detection of small peritoneal implants and omental infiltration, reaching an accuracy rate of 100 % in the correct malignant lesions characterization and of 75 % in staging [23].

Nowadays, a growing attention has been paid to the addition of diffusion-weighted imaging (DWI) supplemented with dynamic contrast-enhanced MR (DCE-MR) to morphologic imaging that improves tumor characterization, as well as peritoneal and lymph node staging [24–27]. DWI is based on the detection of higher cellular density and reduced extracellular space in malignant tumors than benign lesions. Therefore, the characterization of tissues by means of DCE-MR and DWI enables a move from morphologic assessment to characterization of tumor vascularity and cellularity [28].

Standard MRI sensitivity is considerably lower than DWI in the detection of abdominal implants, especially for those smaller than 1 cm and in anatomic areas where small tumor implants are adjacent to tissues with similar signal intensity, such as the right subdiaphragmatic space, omentum, root of the mesentery, and visceral peritoneum of the small bowel and bladder [29]. The combination of functional information with conventional anatomical visualization (DCE-MR) holds promise to characterize peritoneal disease accurately [30] showing a high per-lesion sensitivity (95 %) and specificity (80 %) in the description of peritoneal dissemination [29]. Recent studies have shown a better accuracy (91 %) for the abdominal staging in patients with ovarian cancer when DWI is performed, and the addition of DWI to conventional MRI increases the number of detected peritoneal lesions by 21–29 % [24, 25].

The DWI technique also provides more information about lymph node characterization. MRI lymphonodal status evaluation, based on simple dimensional parameter, has a sensitivity of 64.3 % and specificity of 75 % [29], while the addiction of DWI increases sensitivity up to 77 % and specificity to 91 % [24].

For this reason, the addition of DWI to an MRI protocol could help to reduce inter-center difference in ovarian cancer staging, leading to a good interobserver agreement for primary tumor characterization, and peritoneal and distant staging [24].

Computerized Tomography

CT has a limited role in the primary detection and characterization of ovarian cancer, since the low soft tissue contrast of the CT may affect its reliability to discriminate the benignity or malignancy of an ovarian lesion [31, 32]. Furthermore, the CT appearance of ovarian metastases is indistinguishable from a primary ovarian neoplasm.

On the other hand, CT is the first-choice technique to study advanced ovarian carcinoma, being rapid, highly accurate, and widely available. Moreover, the lower incidence of breathing artifacts and image distortion than MRI allows the assessment of cardiophrenic lymph nodes and pleural effusion. For these characteristics, CT after IV administration of a low-osmolarity contrast medium and eventually oral contrast medium to detect tumor deposits along the small and large bowel serosa [33] is currently the standard preoperative imaging staging in women with advanced ovarian cancer [34, 35].

Overall staging accuracy rate for CT has been reported between 70 and 90 %, but a high PPV for imaging bulky disease makes it useful to identify patients with inoperable disease [36]. Standard CT, however, frequently fails to identify small sites of peritoneal spread [30]. Radiology sensitivity for metastases of 1 cm or smaller (25–50 %) is significantly lower than overall sensitivity (85–93 %) [37], and it decreases up to 14 % in absence of ascites.

Computed tomography, with its low specificity, also lacks accuracy for characterizing lymph nodes when their assessment is based on the short-axis-diameter measure [34]. The addition of morphological criteria may reach a specificity of 100 % but decreases sensitivity to 37.5 % [38]. Good results are obtained by CT scan in the assessment of the liver or omental involvement and mesenteric disease (sensitivity from 95 % to 100 % and from 80 % to 86 %, respectively) [39].

During the last decade, many studies have tried to investigate the ability of CT scan to predict surgical outcome in patients with naïve AEOC, in order to suggest patient's suitability for cytoreductive surgery or neoadjuvant chemotherapy. Nelson et al. [40] scored CT scans on the basis of some radiologic criteria, as cytoreducible (no disease remaining in criteria site) or not cytoreducible (at least one site of disease remaining) by standard surgical techniques. The CT findings accurately predicted surgical outcome (optimal RT <2 cm) with a sensitivity of 92.3 % and a specificity of 79.3 %. In 2000, Bristow et al. [41] proposed another CT-based predictive model based on retrospective analysis of 41 patients by two radiologists without knowledge of the operative findings. Thirteen radiographic features were included and a predictive index score was elaborated. PI score ≥4 had the highest overall accuracy (92.7 %) and identified patients undergoing suboptimal cytoreduction (RT <1 cm) with a sensitivity of 100 %. Nevertheless, a retrospective analysis on 180 patients with advanced disease meeting criteria for non-resectability showed that optimal cytoreduction was still achieved in 92.2 % of cases and complete cytoreduction in 22.2 % [42].

Dowdy et al. [43] published results of a retrospective analysis in which 87 preoperative CT scans were reviewed for 17 criteria indicating disease extent by two radiologists without knowledge of operative outcome. The authors found that a model based on diffuse peritoneal thickening and ascites had 68 % PPV and 52 % sensitivity and was associated with a low rate of optimal cytoreduction (RT <1 cm) (32 %).

Since then, many efforts have been made in order to find a correlation between preoperative findings and final surgical outcome in these patients. The combination of clinical (either CA-125 serum levels or ECOG PS) and radiological features is able to offer the best performances in terms of prediction of residual disease after PDS, as shown in some retrospective series from MSKCC and MD Anderson CC, Mayo Clinic, and Catholic University of Sacred Heart [14, 44, 45]. Unfortunately, these tests need to be validated in an external center.

FDG-PET/CT

PET integrated with CT (PET/CT) is now a well-established noninvasive imaging tool in oncology, and many studies have already shown its usefulness for diagnosis and staging of a recurrent ovarian cancer. However, the role of FDG-PET/CT for the initial evaluation of women with ovarian cancer is limited, especially in women with early stage disease as well as for characterizing adnexal masses [46].

Regarding the assessment of tumor spread in AEOC, PET/CT scan has shown a high false-negative rate for lesions less than 5 mm, such as carcinomatosis, in the presence of diffuse miliary visceral implants mimicking physiological bowel activity and in women with cystic or necrotic lesions or lesions with copious mucinous collections as in mucinous tumors [30, 47]. Recent studies have shown that PET/CT is better than CT in detecting retroperitoneal lymph node metastases, but not peritoneal metastases [48]. Hynninen et al. [49] prospectively studied 41 women with ovarian cancer who underwent preoperative fluorodeoxyglucose (FDG) PET/CT followed by diagnostic high-dose contrast-enhanced CT. The sensitivity of PET/CT and CT in the detection of unresectable disease was poor in certain areas of the peritoneal cavity (64 % for PET/CT and 27 % for CT in the small bowel mesentery; 65 % for PET/CT and 55 % for CT in the right upper abdomen). In the overall site-based analysis, the sensitivity for PET/CT and CT was 51 % and 41 %, respectively, whereas the specificity was 89 % and 92 % and the accuracy was 64 % and 57 %, respectively. Preoperative contrast-enhanced CT suggested extra-abdominal disease spread in 61 % patients and PET/CT in 78 % patients.

Fruscio et al. [50] also evaluated patients with suspected advanced ovarian cancer with preoperative 18-FDG-PET/CT. The patients were divided into three groups on the basis of clinical and PET/CT findings: group A, stage III by both clinical and PET findings; group B, stage III by clinical findings and stage IV by PET/CT; and group C, stage IV by both clinical and PET/CT findings. Twenty-five patients had their disease upstaged to stage IV by PET/CT. The proportion of patients with residual tumor <1 cm was similar in groups B and C and was significantly higher in groups B and C than in group A. Similarly, complete response to adjuvant chemotherapy was achieved more frequently in patients in group A.

In a consecutive series of 343 AEOC, a group of researchers from Korea have developed a nomogram to predict incomplete cytoreduction, including surgical aggressiveness index, positron emission tomography (tumoral uptake ratio = highest SUV max in the upper abdomen/lower abdomen), and computed tomography features (diaphragm, ascites, peritoneal carcinosis, small bowel mesentery). This nomogram had a concordance index of 0.881 (95 % CI = 0.838–0.923), which was confirmed in the validation cohort (concordance index = 0.881; 95 % CI = 0.790–0.932) [51]. In an attempt to compare three different modalities (multidetector CT or MDCT, MRI, PET/CT) to assess peritoneal carcinosis in AEOC patients, MRI showed the highest sensitivity and FDG-PET/CT had the highest specificity, but no significant differences were found between the three techniques. Thus, MDCT, as the fastest, most economical, and most widely available modality, may be considered the examination of choice, if a stand-alone technique is required. If inconclusive, PET/CT or MRI may offer additional insights. Whole-body FDG-PET/CT may be more accurate for supradiaphragmatic metastatic extension [52].

Surgical Scoring System

The possibility to achieve optimal/complete cytoreduction (RT = 0/<1 cm) is related to the extent of disease before surgery [53]. Unfortunately, there is no perfect tool to preoperatively determine whether patients can be optimally debulked or should be proposed for neoadjuvant chemotherapy. To quantify with more precision the intra-abdominal extent of the disease, a number of numerical ranking systems based on the intraoperative tumor assessment have been proposed. The first was PCI (peritoneal cancer index) [54] used to describe peritoneal spread in different malignant tumors. Subsequently, other scores have been proposed by Eisenkop et al. [55], Aletti et al. [4], and Fagotti et al. [56].

Tentes et al. [57] evaluated the role of PCI in ovarian cancer, combining the distribution of the tumor throughout 13 abdominopelvic regions with a lesion size score. Mean survival and 5-year survival rates for patients with a PCI <10 were 80 ± 12 months and 65 %, respectively, while mean survival and 5-year survival rates for patients with a PCI >10 were 38 ± 7 months and 29 %, respectively. Similarly, Eisenkop ranking system reflects the continuum of progressively extensive tumor involvement by ovarian cancer for five anatomic regions [55].

Aletti et al. [4] provided a validated system to track surgical outcomes in gynecologic cancer in order to improve overall patient care. Analyzing 564 patients with stage IIIC and IV epithelial ovarian cancer enrolled by three different US gynecological oncologic centers, they demonstrated that surgical complexity score, based upon complexity and number of surgical procedures performed, primarily influences morbidity and postoperative outcomes in ovarian cancer patients, including the ability to receive chemotherapy.

These systems have some limits: (a) they were actually based on the classical laparotomic approach (all); (b) they were designed for different pathologies [54]; and (c) they were calculated after completing surgery for a different purpose [4].

Another emerging surgical scoring system is based on the use of laparoscopy. Recently, different carcinomatosis scores have been compared to assess their relevance to predict resectability, morbidity, and outcome in 61 patients who had surgical treatment for AEOC. The authors found that the most relevant scoring system to predict postoperative complications was the Aletti score, but PCI and Eisenkop scores were also relevant. The best predictors of chances to achieve complete resection were the Fagotti-modified score and the PCI score [58].

The rationale for a laparoscopic evaluation prior to cytoreductive surgery includes (1) intraperitoneal diffusion of disease can be easily assessed by laparoscopy, and the surgeon may be more confident with a direct visualization of the cancer spread; (2) this approach could spare patients an unnecessary laparotomy resulting in suboptimal cytoreduction; (3) patients deemed not to be candidates for cytoreduction could proceed immediately to neoadjuvant chemotherapy without having to recover from laparotomy-related complications (incisional hernia); and (4) laparoscopy allows collection of tissue for definitive diagnosis and for molecular analyses.

Vergote et al. in 1998 [59] published the first study evaluating laparoscopy prior to cytoreduction in a retrospective analysis of 285 patients with advanced ovarian carcinoma. Then, two Italian studies were published in 2005 and 2006 [60, 61], suggesting a role of laparoscopy in detecting patients with advanced ovarian cancer suitable for NACT versus PDS.

Fagotti et al. [60] reported on the ability to assess by laparoscopy simple parameters in 65 AEOC patients: ovarian masses (unilateral or bilateral), omental cake or nodules, peritoneal and diaphragmatic carcinomatosis, mesenteric retraction, bowel and stomach infiltration, liver metastases, and bulky lymph nodes. Each variable was widely assessed by laparoscopy. The overall accuracy rate of laparoscopy in predicting optimal cytoreduction was 90 %. The NPV of clinical–radiological evaluation was 73 %, whereas the NPV of laparoscopy was 100 % (i.e., in no case when disease was judged incompletely resectable on the basis of laparoscopy findings was disease judged completely resectable at laparotomy). The PPVs of clinical–radiological evaluation and laparoscopy were both 87 %. This work was updated in 2006, when the authors [56] proposed a simple laparoscopy-based scoring system (PIV) to estimate the chances of achieving optimal cytoreduction based on the presence of an omental cake, peritoneal carcinosis, diaphragmatic carcinosis, mesenteric retraction, bowel infiltration, stomach infiltration, and liver metastases. Each parameter was assigned 2 points, if present. A score of greater than eight predicted a suboptimal surgery with a specificity of 100 %, a positive predictive value of 100 %, and a negative predictive value of 70 %. This score was validated in an external cohort of 55 French patients with stage III–IV ovarian cancer [62], showing that a simplified score (excluding omental cake and peritoneal carcinomatosis) could also be used. This represents the first study which supports the ability of an objective quantitative score based on laparoscopy more that on radiologic characteristics to foresee optimal cytoreduction chances for a single patient with advanced ovarian cancer. In 2008, Fagotti et al. [63] reported prospective data on 113 patients who underwent laparoscopy and had the likelihood of optimal cytoreduction evaluated using the PIV score [15]. The results confirmed that at a PIV of ≥8, the probability of optimal cytoreduction (residual tumor ≤1 cm) at laparotomy was 0; 40.5 % of the patients had a PIV of ≥8 and avoided unnecessary exploratory laparotomy. In 2011, the same group of investigators [64] prospectively estimated the learning curve for determining the PIV. The authors compared the scores for each laparoscopic parameter assigned by fellows and senior surgeons showing that fellows in gynecologic oncology with at least 12 months' experience assigned laparoscopy-based scores similar to those of senior surgeons.

A potential concern about implementing preoperative laparoscopic assessment as part of standard practice is the feasibility of this approach not only at major academic institutions but also at other sites. To determine the reproducibility of laparoscopic assessment, Fagotti et al. performed a prospective, multicenter trial (Olympia-MITO 13) [65], in which the application of the laparoscopy-based PIV was evaluated in four satellite centers. A total of 120 patients with clinical suspicion of advanced ovarian, fallopian tube, or primary peritoneal cancer underwent staging laparoscopy at the satellite centers; the procedures were recorded and blindly reviewed at the coordinator center afterward. The most difficult feature to assess was mesenteric retraction, which was not evaluable in 31 of 120 cases (25.8 %). The rate of evaluation of the remaining variables ranged from 99.2 % (peritoneal carcinomatosis) to 90 % (bowel infiltration). An accuracy rate of 80 % or greater was reached in three of the four satellite centers. These studies have validated a laparoscopy-based scoring system that allows surgeons to determine with great accuracy at the time of initial diagnosis of advanced stage ovarian cancer the likelihood that optimal cytoreduction is possible. These studies have also demonstrated that use of this scoring system is reproducible at other institutions.

In order to definitively state the role of staging laparoscopy in advanced ovarian cancer, a last step was needed, which was to investigate if the introduction of such management could negatively influence prognosis in these patients. To this purpose, a retrospective survival analysis on 300 women with FIGO stages IIIC and IV ovarian, fallopian tube, or primary peritoneal carcinoma was published in 2013 [66]. There were no complications related to the laparoscopic procedure. The median PFS in women with R0 resection at primary debulking surgery was 25 months (95 % CI, 15.1–34.8 months), which was significantly longer than the median progression-free survival in patients with less than R0 resection on primary debulking surgery and patients who underwent interval debulking surgery after chemotherapy ($P = 0.0001$). However, other prognostic implications can be ascribed to the laparoscopic score of intraperitoneal diffusion of disease. Vizzielli et al. [67] demonstrated that tumor burden, as assessed by laparoscopic PIV, is an independent prognostic factor together with RT at primary surgery in 348 patients who underwent laparoscopy before primary cytoreductive surgery or neoadjuvant chemotherapy.

Conclusions

A recent Cochrane Review evaluated the accuracy of diagnostic laparoscopy to determine the resectability of disease in patients suspected of having a diagnosis of advanced ovarian cancer [68]. Between 27 and 64 % of patients were considered to have too extensive disease to undergo laparotomy after laparoscopic assessment. They also found that the other 36–73 % were considered suitable for laparotomy and they underwent this surgery. At laparotomy, between 4 and 31 % were found to have residual tumor remaining after surgery, suggesting that they could have been spared a laparotomy. The authors concluded that although diagnostic laparoscopy may seem better than standard diagnostic staging alone, it should not be considered a standard procedure in clinical practice. The authors do recognize that there were several weaknesses in this review including the fact that they could not correct for factors leading to bias. However, most recent NCCN guidelines include Staging-Laparoscopy (S-LPS) as a tool to manage AEOC patients toward PDS or NACT with a IIB level of evidence.

The Laparoscopic-Predictive Index (LPS-PI) was initially designed, and prospectively validated, before the achievement of relevant improvements in the surgical management of AEOC. In fact, the recent introduction of upper abdominal surgery (UAS) in the surgical repertoire of gynecologic oncologists has significantly increased the chance of achieving a complete PDS (RT=0), with significant survival benefit. Therefore, the same authors have hypothesized that some updates are needed to allow a safe application of the LPS-PI in the current therapeutic scenario. In a retrospective analysis, they demonstrated that raising the bar of RT to zero does not impair the reliability of PIV. On the contrary, the updated LPS-PI shows improved discriminating performance, with a lower rate of inappropriate laparotomic explorations at the new established cutoff value of ten [69] (*Gyn Onc*, submitted).

To date, two RCTs are ongoing regarding this issue. One is from the Netherlands [70], with the aim to evaluate the role of laparoscopy prior to primary debulking surgery leaving residual tumor of <1 cm in women with advanced ovarian cancer. Participants are randomized between upfront surgery or diagnostic laparoscopy. Depending on the result of laparoscopy, patients undergo surgery within 3 weeks, followed by six courses of platinum-based chemotherapy, or are treated with neoadjuvant chemotherapy followed by interval debulking 3–4 weeks after three courses of chemotherapy, followed by another three courses of chemotherapy. Primary outcome measure is the proportion of patients with residual <1 cm. The other one is from Italy, the SCORPION trial (NCT01461850) [71], with the aim to compare surgical complications and PFS of primary surgery versus IDS. This trial includes patients with advanced ovarian cancer (FIGO stage IIIC) who have PIV scores of 8 through 12. Patients are randomized to primary debulking surgery followed by adjuvant chemotherapy or neoadjuvant chemotherapy followed by interval debulking surgery and subsequent additional chemotherapy. In this study, all patients undergo diagnostic laparoscopy, and a PIV is assigned.

Capitalizing on the experience of endoscopic preoperative triage assessment, investigators at the University of Texas, MD Anderson Cancer Center, are leveraging laparoscopy as a means of surgical triage, to provide organ-specific tumor sampling (primary tumor, omentum, two additional metastatic sites) and to investigate novel therapeutics [72].

In conclusion, existing studies point to a highly valuable role for laparoscopy for objectively assessing the feasibility of optimal primary and interval cytoreductive surgery for patients with advanced stage ovarian cancer (FIGO stages III and IV). The Fagotti laparoscopy-based score is a useful predictor of optimal cytoreduction. Moreover, standardized use of the Fagotti score should be enforced to ensure that results are concordant across different centers, with a PIV of ≥8 demonstrated to have the best accuracy in identifying disease dissemination and predicting suboptimal cytoreduction. Furthermore, following completion of the ongoing clinical trials, we expect the use of this laparoscopy-based scoring system to become completely standard [73].

References

1. Fathalla MF. Incessant ovulation and ovarian cancer – a hypothesis re-visited. Facts Views Vis Obgyn. 2013;5(4):292–7.
2. Tan D, Agarwal R, Kaye SB. Mechanisms of transcoelomic metastasis in ovarian cancer. Lancet. 2006;7:925–34.
3. Dauplat J, Hacker NF, Nieberg R, et al. Distant metastases in epithelial ovarian carcinoma. Cancer. 1987;60:1561–6.
4. Aletti GD, Santillan A, Eisenhauer EL, Hu J, Aletti G, Podratz KC, Bristow RE, Chi DS, Cliby WA. A new frontier for quality of care in gynecologic oncology surgery: multi-institutional assessment of short-term outcomes for ovarian cancer using a risk-adjusted model. Gynecol Oncol. 2007;107(1):99–106.
5. Barlin JN, Yu C, Hill EK, Zivanovic O, Kolev V, Levine DA, Sonoda Y, Abu-Rustum NR, Huh J, Barakat RR, Kattan MW, Chi DS. Nomogram for predicting 5-year disease-specific mortality after primary surgery for epithelial ovarian cancer. Gynecol Oncol. 2012;125(1): 25–30.
6. Oken MM, Creech RH, Tormey DC, Horton J, Davis TE, McFadden ET, Carbone PP. Toxicity and response criteria of the Eastern Cooperative Oncology Group. Am J Clin Oncol. 1982;5(6):649–55.
7. Rosen DG, Wang L, Atkinson JN, Yu Y, Lu KH, Diamandis EP, Hellstrom I, Mok SC, Liu J, Bast Jr RC. Potential markers that complement expression of CA125 in epithelial ovarian cancer. Gynecol Oncol. 2005;99(2):267–77.
8. Chi DS, Venkatraman ES, Masson V, Hoskins WJ. The ability of preoperative serum CA-125 to predict optimal primary tumor cytoreduction in stage III epithelial ovarian carcinoma. Gynecol Oncol. 2000;77:227–31.
9. Chi DS, Zivanovic O, Palayekar MJ, Eisenhauer EL, Abu-Rustum NR, Sonoda Y, Levine DA, Leitao MM, Brown CL, Barakat RR. A contemporary analysis of the ability of preoperative serum CA-125 to predict primary cytoreductive outcome in patients with advanced ovarian, tubal and peritoneal carcinoma. Gynecol Oncol. 2009;112(1):6–10.
10. Kang S, Kim TJ, Nam BH, Seo SS, Kim BG, Bae DS, Park SY. Preoperative serum CA-125 levels and risk of suboptimal cytoreduction in ovarian cancer: a meta-analysis. J Surg Oncol. 2010;101(1):13–7.
11. Pelissier A, Bonneau C, Chéreau E, de La Motte RT, Fourchotte V, Daraï E, Rouzier R. CA125 kinetic parameters predict optimal cytoreduction in patients with advanced epithelial ovarian cancer treated with neoadjuvant chemotherapy. Gynecol Oncol. 2014;135(3):542–6.
12. Rodriguez N, Rauh-Hain JA, Shoni M, Berkowitz RS, Muto MG, Feltmate C, Schorge JO, Del Carmen MG, Matulonis UA, Horowitz NS. Changes in serum CA-125 can predict optimal cytoreduction to no gross residual disease in patients with advanced stage ovarian cancer treated with neoadjuvant chemotherapy. Gynecol Oncol. 2012;125(2):362–6.
13. Braicu EI, Fotopoulou C, Van Gorp T, Richter R, Chekerov R, Hall C, Butz H, Castillo-Tong DC, Mahner S, Zeillinger R, Concin N, Vergote I, Sehouli J. Preoperative HE4 expression in plasma predicts surgical outcome in primary ovarian cancer patients: results from the OVCAD study. Gynecol Oncol. 2013;128(2):245–51.
14. Suidan RS, Ramirez PT, Sarasohn DM, Teitcher JB, Mironov S, Iyer RB, Zhou Q, Iasonos A, Paul H, Hosaka M, Aghajanian CA, Leitao Jr MM, Gardner GJ, Abu-Rustum NR, Sonoda Y, Levine DA, Hricak H, Chi DS. A multicenter prospective trial evaluating the ability of preoperative computed tomography scan and serum CA-125 to predict suboptimal cytoreduction at primary debulking surgery for advanced ovarian, fallopian tube, and peritoneal cancer. Gynecol Oncol. 2014;134(3):455–61. doi:10.1016/j.ygyno.2014.07.002.
15. Jung DC, Kang S, Kim SC, Kim JW, Nam JH, Ryu SY, Seong SJ, Kim BG. Use of complex surgical procedures, patterns of tumor spread, and CA-125 predicts a risk of incomplete cytoreduction: a Korean Gynecologic Oncology Group study (KGOG-3022). Gynecol Oncol. 2013;131(2):336–40.

16. Tucker SL, Gharpure K, Herbrich SM, Unruh AK, Nick AM, Crane EK, Coleman RL, Guenthoer J, Dalton HJ, Wu SY, Rupaimoole R, Lopez-Berestein G, Ozpolat B, Ivan C, Hu W, Baggerly KA, Sood AK. Molecular biomarkers of residual disease after surgical debulking of high-grade serous ovarian cancer. Clin Cancer Res. 2014;20(12):3280–8.
17. Valentin L. Prospective cross-validation of Doppler ultrasound examination and gray-scale ultrasound imaging for discrimination of benign and malignant pelvic masses. Ultrasound Obstet Gynecol. 1999;14:273–83.
18. Fischerova D, Burgetova A. Imaging techniques for the evaluation of ovarian cancer. Best Pract Res Clin Obstet Gynaecol. 2014;28(5):697–720.
19. Testa AC, Ludovisi M, Savelli L, Fruscella E, Ghi T, Fagotti A, Scambia G, Ferrandina G. Ultrasound and color power Doppler in the detection of metastatic omentum: a prospective study. Ultrasound Obstet Gynecol. 2006;27(1):65–70.
20. Zikan M, Fischerova D, Pinkavova I, Dundr P, Cibula D. Ultrasound-guided tru-cut biopsy of abdominal and pelvic tumors in gynecology. Ultrasound Obstet Gynecol. 2010;36:767–72.
21. Timmerman D, Schwärzler P, Collins WP, et al. Subjective assessment of adnexal masses with the use of ultrasonography: an analysis of interobserver variability and experience. Ultrasound Obstet Gynecol. 1999;13:11–6.
22. Medeiros LR, Stein AT, Fachel J, Garry R, Furness S. Laparoscopy versus laparotomy for benign ovarian tumor: a systematic review and meta-analysis. Int J Gynecol Cancer. 2008; 18(3):387–99.
23. Stevens SK, Hricak H, Stern JL. Ovarian lesions: detection and characterization with gadolinium-enhanced MR imaging at 1.5 T. Radiology. 1991;181(2):481–8.
24. Michielsen K, Vergote I, Op de Beeck K, et al. Whole-body MRI with diffusion-weighted sequence for staging of patients with suspected ovarian cancer: a clinical feasibility study in comparison to CT and FDG-PET/CT. Eur Radiol. 2014;24:889–901.
25. Low RN, Gurney J. Diffusion-weighted MRI (DWI) in the oncology patient: value of breath-hold DWI compared to unenhanced and gadolinium-enhanced MRI. J Magn Reson Imaging. 2007;25:848–58.
26. Low RN, Sebrechts CP, Barone RM, et al. Diffusion-weighted MRI of peritoneal tumors: comparison with conventional MRI and surgical and histopathologic findings–a feasibility study. AJR Am J Roentgenol. 2009;193:461–70.
27. Kyriazi S, Collins DJ, Morgan VA, et al. Diffusion-weighted imaging of peritoneal disease for noninvasive staging of advanced ovarian cancer. Radiographics. 2010;30:1269–85.
28. Wakefield JC, Downey K, Kyriazi S, et al. New MR techniques in gynecologic cancer. AJR Am J Roentgenol. 2013;200:249–60.
29. Ricke J, Sehouli J, Hach C, Hänninen EL, Lichtenegger W, Felix R. Prospective evaluation of contrast-enhanced MRI in the depiction of peritoneal spread in primary or recurrent ovarian cancer. Eur Radiol. 2003;13(5):943–9.
30. Kyriazi S, Kaye SB, deSouza NM. Imaging ovarian cancer and peritoneal metastases–current and emerging techniques. Nat Rev Clin Oncol. 2010;7:381–93.
31. Bharwani N, Reznek RH, Rockall AG. Ovarian cancer management: the role of imaging and diagnostic challenges. Eur J Radiol. 2011;78:41–51.
32. Alt CD, Brocker KA, Eichbaum M, et al. Imaging of female pelvic malignancies regarding MRI, CT, and PET/CT: part 2. Strahlenther Onkol. 2011;187:705–14.
33. Kambadakone AR, Sahani DV. Body perfusion CT: technique, clinical applications, and advances. Radiol Clin North Am. 2009;47(1):161–78.
34. Forstner R, Sala E, Kinkel K, et al. ESUR guidelines: ovarian cancer staging and follow-up. Eur Radiol. 2010;20:2773–80.
35. Mitchell DG, Javitt MC, Glanc P, et al. ACR appropriateness criteria staging and follow-up of ovarian cancer. J Am Coll Radiol. 2013;10:822–7.
36. Forstner R, Hricak H, Occhipinti KA, et al. Ovarian cancer: staging with CT and MR imaging. Radiology. 1995;197(3):619–26.
37. Coakley FV, Choi PH, Gougoutas CA, et al. Peritoneal metastases: detection with spiral CT in patients with ovarian cancer. Radiology. 2002;223:495–9.

38. Kitajima K, Murakami K, Yamasaki E, et al. Diagnostic accuracy of integrated FDG-PET/contrast-enhanced CT in staging ovarian cancer: comparison with enhanced CT. Eur J Nucl Med Mol Imaging. 2008;35:1912–20.
39. Mitchell DG, Hill MC, Hill S, Zaloudek C. Serous carcinoma of the ovary: CT identification of metastatic calcified implants. Radiology. 1986;158(3):649–52.
40. Nelson BE, Rosenfield AT, Schwartz PE. Preoperative abdominopelvic computed tomographic prediction of optimal cytoreduction in epithelial ovarian carcinoma. J Clin Oncol. 1993;11(1):166–72.
41. Bristow RE, Duska LR, Lambrou NC, Fishman EK, O'Neill MJ, Trimble EL, Montz FJ. A model for predicting surgical outcome in patients with advanced ovarian carcinoma using computed tomography. Cancer. 2000;89(7):1532–40.
42. Salani R, Axtell A, Gerardi M, Holschneider C, Bristow RE. Limited utility of conventional criteria for predicting unresectable disease in patients with advanced stage epithelial ovarian cancer. Gynecol Oncol. 2008;108(2):271–5.
43. Dowdy SC, Mullany SA, Brandt KR, Huppert BJ, Cliby WA. The utility of computed tomography scans in predicting suboptimal cytoreductive surgery in women with advanced ovarian carcinoma. Cancer. 2004;101(2):346–52.
44. Ferrandina G, Sallustio G, Fagotti A, Vizzielli G, Paglia A, Cucci E, Margariti A, Aquilani L, Garganese G, Scambia G. Role of CT scan-based and clinical evaluation in the preoperative prediction of optimal cytoreduction in advanced ovarian cancer: a prospective trial. Br J Cancer. 2009;101(7):1066–73.
45. Janco JM, Glaser G, Kim B, McGree ME, Weaver AL, Cliby WA, Dowdy SC, Bakkum-Gamez JN. Development of a prediction model for residual disease in newly diagnosed advanced ovarian cancer. Gynecol Oncol. 2015;138(1):70–7.
46. Rockall AG, Cross S, Flanagan S, et al. The role of FDG-PET/CT in gynaecological cancers. Cancer Imaging. 2012;12:49–65.
47. De Iaco P, Musto A, Orazi L, et al. FDG-PET/CT in advanced ovarian cancer staging: value and pitfalls in detecting lesions in different abdominal and pelvic quadrants compared with laparoscopy. Eur J Radiol. 2011;80:e98–103.
48. Dauwen H, Van Calster B, Deroose CM, Op de Beeck K, Amant F, Neven P, Berteloot P, Leunen K, Vergote I. PET/CT in the staging of patients with a pelvic mass suspicious for ovarian cancer. Gynecol Oncol. 2013;131(3):694–700.
49. Hynninen J, Kemppainen J, Lavonius M, et al. A prospective comparison of integrated FDG-PET/contrast-enhanced CT and contrast-enhanced CT for pretreatment imaging of advanced epithelial ovarian cancer. Gynecol Oncol. 2013;131:389–94.
50. Fruscio R, Sina F, Dolci C, Signorelli M, Crivellaro C, Dell'Anna T, Cuzzocrea M, Guerra L, Milani R, Messa C. Preoperative 18F-FDG PET/CT in the management of advanced epithelial ovarian cancer. Gynecol Oncol. 2013;131(3):689–93.
51. Shim SH, Lee SJ, Kim SO, Kim SN, Kim DY, Lee JJ, Kim JH, Kim YM, Kim YT, Nam JH. Nomogram for predicting incomplete cytoreduction in advanced ovarian cancer patients. Gynecol Oncol. 2015;136(1):30–6.
52. Schmidt S, Meuli RA, Achtari C, Prior JO. Peritoneal carcinomatosis in primary ovarian cancer staging: comparison between MDCT, MRI, and 18F-FDG PET/CT. Clin Nucl Med. 2015;40(5):371–7.
53. Fader AN, Rose PG. Role of surgery in ovarian carcinoma. J Clin Oncol. 2007;25(20):2873–83.
54. Sugarbaker PH, Jablonski KA. Prognostic features of 51 colorectal and 130 appendiceal cancer patients with peritoneal carcinomatosis treated by cytoreductive surgery and intraperitoneal chemotherapy. Ann Surg. 1995;221:124–32.
55. Eisenkop SM, Spirtos NM, Friedman RL, Lin WC, Pisani AL, Perticucci S. Relative influences of tumor volume before surgery and the cytoreductive outcome on survival for patients with advanced ovarian cancer: a prospective study. Gynecol Oncol. 2003;90(2):390–6.
56. Fagotti A, Ferrandina G, Fanfani F, et al. A laparoscopy–based score to predict surgical outcome in patients with advanced ovarian carcinoma: a pilot study. Ann Surg Oncol. 2006;13(8):1156–61.

57. Tentes AA, Tripsiannis G, Markakidis SK, et al. Peritoneal cancer index: a prognostic indicator of survival in advanced ovarian cancer. Eur J Surg Oncol. 2003;29:69–73.
58. Chéreau E, Ballester M, Selle F, et al. Comparison of peritoneal carcinomatosis scoring methods in predicting resectability and prognosis in advanced ovarian cancer. Am J Obstet Gynecol. 2010;202:178.e1–10.
59. Vergote I, De Wever I, Tjalma W, Van Gramberen M, Decloedt J, van Dam P. Neoadjuvant chemotherapy or primary debulking surgery in advanced ovarian carcinoma: a retrospective analysis of 285 patients. Gynecol Oncol. 1998;71(3):431–6.
60. Fagotti A, Fanfani F, Ludovisi M, Lo Voi R, Bifulco G, Testa AC, et al. Role of laparoscopy to assess the chance of optimal cytoreductive surgery in advanced ovarian cancer: a pilot study. Gynecol Oncol. 2005;96:729–35.
61. Angioli R, Innocenza P, Marzio AZ, Natalina M, Ludovico M, Marco C, et al. Diagnostic open laparoscopic in the management of advanced ovarian cancer. Gynecol Oncol. 2006;100:455–61.
62. Brun JL, Rouzier R, Uzan S, Darai E. External validation of a laparoscopic-based score to evaluate resectability of advanced ovarian cancers: clues for a simplified score. Gynecol Oncol. 2008;110:354–9.
63. Fagotti A, Ferrandina G, Fanfani F, Garganese G, Vizzielli F, Carone V, et al. Prospective validation of a laparoscopic predictive model for optimal cytoreduction in advanced ovarian carcinoma. Am J Obstet Gynecol. 2008;199:642.e1–6.
64. Fagotti A, Vizzielli G, Constantini B, Lecca A, Gallota V, Gagliardi ML, et al. Learning curve and pitfalls of a laparoscopic score to describe peritoneal carcinomatosis in advanced ovarian cancer. Acta Obstet Gynecol Scand. 2011;90:1126–31.
65. Fagotti A, Vizzielli G, De Iaco P, Surico D, Buda A, Mandato VD, et al. A multicentric trial (Olympia-MITO13) on the accuracy of laparoscopy to assess peritoneal spread in ovarian cancer. Am J Obstet Gynecol. 2013;209:462.e1-11.
66. Fagotti A, Vizzielli G, Fanfani F, Costantini B, Ferrandina G, Gallotta V, et al. Introduction of staging laparoscopy in the management of advanced epithelial ovarian, tubal and peritoneal cancer: impact on prognosis in a single institution experience. Gynecol Oncol. 2013;131:341–6.
67. Vizzielli G, Costantini B, Tortorella L, Petrillo M, Fanfani F, Chiantera V, et al. Influence of intraperitoneal dissemination assessed by laparoscopy on prognosis of advanced ovarian cancer: an exploratory analysis of a single-institution experience. Ann Surg Oncol. 2014;21:3970–7.
68. Rutten MJ, Leeflang MM, Kenter GG, Mol BW, Buist M. Laparoscopy for diagnosing resectability of disease in patients with advanced ovarian cancer. Cochrane Database Syst Rev. 2014;(2):CD009786.
69. Petrillo M, Vizzielli G, Fanfani F, Gallotta V, Cosentino F, Chiantera V, Legge F, Carbone V, Scambia G, Fagotti A. Definition of a dynamic laparoscopic model for the prediction of incomplete cytoreduction in advanced epithelial ovarian cancer: proof of a concept. Gynecol Oncol. 2015;139(1):5–9.
70. Rutten MJ, Gaarenstroom KN, Van Gorp T, van Meurs HS, Arts HJ, Bossuyt PM, et al. Laparoscopy to predict the result of primary cytoreductive surgery in advanced ovarian cancer patients (LapOvCa-trial): a multicentre randomized controlled study. BMC Cancer. 2012;12:31.
71. Fagotti A, Ferrandina G, Vizzielli G, Fanfani F, Gallotta V, Chiantera V, Costantini B, Margariti PA, Gueli Alletti S, Cosentino F, Tortorella L, Scambia G. Phase III randomised clinical trial comparing primary surgery versus neoadjuvant chemotherapy in advanced epithelial ovarian cancer with high tumour load (SCORPION trial): Final analysis of peri-operative outcome. Eur J Cancer. 2016;59:22–33.
72. Nick AM, Ramirez PT, Sood AK. A framework for personalized surgical approach to ovarian cancer. Nat Rev Clin Oncol. 2015;12(4):239-45. http://dx.doi.org/10.1038/nrclinionc. (in press).
73. Gómez-Hidalgo NR, Martinez-Cannon BA, Nick AM, Lu KH, Sood AK, Coleman RL, Ramirez PT. Predictors of optimal cytoreduction in patients with newly diagnosed advanced-stage epithelial ovarian cancer: time to incorporate laparoscopic assessment into the standard of care. Gynecol Oncol. 2015;137(3):553–8.

Value of Lymphadenectomy

5

Philipp Harter, Florian Heitz, and Andreas du Bois

Abstract

Systematic pelvic and para-aortic lymphadenectomy is a main part of surgical staging in early ovarian cancer and might be indicated in patients with advanced ovarian cancer. In contrast to other tumors like cervical or endometrial cancer, the lymphadenectomy is usually done by median laparotomy. The main reason is not only the appropriate removal from lymph nodes up to the renal veins, it's also the possibility for complete inspection and palpation of the whole abdomen regarding possible peritoneal carcinomatosis, which is not possible by laparoscopy.

Technique of Lymphadenectomy

If pelvic and para-aortic lymphadenectomy is indicated for surgical staging or cytoreduction in women with ovarian cancer, a median laparotomy from the pubic bone up to the xiphoid has to be performed. The retroperitoneal space is opened laterally of the round ligament and is incised cranially on the iliopsoas muscle. The infundibulopelvic ligament is identified cranio-medially, and the ureter is located dorsally. The pelvic lymphadenectomy is started cranially at the bifurcatio aortae, and the ventral portion of the perivascular tissue of the common iliac artery is excised. The tissue is removed laterally to the genitofemoral nerve and medio-dorsal under

P. Harter (✉) • F. Heitz • A. du Bois
Department of Gynecology and Gynecologic Oncology, Kliniken Essen-Mitte, Henricistrasse 92, Essen, Germany
e-mail: p.harter@gmx.de

E. Pujade-Lauraine et al. (eds.), *Ovarian Cancers*,
DOI 10.1007/978-3-319-32110-3_5

the external common iliac vein. The medially located hypogastric plexus should be preserved. At the bifurcation of the common iliac vessels, the common iliac portion of the pelvic lymphadenectomy is cut, and the removal of the tissue surrounding the external vessels is conducted. The caudal resection margin is the Rosenmuller node. The obturator fossa is opened by cutting the fascia of the psoas muscle along the vessel direction and the connecting tissue between the external iliac artery and the psoas fascia, respectively. The caudo-dorsal margin is the obturator nerve, and the cranial margin is the crossing of the ureter. Afterwards, removal of the internal iliac lymph nodes has to be performed.

To perform an adequate para-aortic lymphadenectomy, a complete mobilization of the colon including mobilization of the kidneys and incision of the ligament of Treitz up to the renal vein is indicated. To obtain an optimal exposure of the surgical area, a sufficient retractor must be available to place the bowel on the thoracic wall. The infundibulopelvic ligaments will be ligated at the inferior vena cava on the right side and at the left renal vein. Thereafter, the ureters have to be mobilized completely. Four compartments are going to be dissected during systematic para-aortic lymphadenectomy: (1) paracaval, lateral and dorsal of the inferior vena cava; (2) inter-aortocaval, medial and dorsal of the inferior vena cava and medial and dorsal of the aorta abdominalis; (3) low para-aortic, lateral and dorsal the aorta between the common iliac artery and the inferior mesenteric artery; and (4) high para-aortic, lateral and dorsal of the abdominal aorta and between the inferior mesenteric artery and the renal vessels. The first area for lymphadenectomy is the paracaval space. The paracaval tissue is dissected vertically up to the renal vein. In the next step, the inter-aortic fraction of the lymphatic tissue between the cava and aorta down to the flavum ligament is harvested. The para-aortic tissue is dissected vertically primary between the common iliac artery and the inferior mesenteric artery and in a second step between the inferior mesenteric artery and the renal vein.

Morbidity of Pelvic and Para-aortic Lymphadenectomy

The additional morbidity of this procedure within a complex multivisceral surgery including also multiple other procedures is difficult to define. The only randomized trial regarding additional systematic lymphadenectomy in advanced ovarian cancer reported a statistically significant impact on median operative time (+50 min), median blood loss (+350 ml), and the number of patients undergoing blood transfusions (59 to >72 %). There were no differences regarding the number of hospital days, intraoperative complications, leakage of bowel anastomosis, intestinal fistula, and adhesive small bowel obstructions. Patients in the lymphadenectomy arm had higher perioperative and late morbidity (60 patients vs. 39 patients). The differences were mainly caused by lymphocysts and lymphedema in the lymphadenectomy group [17].

Lymphadenectomy in Early Ovarian Cancer

The open systematic pelvic and para-aortic lymphadenectomy is the gold standard for surgical staging in early invasive ovarian cancer since decades and is implemented in several national guidelines [1, 2]. Systematic lymphadenectomy is not indicated in patients with borderline ovarian tumors, sex cord-stromal tumors, or germ cell tumors in case of clinical/radiological negative nodes. An exception might be very early germ cell tumors without indication for an adjuvant chemotherapy. The goal of this procedure is to remove suspicious and even clinically unsuspicious, but microscopically positive lymph nodes by the technique described above. While this staging procedure aims not only for removal of residual disease in lymph nodes, the histological results will also influence the indication and constitution of adjuvant chemotherapy. It was shown by several authors that complete surgical staging including pelvic and para-aortic lymphadenectomy shows a better prognosis compared to incomplete surgical staging [3, 4]. Despite this definition as standard of care since several years, national quality assurance programs have shown that this procedure was not performed in more than one third of patients resulting in incomplete staging and inferior survival [5]. A prospective study in ovarian cancer limited to the pelvis showed a 22 % rate of lymph node metastasis diagnosed by systematic pelvic and para-aortic lymphadenectomy [6]. It could not be confirmed in this prospective randomized trial that survival was affected; however, the trial was underpowered with respect to survival analysis. Multiple retrospective single-center series have shown that the rate of positive lymph nodes in patients with presumed early stage disease is about 15 % [7, 8]. The rate of positive nodes depends on histologic subtype and grading. Highest rates of positive nodes were reported in serious and high-grade ovarian cancers. The rate of positive nodes in stage IA grade I mucinous ovarian cancer seems to be very low; however, final pathologic results are usually not available during surgery. Therefore, surgical staging should be performed in these tumors, too. In contrast, in patients with complete surgical staging in, e.g., per frozen section diagnosed borderline tumors and later on corrected histological result of a mucinous ovarian cancer, stage FIGO IA, grade I, the indication for a relaparotomy for systematic pelvic and para-aortic lymphadenectomy has to be discussed individually. In contrast, relaparotomy is justified in all other scenarios of an early invasive epithelial ovarian cancer for completion of surgical staging. Complete surgical staging including systematic lymphadenectomy should also be performed in patients with fertility-preserving surgery.

Lymphadenectomy in Advanced Ovarian Cancer

While the indication for lymphadenectomy in early ovarian cancer is defined, its role in advanced ovarian cancer is less clear. Lymphatic spread has been reported to be a common feature of ovarian cancer in advanced stage disease. Unselected series including all FIGO stages reported a 44–53 % rate of lymph node metastasis detected by systematic lymphadenectomy [9, 10]. This rate increases up to nearby 80 % of patients with systematic lymphadenectomy during surgery for advanced ovarian cancer [9]. It was also shown that in patients in advanced stage ovarian cancer with complete resection and systematic and para-aortic lymphadenectomy, not only the status (positive versus negative) but also the lymph node ratio was an important prognostic factor [11]. The general surgical strategy in patients with advanced ovarian cancer is complete tumor resection at primary surgery. If this is not possible, a resection of all tumor larger than 1 cm is recommended to achieve a residual disease status of 1–10 mm. Therefore, three prognostic subgroups have to be distinguished. While in patients with complete resection, the prognosis is good with a median survival of 99 months, it is lower in patients with residual disease of 1–10 mm (median survival 36 months) or in patients with larger residual tumors (median survival 29 months) [12]. The prognostic value of complete and/or optimal debulking has also been reported on several other occasions and confirmed in meta-analyses [13, 14].

The role of lymphadenectomy as part of surgical debulking in advanced ovarian cancer is controversial. Several clinical scenarios of lymphadenectomy in relation to achieved intraperitoneal debulking status can be discussed separately: Patients in whom intraperitoneal debulking could not render resection to so-called optimal, small, or no gross residual disease would not benefit at all from lymphadenectomy with respect to the maximum diameter of residual disease. Patients with bulky nodes but complete or almost complete debulking intraperitoneally could benefit from removal of enlarged metastatic nodes by reducing macroscopic residual tumor. Lymphadenectomy in patients with clinically not suspicious lymph nodes and small residual disease intraperitoneally might not change the residual disease status but may reduce tumor burden in a potential caveat not optimally accessible by chemotherapy [15]. The latter hypothesis was employed by the International Multicenter Lymphadenectomy trial that showed a beneficial impact of systematic lymphadenectomy with respect to progression-free survival [16]. However, no survival benefit was reported in this trial, and some authors concluded that systematic lymphadenectomy should not be considered as standard therapy in advanced ovarian cancer anymore [17]. This conclusion may not be generalized to patients with macroscopically complete resection intraperitoneally, because this subgroup did not substantially contribute to the results of an international multicenter trial. This trial indicated a 28 % rate of clinically not suspicious lymph nodes bearing metastatic disease. The unsatisfactory reliability of intraoperative palpation for diagnosis of lymph node metastasis was confirmed by others [9, 18] and is possibly based on similar size of metastatic and nonmetastatic lymph nodes [19, 20].

Table 5.1 Management of lymph nodes in invasive epithelial ovarian cancer

FIGO stage	Intra-abdominal residual disease	Radiological and clinically negative LN	Positive lymph nodes >1 cm
FIGO I–II	0 >0: stop doing surgery for ovarian cancer	Yes Complete surgical staging	–/–
FIGO III–IV	0	Yes or No?	Yes LN >1 cm ≥TE/LNE →Reduction of residual disease
	1–10 mm	Yes or No?	Yes LN >1 cm ≥TE/LNE →Reduction of residual disease
	>10 mm	No	No

LN lymph node, *TE* tumor extirpation, *LNE* lymphadenectomy

Finally, in patients with intraperitoneally macroscopic complete debulking, systematic lymphadenectomy might theoretically add complete resection of retroperitoneal disease, thus achieving a true macroscopic complete resection status in that proportion of patients who would have undiagnosed residual retroperitoneal disease without lymphadenectomy. Retrospective series and an exploratory analysis of a prospective chemotherapy trial supported this hypothesis by demonstrating an impact of systematic lymphadenectomy on prognosis [21–24]. The latter was supported by an analysis of the SEER database [25]. By analyzing the AGO meta-database, it was reported that lymphadenectomy was associated with superior survival in patients without gross residual disease. The median survival duration was 103 and 84 months; 5-year survival rates were 67.4 and 59.2 % ($p=0.0166$). Multivariate analysis confirmed a significant impact of lymphadenectomy on overall survival ($p=0.0123$). The same analysis in patients with small residual tumor up to 1 cm barely reached significance ($p=0.0497$), and significance was only demonstrated within this subgroup for patients with clinically suspect nodes in whom lymphadenectomy resulted in a 16 % gain in 5-year overall survival [26]. On overview of management of lymph nodes in epithelial ovarian cancer is given in Table 5.1.

Data from prospectively randomized trials evaluating the potential role of systematic lymphadenectomy in advanced ovarian cancer and complete intraperitoneal resection are still pending (LION trial; ClinicalTrials.gov Identifier: NCT00712218; CARACO trial; ClinicalTrials.gov Identifier: NCT01218490).

Table of risk of lymph nodes involvement correlated to FIGO stage.

Authors (years)	*n*	FIGO stage	Risk of lymph nodes involvement (%)
Takeshima (2007)	208	I	20/156 (13 %)
		II	18/37 (49 %)
		III	9/15 (60 %)
Neigishi (2004)	150	I	8/123 (6.5 %)
		II	11/27 (41 %)
Morice (2003)	276	I	17/85 (20 %)
		II	6/15 (40 %)
		III–IV	99/176 (62.5 %)
DiRe (1996)	448	II	17/56 (30.4 %)
		III	142/461 (31 %)
		IV	35/88 (77 %)
Onda (1996)	110	I	7/33 (21.2 %)
		II	6/26 (23.1 %)
		III	29/43 (67.4 %)
		IV	6/8 (75 %)
Burghardt (1991)	180	I	9/37 (24.3 %)
		II	7/14 (50 %)
		III	84/114 (73.7 %)
		IV	11/15 (73.3 %)

References

1. Wagner U, Harter P, Hilpert F, et al. S3-guideline on diagnostics, therapy and follow-up of malignant ovarian tumours: short version 1.0 – AWMF registration number: 032/035OL, june 2013. Geburtshilfe Frauenheilkd. 2013;73(9):874–89.
2. Lhommé C, Morice P, Planchamp F, et al. Clinical practice guidelines 2008 for the surgical treatment, medical first-line and consolidation treatments of patients with epithelial ovarian cancer–update. According to the methodology of Standards, Options: Recommendations (SOR). Bull Cancer. 2008;95(9):881–6.
3. Trimbos JB, Vergote I, Bolis G, et al. Impact of adjuvant chemotherapy and surgical staging in early-stage ovarian carcinoma: european organisation for research and treatment of cancer-adjuvant chemotherapy in ovarian neoplasm trial. J Natl Cancer Inst. 2003;95:113–25.
4. Chan JK, Munro EG, Cheung MK, et al. Association of lymphadenectomy and survival in stage I ovarian cancer patients. Obstet Gynecol. 2007;109:12–9.
5. du Bois A, Rochon J, Lamparter C, Pfisterer J. The quality assurance program of the AGO organkommission OVAR (QS-OVAR): pattern of care and reality in Germany 2001. Zentralbl Gynakol. 2005;127(1):9–17.
6. Maggione A, Benedetti-Panici P, Dell'Anna T, et al. Randomised study of systematic lymph-adenectomy in patients with epithelial ovarian cancer macroscopically confined to the pelvis. Br J Cancer. 2006;95:699–704.
7. Onda T, Yoshikawa H, Yokota H, Yasugi T, Taketani Y. Assessment of metastases to aortic and pelvic lymph nodes in epithelial ovarian carcinoma. A proposal for essential sites for lymph node biopsy. Cancer. 1996;78(4):803–8.
8. Baiocchi G, Grosso G, di Re E, et al. Systematic pelvic and paraaortic lymphadenectomy at second-look laparotomy for ovarian cancer. Gynecol Oncol. 1998;69(2):151–6.

9. Harter P, Gnauert K, Hils R, et al. Pattern and clinical predictors of lymph node metastases in epithelial ovarian cancer. Int J Gynecol Cancer. 2007;17(6):1238–44.
10. Morice P, Joulie F, Camatte S, et al. Lymph node involvement in epithelial ovarian cancer: analysis of 276 pelvic and paraaortic lymphadenectomies and surgical implications. J Am Coll Surg. 2003;197:198–205.
11. Ataseven B, Grimm C, Harter P, et al. Prognostic value of lymph node ratio in patients with advanced epithelial ovarian cancer. Gynecol Oncol. 2014;135(3):435–40.
12. du Bois A, Reuss A, Pujade-Lauraine E, Harter P, Ray-Coquard I, Pfisterer J. Role of surgical outcome as prognostic factor in advanced epithelial ovarian cancer: A combined exploratory analysis of 3 prospectively randomized phase 3 multicenter trials. Cancer. 2009;115(6):1234–44.
13. Bristow RE, Tomacruz RS, Armstrong DK, et al. Survival effect of maximal cytoreductive surgery for advanced ovarian carcinoma during the platinum era: a meta-analysis. J Clin Oncol. 2002;20:1248–59.
14. Winter 3rd WE, Maxwell GL, Tian C, et al. Prognostic factors for stage III epithelial ovarian cancer: a Gynecologic Oncology Group study. J Clin Oncol. 2007;25:3621–7.
15. Morice P, Joulie F, Rey A, et al. Are nodal metastasis in ovarian cancer chemoresistant lesions? Analysis of nodal involvement in 105 patients treated with preoperative chemotherapy. Eur J Gynaecol Oncol. 2004;25:169–74.
16. Benedetti Panici P, Maggione A, Hacker N, et al. Systematic aortic and pelvic lymphadenectomy versus resection of bulky nodes only in optimally debulked advanced ovarian cancer: a randomized clinical trial. J Natl Cancer Inst. 2005;97:560–5.
17. Chambers SK. Systematic lymphadenectomy in advanced epithelial ovarian cancer: two decades of uncertainty resolved. J Natl Cancer Inst. 2005;97:548–9.
18. Spirtos NM, Gross GM, Freddo JL, Ballon SC. Cytoreductive surgery in advanced epithelial ovarian cancer of the ovary: the impact of aortic and pelvic lymphadenectomy. Gynecol Oncol. 1995;56:345–52.
19. Pereira A, Magrina JF, Rex V, Cortes M, Magtibay PM. Pelvic and aortic lymph node metastasis in epithelial ovarian cancer. Gynecol Oncol. 2007;67:10214–21.
20. Tangjitgamol S, Manusirivithaya S, Sheanakul C, et al. Can we rely on the size of lymph node in determining nodal metastases in ovarian cancer. Int J Gynecol Cancer. 2003;13:297–302.
21. Aletti GD, Dowdy S, Podratz KC, Cliby WA. Role of lymphadenectomy in the management of grossly apparent advanced stage epithelial ovarian cancer. Am J Obstet Gynecol. 2006;195:1862–8.
22. di Re F, Baiocchi G, Fontanelli R, et al. Systematic pelvic and paraaortic lymphadenectomy for advanced ovarian cancer: prognostic significance of node metastases. Gynecol Oncol. 1996;62:360–5.
23. Scarabelli C, Gallo A, Visentin MC, Canzonieri V, Carbone A, Zarelli A. Systematic pelvic and para-aortic lymphadenectomy in advanced ovarian cancer patients with no residual intraperitoneal disease. Int J Gynecol Cancer. 1997;7:18–26.
24. Crawford SC, Vasey PA, Paul J, Hay A, Davis JA, Kaye JB. Does aggressive surgery only benefit patients with less advanced ovarian cancer? Results from an international comparison within the SCOTROC-1 trial. J Clin Oncol. 2005;23:8802–11.
25. Chan JK, Urban R, Hu JM, et al. The potential therapeutic role of lymph node resection in epithelial ovarian cancer: a study of 13.918 patients. Br J Cancer. 2007;96:1817–22.
26. du Bois A, Reuss A, Harter P, et al. Potential role of lymphadenectomy in advanced ovarian cancer: a combined exploratory analysis of three prospectively randomized phase III multicenter trials. J Clin Oncol. 2010;28(10):1733–9.

Ovarian Cancer and HIPEC: In the Era of Evidence Based Medicine

6

Jean-Marc Classe, Isabelle Jaffre, Naoual Bakrin, Dominique Berton-Rigaud, Jean-Sébastien Frenel, and Olivier Glehen

Abstract

Patients treated for an advanced ovarian cancer experience inexorably a peritoneal diffusion Hyperthermic Intra Peritoneal Chemotherapy (HIPEC), combining complete cytoreductive surgery and intra peritoneal heated chemotherapy, has been used to treat ovarian cancer patients with the hope of an improvement in survival.

Currently HIPEC remains an experimental procedure in the case of patients treated for an ovarian cancer.

In this review we describe preclinical studies, with hypothesis of hyperthermia synergy with intra peritoneal chemotherapy. Phase I and Phase II clinical series emphasizing the absence of control group in most of clinical series. At last we present ongoing phase III trials aimed to assess survival impact of HIPEC in the treatment of advanced ovarian cancer.

HIPEC is an innovative treatment. Before using it outside clinical trials in the case of initial treatment of advanced ovarian cancer, or in the case of the first relapse, results of large multi-institutionnal randomised trials built to assess impact on survival, are required.

J.-M. Classe (✉) • D. Berton-Rigaud • J.-S. Frenel
Département Chirurgie Oncologique, Institut de cancérologie de l'Ouest, Boulevard du professeur J. Monod, Nantes 44000, France
e-mail: jean-marc.classe@ico.unicancer.fr

I. Jaffre
Département Chirurgie Oncologique, Hospices Civils, Boulevard du professeur J. Monod, Nantes 44000, France

N. Bakrin • O. Glehen
Département Chirurgie Oncologique, Hospices civils, 3 quai des Célestins, Lyon 69002, France

E. Pujade-Lauraine et al. (eds.), *Ovarian Cancers*,
DOI 10.1007/978-3-319-32110-3_6

Introduction

Ovarian cancer is the leading cause of death among women with gynecologic cancer [1].

Without any possibility to build screening programs, ovarian cancer is mainly diagnosed at an advanced stage [2].

Current standard treatment involves complete surgery, with the goal of no macroscopic residual disease, systemic platinum-based bi-chemotherapy, and targeted therapy.

Meta-analysis demonstrates overall survival benefit of complete surgery when compared to the last definition of optimal surgery with a residual or less than 1 cm [3].

Recent randomized trials have shown in case of advanced ovarian cancer an overall survival of 30 months and a disease-free survival of 12 months [4] and in case of the first late relapse, respectively, 33 months and 11.3 months for OS and DFS [5, 6].

Even with the best treatment, 85 % of patients experience a first relapse in a mean period of two years after initial treatment [4].

Ovarian cancer diffusion is mainly limited to peritoneal cavity, peritoneal carcinomatosis, with rare distant metastasis [7]. Patients with FIGO III–IV ovarian cancer with negative peritoneal biopsies at the end of initial treatment experience a 5-year DFS of 40 % [8].

Based on this peritoneal failure, efficiency of intraperitoneal chemotherapy was assessed by randomized trials (IPC). IPC consists of six courses of chemotherapy directly delivered into the abdominal cavity through an intraperitoneal catheter placed by the surgeon. Randomized trials have demonstrated significant improvement of disease-free and overall survival when compared to intravenous standard treatment. A recent meta-analysis of nine trials with 2119 patients confirmed that IPC induces an important improvement of OS and PFS [9]. For example, in the GOG 172 trial, in the subgroup of patients with complete cytoreductive surgery, median overall survival in the IPC group was 127.6 months, and disease-free survival was 60.4 months [10]. Significant improvement of survival was obtained despite poor intraperitoneal diffusion of chemotherapy due to postoperative adhesions and despite a low rate of complete treatment, with approximately 50 % of patients who achieved the full six-course program of IPC. Nevertheless, throughout the world IPC is not currently part of routine practice due to an important rate of morbidity and organizational obstacles.

Today innovative treatments allow less improvement in survival. A recent targeted antiangiogenic therapy, bevacizumab, allowed OS and PFS improvement of ¾ months in adjuvant setting and PFS improvement only in recurrent setting [11].

Hyperthermic intraperitoneal chemotherapy (HIPEC) could be considered as an innovative option with the combination of two leading parameters of survival improvement: complete surgery with no residual and intraperitoneal chemotherapy. HIPEC is performed after complete surgery, during the same surgical procedure, with two different techniques: open, coliseum technique, or closed [12]. HIPEC is not supposed to replace systemic therapy. HIPEC is based on the hypothesis of the treatment of remaining microscopic peritoneal disease even in case of a macroscopic complete surgery classified CC0 by the surgeon. HIPEC is a supplementary treatment to standard complete surgery and systemic standard chemotherapy.

To switch from an innovative hope to a standard option for routine use, HIPEC must follow the known steps of clinical research. After phase I and II trials, HIPEC must be compared with standard treatment in randomized setting. In colorectal carcinomatosis, Verwaal et al. have built a trial comparing complete surgery and HIPEC to palliative surgery and intravenous chemotherapy [13]. With this design it is controversial to conclude that survival benefit was due to HIPEC or to complete surgery. Late results of survival, after prolonged follow-up, median DFS is 22 months in HIPEC group compared to 12 months in palliative group [14].

Our aim was to review scientific proofs of HIPEC impact on survival in ovarian cancer patients considering frontline and relapse treatment.

Preclinical Studies

Considering peritoneal development of ovarian cancer and frequent peritoneal failure, peritoneum is a treatment target and intraperitoneal treatment an alternative to intravenous treatment.

Considering the advantage of the peritoneum/plasma barrier, a water-soluble drug with a high molecular weight could guarantee a high IP drug concentration with a low plasma drug diffusion. Platinum derived peritoneum/plasma ratios 20 times and taxanes derived up to 1000 times [15].

Compared to IPC, HIPEC has some characteristics to be added. Firstly HIPEC does not replace intravenous courses of bi-chemotherapy but is added to this standard treatment.

HIPEC is assimilated to one-shot chemotherapy, in opposition with the fundamental concept of systemic chemotherapy with a succession of courses based on cellular repair mechanisms. Observation of cisplatin-induced DNA adducts demonstrates penetration and antineoplastic activity of IPC [16].

In order to balance the disadvantage of a one-shot treatment, HIPEC combine hyperthermia and intraoperative diffusion of intraperitoneal chemotherapy. Intraoperative drug delivery avoids the problem of postoperative adhesion observed in case of IPC.

Hyperthermia has lethal effects on human neoplastic cells [17]. The main effects can be summarized as follows: direct cytotoxic effect with protein denaturation leading to apoptosis, indirect effect on DNA repair mechanisms, induction of heat shock proteins activating natural cell killers, and increase in tumor penetration of cisplatin [18]. The best tolerated temperature was not defined into clinical phase I studies with escalating steps. Considering SHIN 3 humanized ovarian cancer cells, studying temperature, carboplatinum or cis-platinum concentration, and length of exposure, Muller et al. showed that highest rate of cancer cell death was obtained with a duration of 60 mn at 41 °C [19]. Drugs selected for HIPEC must be heat stable and have a high molecular weight. In clinical series temperature, duration of exposure and kind and concentration of intraperitoneal drugs are heterogeneous parameters (Tables). However, optimal intraperitoneal temperature was never demonstrated in scientific paper.

After first experience of thermal infusion in 15 dogs, Spratt et al. published the first case report of HIPEC in a man with pseudomyxoma [20].

Mortality Morbidity

Jacquet et al., in a retrospective series of 60 patients treated by CRS and HIPEC for a PC from adenocarcinoma of the colon or appendix, described a 35 % rate of morbidity, significantly associated with high HIPEC temperature, duration of surgery, and high number of peritonectomy, with a mortality rate of 5 % [21].

Not any paper compares results of heavy surgery and HIPEC to heavy surgery without HIPEC in the treatment of advanced ovarian cancer. A recent literature search of mortality and morbidity of cytoreductive surgery and HIPEC retained outcome from 24 institutions mainly observational, retrospective, nonrandomized series without control group [22]. In tertiary high-volume centers, the mortality rates ranged from 0.9 to 5.8 %. The common causes of perioperative mortality were sepsis and multi-organ failure as a result of surgical complications. The rate of major or grade III/IV morbidity ranged from 12 to 52 %, with a reoperation rates ranged from 0 to 23 %. Common postoperative complications include sepsis, fistula abscess, ileus, perforation, anastomotic leakage, deep venous thrombosis/pulmonary embolus, hematologic toxicity, and renal insufficiency.

Learning curves of this procedure have been demonstrated. The Dutch group demonstrated that over a period of 10 years, where 323 procedures were performed, the implementation of a patient selection process has resulted in improved rates of complete cytoreduction, decrease in postoperative morbidity rates, and decrease in median duration of hospital stay [23]. Careful patient selection with an optimal level of postoperative care must be advocated to avoid undesirable complications of this treatment.

A recent monocentric retrospective series of 91 patients treated with CRS and HIPEC for a primary advanced ovarian cancer or a relapse found 12 % of grade III–IV complications [24]. In a multivariate analysis, only PCI value >12 and intestinal resection were independent factors linked with major morbidity. Bakrin et al. published the biggest world series of 566 HIPEC for ovarian cancer treatment; advanced primary or relapse, from 13 French centers, showed mortality 0.8 % rate and severe grade III–IV morbidity ranged from 0.8 to 31.3 % [25]. Without a homogeneous system to describe morbidity, it is hard to compare series from each other.

We can distinguish a specific morbidity of HIPEC related to systemic effects of the antimitotic drugs. Hematologic toxicity, grade 3–4 morbidity occurs in 8–31 % of cases, particularly when bone marrow has been previously challenged by previous courses of chemotherapy. Each antimitotic drug presents specific potential adverse effects and needs to be managed specifically. For instance, the use of oxaliplatin increases the risk of postoperative hemoperitoneum; the use of cisplatin is associated with a risk of kidney failure that requires optimal perioperative hydration and close follow-up of kidney function.

Selection of patient, selection of the number of resections and length of surgery, re-nutrition before surgery, and high-volume centers with a resuscitation unit should reduce the mortality and morbidity rates.

Scientific Level of Evidence

Phase I Studies

Phase I trial with escalating doses, with the definition of stopping rules, allows to define the best tolerated dose of a drug. PubMed search for key words HIPEC/ovarian cancer/phase I trial allows to find only four papers. In case of HIPEC, drug must also resist and remain efficient in hyperthermic condition.

Steller et al. published a phase I trial of continuous hyperthermic peritoneal perfusion with high-dose carboplatin as primary treatment of patients with small-volume residual ovarian cancer [26]. The maximum tolerated dose (MTD) for intraperitoneal carboplatin administered as HIPEC was established at 1200 mg/m^2.

Lentz et al. published a phase I study designed to determine the maximum tolerated dose (MTD) of carboplatin used intraoperatively as hyperthermic intraperitoneal chemotherapy (HIPEC) in stage III ovarian cancer patient [27]. The maximum tolerated dose (MTD) for intraperitoneal carboplatin administered as IPHC was established at 1000 mg/m^2.

Harrison et al. published a phase I study to determine the safety and pharmacokinetics of intraperitoneal pegylated liposomal doxorubicin (PLD) used in the context of HIPEC in patients with advanced abdominal-only malignancies, among 21 patients only 3 patients have an ovarian cancer [28]. The maximum dose evaluated in this trial was 100 mg/m^2 and was well tolerated.

Zivanovic et al. published HIPEC ROC I: A phase I study of cisplatin administered as hyperthermic intraperitoneal chemoperfusion followed by postoperative intravenous platinum-based chemotherapy in patients with platinum-sensitive recurrent epithelial ovarian cancer [16]. Cisplatin administered as HIPEC at a dose of 100 mg/m^2 has an acceptable safety profile in selected patients undergoing secondary cytoreductive surgery for platinum-sensitive recurrent EOC.

At present over the world, three phase I studies are ongoing, still recruiting or closed but not published (ClinicalTrials.gov):

Leslie Randal from University of California: This phase I studies the side effects and best dose of heated carboplatin given into the abdomen at the time of surgery in treating patients with stage II–IV ovarian, fallopian tube, or peritoneal cancer.

William Helm from University of Louisville: This is a phase I study of intraperitoneal hyperthermic docetaxel given at the time of second look surgery following frontline normothermic intraperitoneal and intravenous cisplatin/paclitaxel for patients with stage II and III ovarian carcinoma. Sebastien Gouy from Gustave Roussy Institute: This is a phase I trial dose escalation of cisplatin HIPEC in patients with unresectable stage IIIC ovarian, tube, or peritoneal primary adenocarcinoma (CHIPASTIN).

Phase II Studies

PubMed search for key words HIPEC/ovarian cancer/phase II trial allows to find XX papers of prospective studies.

Di Giorgio et al. (2008) published a series of 47 patients, 22 primary advanced ovarian cancer and 25 relapsed, treated with HIPEC (cisplatin 75 mg/m^2 for 60 mn) followed by systemic chemotherapy. Major postoperative morbidity, requiring rehospitalization, intensive care unit admission, or radiological intervention, developed in 21.3 %, and mortality rate was 4.2 %. The mean overall survival was 30.4 months, and mean disease-free survival was 27.4 % [29].

Ceelen et al. (2009) published a series of 42 patients treated for a first relapse >6 months after the end of initial treatment. HIPEC with cisplatin ranges from 100 to 250 mg/m^2 for 90 min or oxaliplatin 460 mg/m^2 for 30 mn. Major morbidity rate was 21 % with no postoperative morbidity. Median overall survival (OS) was 37 months (95 % confidence interval 12.2–61.8), and median progression-free survival was 13 months.

Lim et al. (2009) published a series of 30 patients treated for an advanced ovarian cancer with HIPEC (cisplatin 75 mg/m^2 for 90 mn). Major morbidity rate was 21 % with no postoperative mortality.

Asero 2009.

Pomel et al. (2010) published a study aimed to evaluate the HIPEC (oxaliplatin 460–350 mg/m^2)-related morbidity as consolidation therapy for 31 advanced ovarian cancer patient. Major morbidity rate was 29 % with no postoperative mortality. Two-year disease-free and overall survival were 27 % and 67 %, respectively. As a result of this high level of morbidity, the trial was closed.

Deraco et al. (2011) published a multi-institutional phase II trial to assess overall survival after cytoreductive surgery (CRS) and hyperthermic intraperitoneal chemotherapy (HIPEC) in 26 treatment-naive epithelial ovarian cancer (EOC) with advanced peritoneal involvement. Major morbidity rate was 15 % with 4 % postoperative morbidity. After a median follow-up of 25 months, 5-year overall survival was 60.7 %, and 5-year progression-free survival was 15.2 % (median 30 months).

At present over the world, four phase II studies are ongoing, still recruiting or closed but not published (ClinicalTrials.gov):

Sang-Yoon Park, National Cancer Center, Korea: The phase II study of HIPEC with cisplatin followed by intravenous chemotherapy in patients with ovarian cancer.

Anna Fagotti, Catholic University of Sacred Heart, Roma: This is a phase II study of HIPEC with oxaliplatin in patients with platinum-sensitive recurrent ovarian cancer.

Fernando Figueira, Pernambuco, Brazil: This is a phase II open-label, single-arm clinical trial on safety and efficacy exploring a short-course regimen of intraoperative hyperthermic intraperitoneal chemotherapy (HIPEC) cisplatin as up-front therapy for patients with advanced epithelial ovarian cancer (EOC) undergoing cytoreductive surgery (CRS).

Than Dellinger, City of Hope Medical Center: Cytoreductive surgery with hyperthermic intraperitoneal chemotherapy (HIPEC) and optional postoperative normothermic intraperitoneal (IP) chemotherapy to treat primary or recurrent carcinoma of ovarian, fallopian tube, uterine, or peritoneal origin.

Several retrospective clinical series, either phase I or II but pilot mainly retrospective series, are published aimed to assess efficiency and tolerability of HIPEC for ovarian cancer patients (Table 6.1).

Those studies share some characteristics: heterogeneous drug, with different posology, heterogeneous HIPEC technique open or closed, different temperatures, and duration. Clinical situations are frequently mixed: frontline treatment of advanced disease, progression. Tools to describe postoperative morbidity are heterogeneous limiting accuracy of comparison of published series.

Table 6.1 Published pilot series of ovarian cancer and HIPEC ($n \supseteq 50$ patients, results on survival) without control group

Author (year)	*N* (Period recruitment /year)	Timing	Drug (mg/m²)	Mortality	PFS median months	OS median months
Cotte (2007) [39]	81 (14)	M	Cis (20)	2.5 %	19	28
Pavlov (2009) [40]	56 (12)	M	Doxo (O.1) Cispl (15)	1.8 %	26	43 (primary) 40 (relapse)
Helm (2010) [41]	141	M	Platinum Mito	0.5 %	16.6	30
Roviello (2010) [42]	53 (9)	M	Cispl (100) Mito (25)	0 %	NR	55 % 5 years
Parson (2011) [43]	51 (13)	I	Carbo (1000) Mito (30)	0 %	NR	29
Deraco (2012) [44]	56 (15)	R	Cispl (42) Doxo (15) Cispl (25) Mito (3.3)	5.3 %	10.8	25.7
Bakrin (2013) [25]	566 (19)	M	Cispl Oxaly Doxo Mito	0.8 %	NR	35.4
Robella M (2014) [45]	70 (17)	M	Cispl (100) – Doxo (15.2)	7 %	NR	48 (primary) 28 (relapse)
Konigstrainer (2014) [46]	62 (5)	R	Cispl (50)	0 %	NR	35 (CC0-1) 14 (CC2)
Coccolini (2015) [47]	54 (6.5)	M	Cispl (100) – Pacli (175)	0 %	12.4	32.9
Classe (2015) [33]	314 (10)	R	Cispl Oxaly Doxo Mito	1 %	14 % 5 years	38 % 5 years

N number of patients included. Period of recruitment: period from the first to the last patient included
Timing *I* (Initial), *R* (relapse), *M* (mixed)
NR Not related

Bakrin et al. published the biggest retrospective series of 566 patients treated for a primary advanced ovarian cancer ($n=92$) or a relapse, either first or more relapse ($n=474$). Several main parameters were heterogeneous: step of the disease – primary treatment, first relapse, more than the first relapse – HIPEC parameters – drug, temperature, concentration, duration, completeness of cytoreductive surgery. Grade 3–4 morbidity rates were 0.8 % and 31.3 %, respectively. Median overall survivals were 35.4 and 45.7 months for advanced and recurrent EOC, respectively. A more recent paper, based on an extraction of the latest paper, focuses on a specific selection of patients with a first relapse [30]. Mortality and morbidity rates were, respectively, 1 % and 30.9 %. Median follow-up was 50 months, 5-year overall survival was 38.0 %, with no difference between platinum-sensitive and platinum-resistant patients, and 5-year disease-free survival was 14 %.

In these studies, the lack of control group prevents to point any specific advantage of HIPEC.

Ten studies of HIPEC for an ovarian cancer compared with a control group without HIPEC are already published (Table 6.2). The number of patients in each arm is very low with 14–60 in HIPEC group and 12–84 in no HIPEC group. Those studies share usual limitations as small effective, heterogeneous clinical situation with four studies in the situation of initial treatment and six in the situation of relapse and heterogeneous drug. The reason of the choice of treatment, HIPEC or not, was never due to a randomization.

Munoz-Casares et al. compared 14 patients treated with secondary surgery and HIPEC to 12 patients treated with secondary surgery without HIPEC, included from 1997–2004. Patients underwent second-line chemotherapy after surgery. The surgery was complete, with no gross residual in 64 % of the HIPEC group and 58 % of

Table 6.2 Series with control group

	Stage	HIPEC drug	HIPEC (*n*)	No HIPEC (*n*)
Ryu (2004) [48]	Primary	Carboplatinum	57	60
Gori (2005) [49]	Primary	Cisplatinum	32	19
Bae (2007) [50]	Primary	Paclitaxel (22) Carboplatinum (45)	67	29
Munoz casares (2009) [34]	Relapse	Paclitaxel	14	12
Spilliotis (2011) [51]	Relapse	Cisplat/Pacli	24	24
Warschkow (2012) [52]	Primary	Cisplatinum	21	90
Fagotti (2012) [36]	Relapse	Oxaliplatinum	30	37
Lebrun (2014) [37]	Relapse	Cisplatinum	23	19
Safra (2014) [53]	Primary	Cisplat/Doxo Pacli/Carbo Cisplat/Mito	27	84
Cascales campos (2015) [54]	Relapse	Paclitaxel	32	22

the control group. Overall survival was significantly higher in the HIPEC group when compared to the control group [17].

Spiliotis et al. [19] compared patients treated for a first ovarian cancer relapse (24 patients treated with surgery and HIPEC followed with second-line chemotherapy compared to 24 patients treated with surgery without HIPEC and second-line chemotherapy). The 3-year overall survival was significantly better in the HIPEC group [19]. Complete surgery and peritoneal cancer index were linked with a better survival.

Fagotti et al. [18] compared patients treated for a first ovarian cancer relapse (30 patients treated with complete secondary surgery [cc0–cc1] and HIPEC, followed with second-line chemotherapy to 37 patients treated with second-line chemotherapy alone for 13 patients and second-line chemotherapy and secondary surgery for 24 of them) without information regarding the completeness of the cytoreduction score at the time of secondary surgery for these patients. Disease-free survival and overall survival were significantly better in the HIPEC group [18].

Lebrun JF et al. is the first case-control series with a matching of patients based on the main prognostic factors, with only serous ovarian carcinoma and a complete secondary surgery for each patient in the two groups (23 HIPEC, 19 control group). Patient selection was based on inclusion criteria to reduce bias: only first relapse, complete surgery, only serous carcinoma with no differences considering main prognosis factors. At 4 years OS was 75.6 % in the HIPEC group and 19.4 % in the control group ($p=0.013$) (Le Brun 2014 #45).

Phase III Studies

Currently, four prospective European trials are ongoing testing the impact of complete surgery and HIPEC with cis-platinum on first platinum-sensitive relapse of epithelial ovarian cancer.

CHORINE, an Italian randomized trial stage IIIC unresectable epithelial ovarian/tubal cancer with partial or complete response after first-line neoadjuvant chemotherapy (three cycles CBDCA + paclitaxel): a phase 3 prospective randomized study comparing cytoreductive surgery + hyperthermic intraperitoneal chemotherapy (CDDP + paclitaxel) + three cycles CBDCA + paclitaxel vs cytoreductive surgery alone + three cycles CBDCA + paclitaxel (ClinicalTrials.gov/NCT01628380). DFS 2 years. Ansaloni OVHIPEC, a Netherland randomized trial, phase III randomized clinical trial for stage III ovarian carcinoma randomizing between secondary debulking surgery with or without hyperthermic intraperitoneal chemotherapy, DFS, Van Driel. Clinicaltrials.gov NCT00426257.

HORSE, an Italian randomized multicenter trial comparing interval surgery plus HIPEC *versus* interval surgery alone, aimed to assess relapse-free survival (available at http://clinicaltrials.gov/show/NCT01539785).

CHIPOR, a French prospective multicenter randomized trial comparing, after six courses of second-line chemotherapy, surgery plus HIPEC *versus* surgery alone, aimed to assess overall survival (available at http://clinicaltrials.gov/show/NCT01376752).

Guidelines

At the present time, HIPEC is not part of standard treatment of ovarian cancer patients and does not appear even as an option, in any international guideline. As recent editorials, the cooperative German group AGO published a statement which declared that HIPEC is unwarranted in routine use outside of controlled clinical trials (Harter 2013 #42).

Conclusion

HIPEC is rational considering both ovarian cancer peritoneal failure and already proved intraperitoneal treatment efficiency.

Scientific literature contains few phase I trials, weak phase II trial mainly retrospective without control group, and not any published results of randomized phase III trial allowing to point efficiency of HIPEC randomly compared to standard treatment.

Ongoing phase III trials will bring first responses.

At present scientific proofs of efficiency are too weak to propose routinely HIPEC for ovarian cancer patient. Inclusion in clinical trials, prospective evaluations, must be privileged.

Teams involved in HIPEC share the responsibility to participate in the recruitment of patients in ongoing trial to switch for the current status of HIPEC as a simple hypothesis to the demonstration of its real efficiency.

We all owe this effort to our patients.

References

1. Siegel R, Naishadham D, Jemal A. Cancer statistics, 2012. CA Cancer J Clin. 2012;62:10–29.
2. Hennessy BT, Coleman RL, Markman M. Ovarian cancer. Lancet. 2009;374:1371–82.
3. Elattar A, Bryant A, Winter-Roach BA, et al. Optimal primary surgical treatment for advanced epithelial ovarian cancer. Cochrane Database Syst Rev 2011;(8):CD007565.
4. Vergote I, Trope CG, Amant F, et al. Neoadjuvant chemotherapy or primary surgery in stage IIIC or IV ovarian cancer. N Engl J Med. 2010;363:943–53.
5. Wagner U, Marth C, Largillier R, et al. Final overall survival results of phase III GCIG CALYPSO trial of pegylated liposomal doxorubicin and carboplatin vs paclitaxel and carboplatin in platinum-sensitive ovarian cancer patients. Br J Cancer. 2012;107:588–91.
6. Pujade-Lauraine E, Wagner U, Aavall-Lundqvist E, et al. Pegylated liposomal Doxorubicin and Carboplatin compared with Paclitaxel and Carboplatin for patients with platinum-sensitive ovarian cancer in late relapse. J Clin Oncol. 2010;28:3323–9.
7. Cannistra SA. Cancer of the ovary. N Engl J Med. 2004;351:2519–29.
8. Rubin SC, Randall TC, Armstrong KA, et al. Ten-year follow-up of ovarian cancer patients after second-look laparotomy with negative findings. Obstet Gynecol. 1999;93:21–4.
9. Jaaback K, Johnson N, Lawrie TA. Intraperitoneal chemotherapy for the initial management of primary epithelial ovarian cancer. Cochrane Database Syst Rev 2011;(11):CD005340.
10. Armstrong DK, Bundy B, Wenzel L, et al. Intraperitoneal cisplatin and paclitaxel in ovarian cancer. N Engl J Med. 2006;354:34–43.

11. Zhou M, Yu P, Qu X, et al. Phase III trials of standard chemotherapy with or without bevacizumab for ovarian cancer: a meta-analysis. PLoS One. 2013;8:e81858.
12. Helm CW, Bristow RE, Kusamura S, et al. Hyperthermic intraperitoneal chemotherapy with and without cytoreductive surgery for epithelial ovarian cancer. J Surg Oncol. 2008;98: 283–90.
13. Verwaal VJ, van Ruth S, de Bree E, et al. Randomized trial of cytoreduction and hyperthermic intraperitoneal chemotherapy versus systemic chemotherapy and palliative surgery in patients with peritoneal carcinomatosis of colorectal cancer. J Clin Oncol. 2003;21: 3737–43.
14. Verwaal VJ, Bruin S, Boot H, et al. 8-year follow-up of randomized trial: cytoreduction and hyperthermic intraperitoneal chemotherapy versus systemic chemotherapy in patients with peritoneal carcinomatosis of colorectal cancer. Ann Surg Oncol. 2008;15:2426–32.
15. Markman M. Intraperitoneal drug delivery of antineoplastics. Drugs. 2001;61:1057–65.
16. Zivanovic O, Abramian A, Kullmann M, et al. HIPEC ROC I: a phase I study of cisplatin administered as hyperthermic intraoperative intraperitoneal chemoperfusion followed by postoperative intravenous platinum-based chemotherapy in patients with platinum-sensitive recurrent epithelial ovarian cancer. Int J Cancer. 2015;136:699–708.
17. Giovanella BC, Stehlin Jr JS, Morgan AC. Selective lethal effect of supranormal temperatures on human neoplastic cells. Cancer Res. 1976;36:3944–50.
18. de Bree E, Rosing H, Filis D, et al. Cytoreductive surgery and intraoperative hyperthermic intraperitoneal chemotherapy with paclitaxel: a clinical and pharmacokinetic study. Ann Surg Oncol. 2008;15:1183–92.
19. Muller M, Cherel M, Dupre PF, et al. The cytotoxic effect of combined hyperthermia and taxane chemotherapy on ovarian cancer cells: results of an in vitro study. Eur Surg Res. 2012;48:55–63.
20. Spratt JS, Adcock RA, Muskovin M, et al. Clinical delivery system for intraperitoneal hyperthermic chemotherapy. Cancer Res. 1980;40:256–60.
21. Jacquet P, Stephens AD, Averbach AM, et al. Analysis of morbidity and mortality in 60 patients with peritoneal carcinomatosis treated by cytoreductive surgery and heated intraoperative intraperitoneal chemotherapy. Cancer. 1996;77:2622–9.
22. Chua TC, Yan TD, Saxena A, Morris DL. Should the treatment of peritoneal carcinomatosis by cytoreductive surgery and hyperthermic intraperitoneal chemotherapy still be regarded as a highly morbid procedure? A systematic review of morbidity and mortality. Ann Surg. 2009;249:900–7.
23. Smeenk RM, Verwaal VJ, Zoetmulder FA. Learning curve of combined modality treatment in peritoneal surface disease. Br J Surg. 2007;94:1408–14.
24. Cascales Campos P, Gil J, Parrilla P. Morbidity and mortality outcomes of cytoreductive surgery and hyperthermic intraperitoneal chemotherapy in patients with primary and recurrent advanced ovarian cancer. Eur J Surg Oncol. 2014;40:970–5.
25. Bakrin N, Bereder JM, Decullier E, et al. Peritoneal carcinomatosis treated with cytoreductive surgery and Hyperthermic Intraperitoneal Chemotherapy (HIPEC) for advanced ovarian carcinoma: a French multicentre retrospective cohort study of 566 patients. Eur J Surg Oncol. 2013;39:1435–43.
26. Steller MA, Egorin MJ, Trimble EL, et al. A pilot phase I trial of continuous hyperthermic peritoneal perfusion with high-dose carboplatin as primary treatment of patients with small-volume residual ovarian cancer. Cancer Chemother Pharmacol. 1999;43:106–14.
27. Lentz SS, Miller BE, Kucera GL, Levine EA. Intraperitoneal hyperthermic chemotherapy using carboplatin: a phase I analysis in ovarian carcinoma. Gynecol Oncol. 2007;106: 207–10.
28. Harrison LE, Bryan M, Pliner L, Saunders T. Phase I trial of pegylated liposomal doxorubicin with hyperthermic intraperitoneal chemotherapy in patients undergoing cytoreduction for advanced intra-abdominal malignancy. Ann Surg Oncol. 2008;15:1407–13.

29. Di Giorgio A, Naticchioni E, Biacchi D, et al. "http://www.ncbi.nlm.nih.gov.gate2.inist.fr/pubmed/18473354" Cytoreductive surgery (peritonectomy procedures) combined with hyperthermic intraperitoneal chemotherapy (HIPEC) in the treatment of diffuse peritoneal carcinomatosis from ovarian cancer. Cancer. 2008 Jul 15;113(2):315–25.
30. Classe JM, Glehen O, Decullier E, et al. French Oncologic and Gynecologic HIPEC Group. "http://www.ncbi.nlm.nih.gov.gate2.inist.fr/pubmed/26254399" Cytoreductive Surgery and Hyperthermic Intraperitoneal Chemotherapy for First Relapse of Ovarian Cancer. Anticancer Res. 2015 Sep;35(9):4997–5005.

Oncofertility Applied to Epithelial Ovarian Cancer

7

Enrica Bentivegna, Sebastien Gouy, Catherine Uzan, Marcos Ballester, Catherine Poirot, Emile Daraï, and Philippe Morice

Abstract

Conservative treatment, consisting in uterine preservation with unilateral salpingo-oophorectomy, can be proposed to selected patients with early epithelial ovarian cancer, with a desire for pregnancy after a histological review and surgical staging.

This procedure can be safely proposed for common histological subtype (mucinous, serous and endometrioid), for stage IA grade 1 and 2, for stage IC1 grade 1 disease.

The literature review of oncological and fertility outcomes after fertility sparing surgery in patients with epithelial ovarian cancer shows: an overall recurrence rate of 12%, a median overall survival of 94% at 5 years, a rate of 43% patients willing a pregnancy of which 66% become pregnant.

Assisted conception procedures after conservative treatment are actually contraindicated, nevertheless many techniques for fertility preservation are now developed.

E. Bentivegna (✉)
Service de Chirurgie Gynécologique, Gustave-Roussy Cancer Campus, 114 rue Edouard-Vaillant, Villejuif Cedex 94805, France
e-mail: enrica.bentivegna@gustaveroussy.fr

S. Gouy • P. Morice
Gustave Roussy Cancer Campus, Villejuif, France
e-mail: Philippe.MORICE@gustaveroussy.fr

C. Uzan
Hôpital de la Pitié-Salpétrière, Paris, France

M. Ballester • E. Daraï
Hôpital Tenon, Paris, France

C. Poirot
Hôpital de Poissy, Poissy, France

E. Pujade-Lauraine et al. (eds.), *Ovarian Cancers*,
DOI 10.1007/978-3-319-32110-3_7

Follow-up is based on a clinical examination, an analysis of tumour markers and the use of systematic imaging, at least every 4 months for the first 2 years, then every 6 months until 5 years and every year thereafter. Test for BRCA1-2 mutations is indicated.

Completion surgery after childbearing, or after 40 years of age in patients who have not become pregnant, is recommended.

Introduction

Conservative and functional surgery is increasingly used in surgical oncology. Its aim is to preserve organs' functionality and to reduce radical resection to allow pregnancy in patients of child-bearing age. Development of new minimally invasive procedures in oncological gynaecologic surgery is a perfect example of this evolution. Although radical surgery remains the gold standard in the treatment of epithelial ovarian cancer (EOC), fertility-sparing surgery (FSS) can be considered in patients with early-stage disease (stage I FIGO [1]), in order to preserve their fertility function and to improve their quality of life. These procedures can be proposed only to selected patients, depending on stage, grade, histological subtypes and prognostic factors. However a consensus for selected criteria is not yet done in literature, despite this topic being discussed since the last two decades.

The aim of this chapter is to clarify the selected criteria for FSS in EOC, the outcome and the fertility rate of these patients by summarising the main data on literature.

Indications of Fertility-Sparing Surgery

The indication of FSS in EOC needs first of all to satisfy some requirements: patient of child-bearing age (not older than 40 years), information on oncological and fertility outcome given to the patient, acceptation of strict follow-up, histological review of ovarian tumour by a designated gynaecologic pathologist and a correct disease staging [2].

The standard surgical procedure in EOC is radical (hysterectomy with bilateral salpingo-oophorectomy). This procedure has to be associated with a surgical staging (peritoneal cytology, omentectomy, complete bilateral pelvic and para-aortic lymphadenectomy, multiple peritoneal biopsies). The aim of surgical staging is to define the stage of disease and to adapt complementary treatment.

A conservative approach, defined as the preservation of at least a part of one ovary and the uterus, should be considered only in patients with early-stage disease.

The indications concerning conservative management of EOC are difficult to analyse in literature, because many reported series are either mixed dealing with conservative treatment in epithelial and non-epithelial ovarian cancer or include invasive and borderline ovarian tumours, considering them as epithelial. Some series reported the results of conservative management but mixing epithelial, borderline and non-epithelial tumours.

Few series reported about conservative treatment exclusively in EOC. DiSaia [3] is one of the first authors to propose conservative treatment for EOC, but with selected inclusion criteria: patients with fertility desire, willing to undergo close gynaecologic follow-up, stage IA, well-encapsulated ovarian cancer without peritumoural adhesions, no invasion of the ovarian capsule, lymphatic channels and\or the mesovarium and negative peritoneal washings.

To start the analysis of literature on FSS in EOC, we selected seven main retrospective series [4–11], including only EOC, with more than ten patients and with precise details concerning the tumour grade distribution for stage IA and IC disease (Table 7.1).

- Colombo et al. [4] in 1994 and Zanetta et al. [5] in 1997 have published the first series specifically dedicated to EOC. Their series involved 56 patients and the authors allow FSS in selected cases: stage IA to IC and any grade disease.
- An American multicentre study involving 52 patients was reported in 2002 [6]. The estimated overall survival in this study for patients with early-stage EOC who underwent FSS was 98 % at 5 years and 93 % at 10 years. The authors suggested FSS in stage I any grade EOC.
- A French multicentre study was published in 2005 [7]: a series involving 34 patients with strict inclusion criteria (systematic review of slides, complete staging surgery and chemotherapy for patients with stage ≥ IC). The authors declare safe FSS only in stage I grade 1 EOC.
- The study of Park et al. in 2008 [8] included 62 patients with EOC, of whom 59 have early stage. Patients with stage IC or grade 3 tumour have significantly poorer survival. FSS can be considered in young patients with stages IA–C grades 1–2.
- An Argentine series [9] included 16 patients with early-stage EOC and 2 patients with advanced stage which were treated conservatively. Disease-free survival (DFS) and overall survival (OS) were, respectively, 83.2 % and 94.4 %. The authors accorded FSS in any stage I with any grade.
- A Japanese multicentre study [10] included a total of 211 patients from 30 institutions undergoing FSS for EOC. The authors recommended FSS in stage IA either with favourable histological subtype or clear cell histology and in stage IC only with favourable histology; in case of grade 3, FSS is to be avoided.
- The largest series was recently published by Fruscio et al. [11]: an Italian retrospective study that evaluated 240 patients treated with FSS. The authors concluded that conservative treatment can be proposed to all young patients when tumour is limited to the ovaries. In case of grade 3, distance recurrences are more frequent and the patients must be monitored closely.

Results reported by those seven series (Table 7.1) suggested that such conservative surgery could be safely performed in patients with stage IA grade 1 and probably grade 2 diseases, respectively, 6 % and 13 % of recurrence rate. In 33 patients with stage IA grade 3 disease, 14 recurrences were observed (42 %) suggesting that conservative management should not be performed in such situations.

Table 7.1 Literature review of oncological outcome after fertility-sparing surgery in epithelial ovarian cancer in relation with stage, grade and histology of disease (representative series including >10 cases)

Author	Year of publication	Patients *n*	Relapses *n* (%)	FIGO stage IA			FIGO stage IC			Histological type			
				Grade 1	Grade 2	Grade 3	Grade 1	Grade 2	Grade 3	Serous	Mucinous	Endometrioid	Clear cell
Colombo et al. Zanetta et al. [4, 5]	1994 1997	56	5 (9 %)	1/24	2/8	1/4	0/10	1/6	0/3	2/18	1/23	2/13	nr
Schilder et al. [6]	2002	52	5 (10 %)	2/33	2/6	0/3	0/5	1/3	0/2	2/10	2/25	1/10	0/5
Morice et al. [7]	2005	34	10 (29 %)	1/13	4/14	1/3	2/2	nr	1/1	2/3	5/21	1/5	1/2
Park et al. [8]	2008	62	11 (18 %)	1/29	0/3	4/4	1/15	1/2	2/2	0/7	7/41	1/8	2/4
Anchezar et al. [9]	2009	18	3 (17 %)	1/10	nr	1/1	0/3	0/1	0/1	0/2	1/9	1/5	0/2
Satoh et al. [10]	2010	211	18 (8 %)	5/95	0/13	2/3	5/65	0/2	1/3	3/27	6/126	4/27	5/30
Fruscio et al. [11]	2013	240	27 (11 %)	7/84	2/31	5/15	6/54	4/37	2/14	11/62	8/99	6/60	2/17
TOTAL		**673**	**79/673 12 %**	**18/288 6 %**	**10/75 13 %**	**14/33 42 %**	**14/154 9 %**	**7/51 14 %**	**6/26 23 %**	**20/128 16 %**	**30/344 9 %**	**16/128 12 %**	**10/60 17 %**

nr data not reported

Controversy Over Stage IC2

Many discussions had concerned stage IC disease because results in the seven series reported different outcomes for patients treated conservatively for stage IC disease, and not all the authors suggested FSS in this case. Probably the key to the discussion in order to explain such potential differences is the heterogeneity of patients having stage IC according to the 1988 FIGO classification [12]: patients are classified as having stage IC disease in case of uni- or bilateral tumour with (a) spread of the tumour on the surface of the ovary (excrescences) and/or (b) ascites containing malignant cells or positive cytology after positive washing and/or (c) capsular rupture. So, patients included as having a stage IC disease were not probably "similar" in terms of criteria used to classify disease as stage IC in those patients. Furthermore, the histological subtype is perhaps somewhat different in those seven series concerning this substage of disease. Such fine difference could explain the absence of homogeneity in the literature until the new 2014 FIGO staging system [1]. Nevertheless, summarising the seven series, conservative management could be probably accorded in stage IC grade 1 disease (9 % of recurrence) but should not be performed in grade 2 or 3 disease, respectively, 14 % and 23 % of recurrence (Table 7.1).

Kajiyama et al. [13] explored recently recurrence predicting prognostic factors after FSS in patients with EOC. In a multicentre study, they included 94 patients on stage I EOC treated conservatively. In accord to the new FIGO classification [1], IC substage was defined: intraoperative spillage (IC1), preoperative capsule rupture or surface invasion (IC2) and positive cytology (IC3). They found 14 recurrences (14.9 %) and the overall recurrence-free survival (RFS) was 84.3 %. There was no significant difference in RFS between patients with stage IC1 and those with stage IA disease. In contrast this significant difference was found between IC2/3 and stage IA. Moreover they showed a significant poorer RFS of patients with grade 1 than grade 2–3 disease. FSS is not recommended for patients with preoperative capsule rupture or surface invasion (IC2), positive cytology (IC3) and grade 2 and 3 disease.

In a recent study about 18 patients [14] only on stage IC (14 grade 1 and 4 unknown), the authors find 5 recurrences (28 %) after FSS, and tumour histology did not exert a statistically significant effect. In terms of fertility outcome, of 10 patients who attempted to conceive, 7 singleton pregnancies were recorded for 5 women. The authors, based on their favourable fertility outcomes in spite of an elevated recurrence rate, suggest that FSS could be considered for EOC patients other than just those with FIGO stage IA grade 1 disease.

The analysis of the SEER (Surveillance, Epidemiology and End Results) database reports the absence of impact on the survival of preservation of the ovary in stage IA or IC disease [15]. Nevertheless, as stated by the authors, "to detect a 20 % difference in survival for pts with stage IC disease, a cohort of 1282 pts with 52 deaths is required". So, as none of the series published involved such a large number of patients, it is not possible to conclude definitively about the safety of conservative management in this situation.

Controversy Over Grade 3

The recommendations of the Fertility Task Force of the European Society of Gynecologic Oncology (ESGO) [2] indicated a safe FSS in EOC for stage IA and IC grade 1, stage IA grade 2 and "conventional histological subtypes". FSS is discussed in stage IC grade 2 and in stage IA clear cell subtype. FSS is contraindicated for grade 3 tumour, stage > I, histologically aggressive tumour.

The large recent Italian series, including 240 patients treated conservatively for EOC, support these recommendations; in particular regarding grade of disease, the authors find that grade 3 disease is an independent worst prognostic factor for RFS and OS compared with grade 1 and grade 2 disease [11].

In the same direction goes the result of the recent retrospective study of Ditto et al. [16]. The authors compared 70 patients treated conservatively for EOC versus 237 treated radically for EOC. In the FSS group 38 (54.3 %) and 32 (45.7 %) patients were at low risk (FIGO stage IA grade 1–2) and high risk (FIGO stage IA grade 3 or more), respectively. On multivariable analysis only stage of disease correlated with DFS: patients affected by FIGO stage IC or more advanced stage experienced a 4.7-fold increased risk of developing recurrences in comparison to patients affected by FIGO stage IA–IB. The FIGO grade 3 is associated with worse OS in multivariable analysis.

Controversy Over Stage II

It appears obviously that for disease extending beyond the ovaries, FSS is avoided because of the major risk of recurrences [7, 8]. Nevertheless there are in literature some cases reported that have been analysed in the recent review of Petrillo et al. [17]. The authors identified 21 patients with stage II–III disease receiving FSS. Recurrent disease was observed in 9 patients (42.8 %) and 23.8 % of the 21 patients died of disease. Radical surgery remains the standard for advanced EOC.

Controversy Over Histological Types

Histological type plays a great role in inclusion criteria: only serous, mucinous and endometrioid EOC should be considered for conservative management.

The data of the seven series (Table 7.1) showed a lower recurrence rate for mucinous subtype (9 %), 12 % of recurrence for endometrioid subtype and 16 % and 17 % for serous and clear cell disease, respectively.

In a recent retrospective series, Lee et al. [18] investigated the outcome of 90 patients treated for a mucinous epithelial ovarian cancer confined to the ovaries: 35 conservatively and 55 radically. There was no statistical difference between the two groups in DFS suggesting that FSS is safe in this histological subtype that occurs commonly in younger women.

Kajiyama et al. [19] compared two groups of patients with stage I clear cell carcinoma: 16 were treated with conservative surgery and 205 with radical surgery.

The OS and DFS were not statistically different between the two groups, and furthermore patients with clear cell carcinoma who underwent FSS did not show a poorer OS and DFS than patients with other histological subtypes. In spite of the small number of patients included, the authors suggested that such management could be proposed in clear cell tumour. The evolution of clear cell disease is different between Asia and Europe and this is probably the reason for such good results. Nevertheless, waiting furthers studies concerning such histological subtype considered as a high-grade disease, patients with clear cell (at least in Europe) and anaplastic EOC must not be considered for conservative treatment, because of the high risk of relapse on the remaining ovary.

Oncological Outcomes

The literature review (Table 7.2) of overall recurrences after FSS in patients with EOC showed a large range between 5 and 29 %, in relation with the heterogeneity of patients included in the different series. The median 5-year OS of all the series is good (94 %) as we expected for an early-stage disease, but it will be interesting to know the 10-year OS probably most influenced by recurrence, but the limited follow-up of these studies not allowed these data.

The prognosis of recurrent patients after conservative surgery for EOC remains poor, particularly in the case of recurrent disease outside from the preserved ovary [26].

Two interesting recent reviews investigated oncological outcomes of FSS in EOC.

The first one published by Du Bois et al. [27] included 15 studies comprising 913 patients. The authors found 11.4 % of global recurrences within a median observation time of 6 years: stage IB/C recurred nearly twice compared to stage IA (OR 1.72, 95 % confidence interval 1.12–2.64, $p < 0.05$), and the risk of recurrence was four times higher in grade 2–3 compared to grade 1 disease (OR 4.26, 95 % confidence interval 2.31–7.86, $p < 0.0001$). There was no statistical difference in recurrences between stage IC/grade 1 and stage IA/grade 1. The authors concluded that FSS is only advisable for unilateral grade 1 tumours.

The second one published by Zapardiel et al. [28] collected the pattern of recurrences of all studies that included more than 30 patients treated conservatively for early-stage EOC (total of 683 patients). They find an overall recurrence rate of 11.5; 4.8 % of the patients presented an isolated relapse in contralateral ovary. Overall survival at 5 years exceeds 90 and 4.4 % of patients died of disease. The authors suggested that it may be reasonable to broaden the indication of FSS to mostly grade 2 and occasionally to grade 3 or stage IC disease.

The pattern of relapse, ovarian or extraovarian recurrence, may influence the prognostic of these patients. In fact ovarian isolated relapse is correlated with the possibility of a new completed surgical treatment and very rarely leads patients to death. In the other and the extraovarian recurrence is more difficult to cure and is significantly associated with a higher risk of death than isolated ovarian recurrences [11].

Table 7.2 Literature review of overall rate of recurrence and fertility outcomes after fertility-sparing surgery in epithelial ovarian cancer (representative series including >10 cases)

Reference	Year of publication	Patients *n*	Relapses *n* (%)	5-year OS	Patients wishing for pregnancy *n* (%)	Patients that became pregnant *n* (%)	Total conception *n*	Non evolutive pregnancy *n*	Live births *n*
Colombo et al. Zanetta et al. [4, 5]	1994 1997	56	5 (9 %)	96 %	nr	20	27	10	17
Raspagliesi et al. [20]	1997	10[a]	0	100 %	9 (90 %)	3 (33 %)	3	1	2
Schilder et al. [6]	2002	52	5 (10 %)	98 %	24 (46 %)	17 (71 %)	32	5	26
Morice et al. [7]	2005	34	10 (29 %)	84 %	nr	9	10	1	6
Borgfeldt et al. [21]	2007	11	1 (9 %)	100 %	nr	7	14	0	14
Park et al. [8]	2008	62[b]	11 (18 %)[1]	88 %	19 (30 %)	15 (79 %)	24	2	22
Schlaerth et al. [22]	2009	20	3 (15 %)	84 %	15 (75 %)	6 (40 %)	9	0	9
Anchezar et al. [9]	2009	18[c]	3 (17 %)	94 %	nr	6	7	0	7
Kwon et al. [23]	2009	21	1 (5 %)	100 %	5 (24 %)	5 (100 %)	5	0	5
Satoh et al. [10]	2010	211	18 (8 %)	93 %	84 (40 %)	45 (53 %)	65	9	56

Kajiyama et al. [13, 24]	2010	60	8 (13 %)	89.8 %	nr	9	13	3	10
	2014	94	14 (15 %)	84.3 %[d]	nr	nr	nr	nr	nr
Cheng et al. [25]	2012	17[e]	1 (6 %)	100 %	8 (47 %)	5 (62 %)	7	1	6
Fruscio et al. [11]	2013	240	27 (11 %)	99 %	105 (44 %)	84 (80 %)	107	16	91
Kashima et al. [14]	2013	18[f]	5 (28 %)	nr	10 (55 %)	5 (50 %)	nr	nr	7
Ditto et al. [16]	2015	70	nr	98 %	nr	nr	nr	nr	nr
Lee et al. [18]	2015	35	6	91 %	nr	nr	nr	nr	nr
TOT		*969*	*110/899 (12 %)*	*1415/15 (94 %)*	*279/651 (43 %)g*	*185/279 (66 %)g*			*224g*

[a]Six patients in stage III disease
[b]Two patients in stage III disease
[c]One patient in stage III disease
[d]DFS (disease-free survival)
[e]One patient in stage III disease
[f]Only stage IC disease
[g]Data concerning only [6, 8, 10, 11, 14, 20, 22, 23, 25]
nr data not reported

Surgical Procedure for Conservative Surgery

Conservative surgery must be considered only after an adequate surgical staging. This staging must include peritoneal washings, excision of any suspicious peritoneal lesion, multiple peritoneal biopsies and omentectomy. Endometrial curettage should be performed in endometrioid subtype because a concomitant endometrial cancer may be discovered. A pelvic and para-aortic lymph node dissection is recommended but still discussed in patients with stage I disease in mucinous subtype or in serous grade I subtypes, because a nodal spread is very uncommon in these cases [29–31].

The fertility-sparing surgery in EOC consists in uterine preservation with unilateral salpingo-oophorectomy. In patients with "limit" indication for conservative surgery (stage IA grade 3 disease, stage IB or IC grade 2 or 3 disease, stage IC2 and IC3 disease), another option could be considered: the removal of both ovaries but with uterine preservation (with the absence of positive uterine curettage at the time of staging surgery) to preserve a potential possibility of "fertility" (oocyte donation or other procedures). Such proposal has never been explored in EOC, but should be evaluated.

In a conservative approach, Munnell [32] proposed to associate a systematic biopsy of the remaining ovary, because on his data a contralateral microscopic involvement existed in 12 % of cases of EOC. Nevertheless, systematic biopsies of contralateral ovarian cancer can induce infertility by provoking postoperative adhesions with the remaining ovary. Moreover, many authors have not found any microscopic implants in a macroscopically normal ovary [4, 6]. On the other hand, Benjamin et al. [33] have reported on a series of 118 patients with stage I EOC a microscopic localisation in the contralateral ovary in 3 patients (2.5 %), with normal macroscopic aspect of the ovary. But these 3 patients had grade 3 tumours and none of the patients with stage I grade 1 or 2 disease had occult metastasis on contralateral ovary. In consequence, a routine biopsy on the contralateral ovary is not recommended if a preoperative vaginal ultrasonography did not reveal deep parenchymatous abnormalities in the contralateral ovary to the tumour and if it seems macroscopically normal during the surgical procedure.

Concerning surgical approach in EOC, laparotomy is the conventional technique that permitted complete and accurate exploration of the abdominal cavity and safe and adequate exposition for debulking surgery in advanced ovarian disease. On the other hand, laparoscopy should be the indicated approach in early-stage ovarian disease with particular regard for patients that may undergo fertility-sparing surgery. In fact laparoscopy has many advantages in this context, lower bleeding, lower contamination, less tissue and organ handling, minimal scars and especially lower postoperative adhesion, that can impact fertility.

In the conservative management of EOC, many authors agree that laparoscopy staging performed by an experienced gynaecologic oncologist is feasible, adequate and safe, without difference in surgicopathologic results and survival outcomes compared with laparotomy approach [34–39]

Recently the first two cases of robotic-assisted FSS for early ovarian cancer have been reported: the first one concerning a 29-year-old woman who developed a well-differentiated endometrioid carcinoma stage IC and the second one concerning a 31-year-old woman with an immature grade 1 teratoma. For the patient with an EOC, a completed staging was performed without complication [40].

Fertility Results After Conservative Surgery

After FSS in EOC few fertility results are available in the literature. The review of these data is shown in Table 7.2. Considering the nine series [6, 8, 10, 11, 14, 20, 22, 23, 25] with available details of fertility outcomes, we found that 43 % (279) of patients with early-stage EOC wished for pregnancy after FSS and 66 % (185) became pregnant with 224 live births (Table 7.2).

Zanetta et al. reported 27 pregnancies in 20 patients [5]. In the American series 24 patients attempted pregnancy and 17 conceived. These 17 patients had 26 term pregnancies and 5 spontaneous abortions [6]. In a French series, 10 pregnancies were observed in 9 patients [7]. Park et al. reported 15 pregnancies in 19 attempted patients that had 22 term pregnancies and 2 spontaneous abortions [8]. Anchezar et al. reported 7 pregnancies in 6 patients out of 18 patients included in the study [9]. In the series of Satoh et al., of the 195 patients who gave reproductive outcomes, 55 achieved 76 pregnancies [10]. In the recent Italian series including 240 patients treated conservatively for EOC, 105 tried to become pregnant and 84 were successful: 16 had one or more spontaneous abortions and 68 had at least one child. The authors find an inverse correlation between tumour grade and willing pregnancy: significantly more patients with grade 1 and 2 disease tried to conceive compared with patients with grade 3 disease [11].

Fertility Preservation and Assisted Conception Procedures

In the last decade different strategies have been developed to preserve ovarian germ cell in young patients treated for cancer. Even in the case of fertility-sparing surgery, completion treatment as chemotherapy and radiotherapy may impact the ovarian germ cell reserve and hormonal function. Before a cancer treatment, if the prognostic disease is favourable, three solutions can be proposed in women of child-bearing age: cryopreservation of a part of the ovarian cortex that can be reimplanted [41], cryopreservation of mature oocytes after a controlled ovarian stimulation [42] or retrieval and storage of immature or in vitro matured oocytes (IVM) [43]. IVM is an attractive alternative for fertility preservation in cancer patients because it does not require ovarian stimulation and is the preferable solution for those tumours with hormonal sensitivity [44].

Nevertheless, after an FSS in EOC, if infertility persists, ovarian stimulation or IVM remains contraindicated. Even if there are not sufficient data in the literature, any hormonal stimulation may increase recurrence rates. Bandera et al. [45] reported a case of a woman with stage IC grade 1 mucinous epithelial ovarian cancer treated conservatively, who underwent the next 3 years 2 cycles of ovulation induction with exogenous gonadotropins. Five months after the second cycle, the patient presented extensive recurrence of disease and she died 2 months later despite extensive surgical debulking followed by chemotherapy.

Moreover ovarian cryopreservation is not a good procedure for patients with EOC, because of the risk to reimplant a part of the ovary containing malignant cells as suspected for auto-transplantation of ovarian tissue in women having suffered from systematic haematological malignancies [46].

In literature there are very few cases reported about fertility-assisted procedure in EOC.

In a multicentre national retrospective study, 40 patients treated conservatively for ovarian tumours (only 3 EOC) were submitted to a fertility-assisted procedure. Seventeen pregnancies were obtained and among these one had an EOC. Only three patients treated for borderline ovarian tumour have a recurrence after induction of ovulation [47].

Fadini et al. [48] reported a case report about a 38-year-old woman with a previous history of infertility, treated for an EOC stage IIC grade 2. Following the strong desire of parenthood by the patient, immature oocytes were collected during surgical procedures. Vitrification and successive warming was carried out. About 1 year after adjuvant treatment finished, the patient had an embryo transfer after ICSI (intracytoplasmic sperm injection) with her cryopreserved in vitro matured oocytes. The procedure didn't evolve in viable pregnancy.

In a recent study about obstetric outcome after orthotopic transplantation of cryopreserved ovarian tissue, among the 20 patients previously treated for malignant disease, only one had an EOC. She became pregnant spontaneously after transplantation, realised 5 years after the end of treatment [49]. Nevertheless, in our practice, for patients treated conservatively for EOC, this procedure remained contraindicated.

Very few data are available in literature on this subject, and more investigations are required to know the real benefit and relative relapse risk of fertility-assisted procedures in patients treated conservatively for early-stage EOC. A new speciality called oncofertility is now developed, and the specialist should be introduced in the multidisciplinary management of patients eligible for FSS.

Follow-Up

After a conservative management of early-stage EOC, a careful follow-up is crucial in order to discover ovarian or extraovarian relapse. Moreover the acceptation of a strict follow-up is one of the criteria to allow FSS.

Follow-up is conventionally based on clinical examination, analysis of tumour markers and the use of a systematic imaging (abdominopelvic ultrasonography), at least every 4 months for the first 2 years and then every 6 months until 5 years and every year thereafter.

These young patients (<40 years old) that undergo an FSS should be tested for BRCA 1–2 mutations in order to adapted the screening of breast cancer.

The use of completion surgery after child-bearing, or in patients who have not been pregnant after 40 years of age, remains to be discussed. Nevertheless, cases of relapsing EOC 10 years after conservative treatment like reported in literature [11, 50] could suggest discussing the removal of the remaining ovary, in order to reduce the risk of recurrence on the spared ovary.

Conclusions

In patients of child-bearing age with early EOC, conservative surgery of one ovary and the uterus can be considered in order to preserve their fertility function and to improve their quality of life. To allow FSS some requirements are necessary: patients not older than 40 years who wish for pregnancy, acceptation of strict follow-up, histological review of ovarian tumour and a complete disease staging.

Ideally, to validate this practice, a randomised trial should be performed to compare FSS and radical surgery in patients with early-stage EOC, but it will be ethically incorrect to propose a radical treatment to young patients of child-bearing age because many studies reported that FSS is a safe management in selected cases. Furthermore, EOC is a rare disease and a randomised trial is technically unrealisable because in a large number of cases, it will be necessary to observe a statistical difference in DFS and OS.

Concerning stage and grade disease, conservative treatment can be safely proposed in stage IA grades 1 and 2 and in stage IC1 grade 1; this procedure is still discussed for stage IC1 grade 2 and is contraindicated in case of bilateral involvement of the ovary, stage IB, IC2/IC3 and grade 3 disease.

Concerning histological subtype, conservative treatment can be safely proposed in mucinous, serous and endometrioid disease; in case of clear cell disease, the indication of FSS is still discussed, and it must be considered the different evolutions of this subtype between Asia and Europe; FSS is contraindicated for anaplastic and neuroendocrine tumour.

The literature review showed an overall rate of recurrences after FSS in patients with EOC of 12 % and a median 5-year overall survival of 94 % (Table 7.2).

Conservative surgery must be considered only after an adequate surgical staging that must include peritoneal washings, excision of any suspicious peritoneal lesion, multiple peritoneal biopsies, omentectomy and pelvic and para-aortic lymphadenectomy. The laparoscopic approach is feasible, adequate and safe, without difference in surgicopathologic results and survival outcomes compared with laparotomy approach, and leads to less postoperative adhesion; this is the surgical approach that might be the best choice.

The literature review of fertility outcomes showed 43 % of patients with early-stage EOC wishing for pregnancy after FSS and 66 % of these patients became pregnant (Table 7.2). Actually fertility-assisted procedure after FSS for early EOC is contraindicated because of elevated risk of recurrence. Fertility improvement should be discussed with multidisciplinary staff including gynaecologic oncologists, pathologists and specialists trained in oncofertility.

The patients should be tested for BRCA 1–2 and carry out a careful follow-up based on clinical examination, analysis of tumour markers and the use of a systematic imaging (abdominopelvic ultrasonography).

The use of completion surgery after child-bearing, or after 40 years old in patients who have not been pregnant, is recommended.

References

1. Prat J, FIGO Committee on Gynecologic Oncology. Staging classification for cancer of the ovary, fallopian tube, and peritoneum. Int J Gynaecol Obstet. 2014;124:1–5.
2. Morice P, Denschlag D, Rodolakis A, et al. Recommendations of the Fertility Task Force of the European Society of Gynecologic Oncology about the conservative management of ovarian malignant tumors. Int J Gynecol Cancer. 2011;21:951–63.
3. DiSaia PJ. Conservative management of the patient with early gynecologic cancer. CA Cancer J Clin. 1989;39:135–54.
4. Colombo N, Chiari S, Maggioni A, Bocciolone L, Torri V, Mangioni C. Controversial issues in the management of early epithelial ovarian cancer: conservative surgery and role of adjuvant therapy. Gynecol Oncol. 1994;55:S47–51.
5. Zanetta G, Chiari S, Rota S, et al. Conservative surgery for stage I ovarian carcinoma in women of childbearing age. Br J Obstet Gynaecol. 1997;104:1030–5.
6. Schilder JM, Thompson AM, DePriest PD, et al. Outcome of reproductive age women with stage IA or IC invasive epithelial ovarian cancer treated with fertility-sparing therapy. Gynecol Oncol. 2002;87:1–7.
7. Morice P, Leblanc E, Rey A, et al. Conservative treatment in epithelial ovarian cancer: results of a multicentre study of the GCCLCC (Groupe des Chirurgiens de Centre de Lutte Contre le Cancer) and SFOG (Société Francaise d'Oncologie Gynécologique). Hum Reprod. 2005;20:1379–85.
8. Park JY, Kim DY, Suh DS, et al. Outcomes of fertility-sparing surgery for invasive epithelial ovarian cancer: oncologic safety and reproductive outcomes. Gynecol Oncol. 2008;110:345–53.
9. Anchezar JP, Sardi J, Soderini A. Long-term follow-up results of fertility sparing surgery in patients with epithelial ovarian cancer. J Surg Oncol. 2009;100:55–8.
10. Satoh T, Hatae M, Watanabe Y, et al. Outcomes of fertility-sparing surgery for stage I epithelial ovarian cancer: a proposal for patient selection. J Clin Oncol. 2010;28:1727–32.
11. Fruscio R, Corso S, Ceppi L, et al. Conservative management of early-stage epithelial ovarian cancer: results of a large retrospective series. Ann Oncol. 2013;24:138–44.
12. Shepherd JH. Revised FIGO staging for gynaecological cancer. Br J Obstet. 1989;96(8):889–92.
13. Kajiyama H, Mizuno M, Shibata K, et al. Recurrence-predicting prognostic factors for patients with early-stage epithelial ovarian cancer undergoing fertility-sparing surgery: a multi-institutional study. Eur J Obstet Gynecol Reprod Biol. 2014;175:97–102.
14. Kashima K, Yahata T, Fujita K, Tanaka K. Outcomes of fertility-sparing surgery for women of reproductive age with FIGO stage IC epithelial ovarian cancer. Int J Gynaecol Obstet. 2013;121(1):53–5.
15. Wright JD, Shah M, Mathew L, et al. Fertility preservation in young women with epithelial ovarian cancer. Cancer. 2009;115(18):4118–26.

16. Ditto A, Martinelli F, Bogani G, et al. Long-term safety of fertility sparing surgery in early stage ovarian cancer: Comparison to standard radical surgical procedures. Gynecol Oncol. 2015;138(1):78–82.
17. Petrillo M, Legge F, Ferrandina G, et al. Fertility-sparing surgery in ovarian cancer extended beyond the ovaries: a case report and review of the literature. Gynecol Obstet Invest. 2014;77:1–5.
18. Lee JY, Jo YR, Kim TH, et al. Safety of fertility-sparing surgery in primary mucinous carcinoma of the ovary. Cancer Res Treat. 2015;47(2):290–7.
19. Kajiyama H, Shibata K, Suzuki S, et al. Is there any possibility of fertility-sparing surgery in patients with clear-cell carcinoma of the ovary? Gynecol Oncol. 2008;111:523–6.
20. Raspagliesi F, Fontanelli R, Paladini D, di Re EM. Conservative surgery in high-risk epithelial ovarian carcinoma. J Am Coll Surg. 1997;185(5):457–60.
21. Borgfeldt C, Iosif C, Måsbäck A. Fertility-sparing surgery and outcome in fertile women with ovarian borderline tumors and epithelial invasive ovarian cancer. Eur J Obstet Gynecol Reprod Biol. 2007;134(1):110–4.
22. Schlaerth AC, Chi DS, Poynor EA, Barakat RR, Brown CL. Long-term survival after fertility-sparing surgery for epithelial ovarian cancer. Int J Gynecol Cancer. 2009;19(7):1199–204.
23. Kwon YS, Hahn HS, Kim TJ, et al. Fertility preservation in patients with early epithelial ovarian cancer. J Gynecol Oncol. 2009;20(1):44–7.
24. Kajiyama H, Shibata K, Suzuki S, et al. Fertility-sparing surgery in young women with invasive epithelial ovarian cancer. Eur J Surg Oncol. 2010;36(4):404–8.
25. Cheng X, Cheng B, Wan X, Lu W, Xie X. Outcomes of conservative surgery in early epithelial ovarian carcinoma. Eur J Gynaecol Oncol. 2012;33(1):93–5.
26. Marpeau O, Schilder J, Zafrani Y, et al. Prognosis of patients who relapse after fertility-sparing surgery in epithelial ovarian cancer. Ann Surg Oncol. 2008;15:478–83.
27. Du Bois A, Heitz F, Harter P. Fertility-sparing surgery in ovarian cancer: a systematic review. Onkologie. 2013;36(7–8):436–43.
28. Zapardiel I, Diestro MD, Aletti G. Conservative treatment of early stage ovarian cancer: oncological and fertility outcomes. Eur J Surg Oncol. 2014;40:387–93.
29. Morice P, Joulie F, Camatte S, et al. Lymph node involvement in epithelial ovarian cancer: analysis of 276 pelvic and paraaortic lymphadenectomies and surgical implications. J Am Coll Surg. 2003;197:198–205.
30. Cho YH, Kim DY, Kim JH, et al. Is complete surgical staging necessary in patients with stage I mucinous epithelial ovarian tumors? Gynecol Oncol. 2006;103:878–82.
31. Schmeler KM, Tao X, Frumovitz M, et al. Prevalence of lymph node metastasis in primary mucinous carcinoma of the ovary. Obstet Gynecol. 2010;116(2 Pt 1):269–73.
32. Munnell EW. Is conservative therapy ever justified in stage I (IA) cancer of the ovary ? Am J Obstet Gynecol. 1969;103:641–50.
33. Benjamin I, Morgan MA, Rubin SC. Occult bilateral involvement in stage I epithelial ovarian cancer. Gynecol Oncol. 1999;72:288–91.
34. Leblanc E, Querleu D, Narducci F, Occelli B, Papageorgiou T, Sonoda Y. Laparoscopic staging of early stage invasive adnexal tumors: a 10-year experience. Gynecol Oncol. 2004;94:624–9.
35. Nezhat FR, Ezzati M, Chuang L, Shamshirsaz AA, Rahaman J, Gretz H. Laparoscopic management of early ovarian and fallopian tube cancers: surgical and survival outcome. Am J Obstet Gynecol. 2009;200:83.
36. Ghezzi F, Malzoni M, Vizza E, et al. Laparoscopic staging of early ovarian cancer: results of a multi-institutional cohort study. Ann Surg Oncol. 2012;19:1589–94.
37. Tozzi R, Köhler C, Ferrara A, Schneider A. Laparoscopic treatment of early ovarian cancer: surgical and survival outcomes. Gynecol Oncol. 2004;93:199–203.
38. Schreuder HW, Pattij TO, Zweemer RP, van Baal MW, Verheijen RH. Increasing experience in laparoscopic staging of early ovarian cancer. Gynecol Surg. 2012;9:89–96.

39. Montanari G, Di Donato N, Del Forno S, et al. Laparoscopic management of early stage ovarian cancer: is it feasible, safe, and adequate? A retrospective study. Eur J Gynaecol Oncol. 2013;34(5):415–8.
40. Finger TN, Nezhat FR. Robotic-assisted fertility-sparing surgery for early ovarian cancer. JSLS. 2014;18(2):308–13.
41. Donnez J, Silber S, Andersen CY, et al. Children born after autotransplantation of cryopreserved ovarian tissue. A review of 13 live births. Ann Med. 2011;243:437–50.
42. Noyes N, Labella PA, Grifo J, Knopman JM. Oocyte cryopreservation: a feasible fertility preservation option for reproductive age cancer survivors. J Assist Reprod Genet. 2010;27: 495–9.
43. Huang JYJ, Chian RC, Gilbert L, et al. Retrieval of immature oocytes from unstimulated ovaries followed by in vitro maturation and vitrification: a novel strategy of fertility preservation for breast cancer patients. AJS. 2010;200:177–83.
44. Berwanger AL, Finet A, El Hachem H, le Parco S, Hesters L, Grynberg M. New trends in female fertility preservation: in vitro maturation of oocytes. Future Oncol. 2012;8(12): 1567–73.
45. Bandera CA, Cramer DW, Friedman AJ, Sheets EE. Fertility therapy in the setting of a history of invasive epithelial ovarian cancer. Gynecol Oncol. 1995;58(1):116–9.
46. Grynberg M, Poulain M, Sebag-Peyrelevade S, le Parco S, Fanchin R, Frydman N. Ovarian tissue and follicle transplantation as an option for fertility preservation. Fertil Steril. 2012;97(6):1260–8.
47. Fortin A, Hazout A, Thoury A, Alvès K, Bats AS, Dhainaut C, Madelenat P. Assisted reproductive technologies after conservative management of borderline or invasive ovarian tumours. Gynecol Obstet Fertil. 2005;33(7–8):488–97.
48. Fadini R, Dal Canto M, Mignini Renzini M, et al. Embryo transfer following in vitro maturation and cryopreservation of oocytes recovered from antral follicles during conservative surgery for ovarian cancer. J Assist Reprod Genet. 2012;29(8):779–81.
49. Dittrich R, Hackl J, Lotz L, Hoffmann I, Beckmann MW. Pregnancies and live births after 20 transplantations of cryopreserved ovarian tissue in a single center. Fertil Steril. 2015; 103(2):462–8.
50. Moore MM, Tewari K, Rose GS, Fruehauf JP, DiSaia PJ. Long-term consequences following conservative management of epithelial ovarian cancer in an infertile patient. Gynecol Oncol. 1999;73(3):452–4.

First-Line Systemic Therapy (Chemo/Antiangiogenics)

8

Sandro Pignata and Sabrina Chiara Cecere

Abstract

Epithelial ovarian cancer (EOC) is often diagnosed in advanced stage. Optimal cytoreductive surgery followed by a platinum–taxane combination has been the cornerstone of treatment for more than 15 years. Despite the best upfront treatment, about 80 % of women with advanced disease achieve an objective response, and 10–20 % are cured with this regimen; nevertheless, disease recurrence occurs in most patients. Delaying progression or recurrence is one of the main goals of current ongoing clinical studies. In the last decade, several trials have investigated new therapeutic strategies such as dose-dense chemotherapy, intraperitoneal therapies (IP), and the integration of standard chemotherapy with biological agents. Bevacizumab, targeting angiogenesis, has been the first biological agent reaching the clinical practice. The GOG218 and the ICON7 trials demonstrated that bevacizumab prolongs progression-free survival in patients with FIGO stages IIIb–IV in combination with platinum-based chemotherapy and, most importantly, as maintenance. Other biological drugs, such as pazopanib, olaparib, and trebananib, showing impressive results in the recurrent setting, have been investigated in the first line, pending definitive results. The ovarian cancer is still considered a unique entity. A better molecular characterization will help researchers to develop some more tailored therapeutic strategies according to different molecular subtypes.

S. Pignata (✉) • S.C. Cecere
Division of Medical Oncology, Department of Uro-Gynaecological Oncology, Istituto Nazionale Tumori Fondazione G Pascale – IRCCS, Naples, Italy
e-mail: s.pignata@istitutotumori.na.it; sabrinacecere@hotmail.it

E. Pujade-Lauraine et al. (eds.), *Ovarian Cancers*,
DOI 10.1007/978-3-319-32110-3_8

Introduction

Ovarian cancer is the seventh most common cancer among women up to 64 years of age. Worldwide there are more than 200,000 new cases of ovarian cancer each year, accounting for around 4 % of all tumors diagnosed in women with a cumulative lifetime risk of ovarian cancer of 0.5 % [23]. In Europe, ovarian cancer is the leading cause of gynecological cancer death, with an estimated 65,697 new cases and 41,448 deaths each year and with just over a third of women alive 5 years after diagnosis [23]. Early diagnosis is considered one of the most important factors that affect prognosis. Unfortunately, the lack of standardized and validated screening procedures and the absence of specific symptoms until advanced stages make difficult to diagnose the disease at a time when a curative approach is still feasible. Epithelial ovarian cancer is a highly chemosensitive tumor, with response rates to primary treatment that reach approximately 75 %; however, also recurrence rates are very high, particularly in the first 2 years after surgery. Approximately, 15 % of cases are localized to the ovaries. In this group 5-year survival is more than 90 %. The majority of diagnoses identify women with advanced disease (International Federation of Gynecology and Obstetrics [FIGO] stages III–IV) which are characterized by a 5-year survival of less than 30 %. Epithelial ovarian cancer is not a unique disease and, morphologically, is classified into five main histologic subtypes: high-grade serous, which accounts for 70 % of all epithelial cancer, low-grade serous (5 %), endometrioid (10 %), mucinous (3–5 %), and clear-cell tumors (10 %) [63]. These different ovarian cancer subtypes show a distinct biological and genetic mutational spectrum: high-grade serous ovarian cancers are characterized by mutations of TP53 in about 96 % of cases and in 20 % of cases by BRCA 1/2 mutations, including a combination of germline and somatic mutations [73]. Low-grade serous ovarian cancer is often associated with K-RAS, B-RAF, and ERB-B2 mutations, while TP53 is rarely mutated [46]. Clear-cell ovarian cancers have less frequent TP53 mutations but have recurrent ARID1A and PIK3CA mutations. Endometrioid ovarian carcinomas have a similar pattern of genetic aberrations, with a low rate of TP53 mutations and prevalent ARID1A, PIK3CA, and CTTNB1 mutations. Mucinous ovarian tumors show K-RAS mutations [73]. These genetic characteristics likely reflect a distinct pathogenesis and lead to different biological behaviors, with impact on prognosis and on response to antineoplastic treatments. Literature data and the growing knowledge of biological features of ovarian cancer lead us to consider as inadequate the prognostic characterization of ovarian cancer based on clinical and pathological parameters (FIGO stage of disease, histological type, degree of differentiation, residual disease after surgery). One recent attempt to view differently this type of tumor was recently proposed. According to the pathogenesis of ovarian cancer, a dualistic model has been formulated that divides EOC into two categories called type I and type II [17, 34, 35, 69]. Type I ovarian cancers tend to be low grade and to have an indolent biological behavior, with characteristic genetic mutations, including low-grade serous, endometrioid, mucinous, and clear-cell ovarian carcinoma [46]. On the contrary, type II ovarian tumors, including high-grade serous, high-grade [68] endometrioid, malignant mixed mesodermal, and undifferentiated ovarian tumors, have an aggressive phenotype and an unstable genome. These subtypes show different prognoses, patterns of spread, and responses to chemotherapy [46]. This variability is still not taken into account in our therapeutic algorithm.

Postoperative Chemotherapy in Early-Stage Ovarian Cancer

Surgery is the cornerstone of EOC, and it is considered curative in most of the cases of women with early-stage tumors. Early-stage ovarian cancer includes FIGO stages Ia, Ib, and Ic [64]. An adequate cytoreductive surgery should be offered both to remove the disease and to provide accurate staging, which is a key factor also for the decision to undergo an adjuvant therapy. The prognosis of early-stage ovarian cancer is good, with a 5-year survival rate of 70–90 % [1]. Although surgery is curative in many cases, about 30 % of the patients recur and require further therapy.

The rationale of adjuvant chemotherapy after complete removal of the disease and adequate surgical staging is to eradicate any residual microscopic deposits of cancer cells responsible of potential recurrence of disease. In order to make an appropriate treatment choice, it is, therefore, important to understand what factors in early stages of ovarian cancer influence the prognosis and the risk of recurrence and, therefore, which patients would benefit most from additional treatment. Uncontrolled retrospective studies identified prognostic factors in this setting. A multivariate analysis of 1545 patients with stage I EOC confirmed tumor grade to be the single most important determinant of survival [78]. Other important independent prognostic factors are age, FIGO stage, substage (capsular involvement or cyst rupture, FIGO stage Ic), histological subtype (e.g., worse prognosis in the undifferentiated tumors), and the presence of ascites. According to literature data, early stages of epithelial ovarian cancer are divided into three different risk categories. Low-risk patients have tumors at FIGO stages Ia and Ib with well-differentiated disease and with no clear-cell histology; in such conditions, surgery is resolutive in 95 % of cases in the absence of evidences that demonstrate a benefit of a subsequent adjuvant chemotherapy [39]. The patients with FIGO stage Ia–Ib moderately differentiated belong to intermediate risk. Poorly differentiated tumors or stages Ic–II are considered high risk as associated with a recurrence rate of 25–40 % and, therefore, are candidates for adjuvant chemotherapy [75]. The patients with intraoperative rupture of the tumor within the abdomen fall into this group. A number of evidences support the use of adjuvant chemotherapy in early-stage ovarian cancer,however the optimal regimen, and duration is still debated [16, 29, 70]. A Cochrane meta-analysis assessed the survival advantage of adjuvant chemotherapy in early-stage ovarian cancer [79]. Five randomized clinical trials were included in the analysis. While the earliest three trials lacked enough events to demonstrate a possible impact of adjuvant treatment, on the contrary, the ICON1 and the ACTION trial [75] included a larger number of patients and had a sufficient power to demonstrate a treatment effect. These two trials randomized patients with serous, mucinous, endometrioid, clear-cell, and undifferentiated ovarian carcinomas to receive platinum-based chemotherapy or no chemotherapy. The 5-year and the updated 10-year overall survival rate was significantly better for women receiving adjuvant chemotherapy compared with the control group. Similar findings were reported for progression-free survival [79]. Additionally, these two trials address the question of which patients with early-stage ovarian cancer benefit more from adjuvant chemotherapy. The ICON1 trial stratified patients in low/intermediate risk (FIGO stage Ia, G1–G2, or FIGO stages Ib–Ic, G1) and high risk (FIGO stage Ia, G3, and Ib/Ic, G2–G3, any clear cell). Both overall and progression-free survival were better in high-risk patients, but no difference was observed among treated and non-treated low- to intermediate-risk patients at 5- and 10-year follow-up [72]. Conversely, the ACTION trial strongly recommended a complete surgical staging and planned a subgroup analysis on suboptimally and optimally staged patients. Patients with FIGO stage Ia/Ib, G2–G3, and FIGO stage Ic/IIa were included. Among the suboptimally staged women, adjuvant chemotherapy increased the overall (OS) and disease-free survival (DFS), whereas in the optimally staged patients, no difference was observed between the treated group and the control group. At a median follow-up of 10 years, earlier data were confirmed [79]. These results may suggest that there is a subgroup of good-prognosis patients who apparently do not benefit from adjuvant chemotherapy. In particular, it is hypothesized that chemotherapy impacts only on occult disease in suboptimally staged patients. Nonetheless, a benefit in optimally staged tumor cannot be excluded. In summary, adjuvant chemotherapy may be avoided only for low-risk, optimally staged, stage I patients (FIGO stage Ia/Ib, G1–G2); chemotherapy is indicated after surgery for patients with high-risk stage I disease (FIGO stage Ic, G3). In case of suboptimal surgical staging of low-risk stage I patients, benefits and effects of adjuvant chemotherapy should be discussed with each individual patient [1, 53, 54]. Regarding the chemotherapy regimen in this setting, studies comparing carboplatin plus paclitaxel versus carboplatin alone are not available. Indirect suggestions of greater efficacy of the carboplatin–taxane combination are gathered by results in advanced-stage disease. In the absence of clear recommendations, single-agent carboplatin can be considered a reasonable alternative to the doublet in intermediate- and high-risk early-stage ovarian cancer patients [1, 39, 53, 54]. The optimal duration of adjuvant chemotherapy remains a matter of investigation. A randomized trial which compared three versus six cycles of platinum plus paclitaxel for early-stage ovarian cancer revealed a nonstatistically significant 24 % reduction in recurrence rate in patients who underwent six courses of chemotherapy [6]. A subgroup analysis stratifying patients on the basis of clinical and pathological features showed a statistically significant benefit of six versus three cycles of chemotherapy only in serous tumors, while outcome for non-serous was not influenced by the duration of chemotherapy [14]. Again, there may be a subgroup of patients who do not benefit from intensive adjuvant chemotherapy and future research is needed to confirm these hypotheses. Recently the Cochrane review has been updated including mature data (10-year follow-up) of the same trials [36]. The conclusion is that adjuvant platinum-based chemotherapy is effective in prolonging survival in women with early-stage (FIGO stage I/IIa) epithelial ovarian cancer. It remains uncertain whether women with low- and intermediate-risk early-stage disease will benefit as much from adjuvant chemotherapy as women with high-risk disease. Decisions to use adjuvant chemotherapy in these women should be individualized to take into account individual factors.

Also, the choice to prescribe adjuvant chemotherapy in the early stages of the type I tumors including the less common clear-cell, mucinous, and low-grade serous carcinoma [34] is object of debate. Comparing the outcome for different histologic subtypes in large randomized trials evaluating paclitaxel/carboplatin in advanced ovarian cancer, it seems that clear-cell and mucinous carcinomas are more chemo-resistant than serous carcinomas [25, 57]. Adjuvant chemotherapy is usually not given for stage I mucinous tumors, while this topic is still debated for clear-cell cancers. On the contrary, stage Ic tumors, that have poorer prognosis, are usually treated as for the other hystotypes.

First-Line Treatment in Advanced Stages: Stages III–IV According to FIGO 2009 Classification

Both the American and European guidelines recommend surgery as the initial approach to ovarian malignancies [1, 39, 53, 54]. The actual treatment of ovarian cancer at an advanced stage (FIGO stages III–IV) is based on the proper integration of surgery and medical approach. The goal of primary surgery, defined as optimal cytoreduction, is the absence of residual cancer. For more than 20 years, tumor debulking surgery followed by platinum/taxane combination chemotherapy has remained the standard first-line treatment. Currently, the first-line treatment of ovarian cancer consists of the combination of carboplatin AUC 5.0–7.5 and paclitaxel 175 mg/m^2 with three-weekly schedule. This choice comes from the results of several trials that demonstrated the superiority of paclitaxel-based chemotherapy regimens and the equal effectiveness of carboplatin compared to those containing cisplatin (GOG111, GOG 114, GOG 158, AGO-OV.2, AGO-OV.104) [47, 52, 55, 60]. The shift from cisplatin to carboplatin was based on safety considerations and easier handling use. As expected, paclitaxel/carboplatin was associated with significantly different toxicity profiles consisting in less nausea, vomiting, and neuropathy, but greater myelosuppression that was overall manageable. Furthermore, the analysis of quality of life, assessed by the EORTC QLQ-C30 questionnaire, demonstrated significantly better scores for the paclitaxel/carboplatin arm when compared with the cisplatin-based treatment. Given the evidence of a more favorable toxicity profile and ease of delivery, the carboplatin/paclitaxel combination has been considered for years the standard of care in epithelial ovarian cancer treatment. However, although the initial response rates are high, most patients (75–80 %) with advanced-stage ovarian cancer relapse within 18 months and eventually die from the disease within a median of 32–57 months.

New strategies have been studied to improve the outcome of this first-line therapy. Moreover, a safety profile of carboplatin and paclitaxel combination, mainly alopecia and neurotoxicity, has prompted researchers to look for new doublets potentially better tolerated and equally or more effective. Several efforts have focused on further intensifying the chemotherapy regimens with the addition of a third or fourth cytotoxic agent; however, attempts in this regard have consistently been disappointing, producing suboptimal responses with no survival advantage and higher toxicities [9, 28]. The SCOTROC1 trial [77] was a Scottish randomized phase III trial, which included more than 1000 women with stage Ic–IV EOC; it compared the carboplatin/docetaxel doublet to the combination of carboplatin and paclitaxel. No efficacy differences were founded between both arms at final analysis. The biggest difference that emerged was related to the toxicity profile of the two treatment regimens. A higher rate of myelosuppression (including complicated grade 3–4 neutropenia) was found with carboplatin/docetaxel, whereas a higher rate of neurotoxicity has been described in patients treated with carboplatin/paclitaxel. According to these data, docetaxel and carboplatin could be considered as a valid alternative to carboplatin/paclitaxel in some selected cases. In the MITO-2 trial [61], carboplatin AUC 5 in combination with pegylated liposomal doxorubicin (PLD) at a dose of 30 mg/m^2 every 3 weeks for six cycles was compared to the standard carboplatin/paclitaxel combination in 820 patients with FIGO stage Ic–IV EOC. Once again the alternative doublet (carboplatin/PLD) failed to show a greater efficacy compared to standard-of-care chemotherapy in terms of PFS, OS, and response rate (PFS, 19 vs. 16.8 months; $p = 0.58$; median OS, 61.6 vs. 53.2 months; $p = 0.32$; response rate, 57 vs. 59 %; $p = 0.76$). Regarding toxicity profile, thrombocytopenia, anemia, stomatitis, and skin toxicity were significantly more frequent in the PLD arm, whereas neuropathy, diarrhea, and hair loss were most frequent in those treated with paclitaxel. These results let us to consider carboplatin/PLD as a reasonable alternative to carboplatin/paclitaxel, particularly in patients who experienced hypersensitivity to paclitaxel, asked to avoid alopecia, or are at risk of peripheral neuropathy.

Dose-dense therapy has been investigated as another alternative to improve first-line efficacy treatment. Literature data show that weekly administration of antineoplastic agents may have potentially enhanced antitumor activity and decreased toxicity due to extended exposure but fairly low concentration of the drugs [43].

Studies in breast cancer demonstrated a greater activity of paclitaxel administered at low doses every week compared to standard three-weekly schedule. This difference was supposed to be also related to an antiangiogenic effect associated to dose-dense administration. These results prompted to the JGOG 3016 trial [33]. This multicentric Japanese phase III study randomized more than 600 women with FIGO stage II–IV EOC to receive weekly paclitaxel (80 mg/m^2, days 1, 8, and 15) in combination with three-weekly carboplatin (AUC6, day 1) or a standard three-weekly regimen into first-line ovarian cancer treatment. The results showed an impressive superiority of the dose-dense paclitaxel and carboplatin regimen in terms of PFS (28.2 vs. 17.5 months; HR, 0.76; 95 % CI, 0.62–0.91; $p = 0.0037$) and OS (100.5 vs. 62.2 months; HR, 0.79; 95 % CI, 0.63–0.99; $p = 0.039$), but with increased toxicity leading to more frequent early discontinuation of treatment in the dose-dense arm (53 vs. 37 %). The role of weekly chemotherapy was further evaluated in a European study, the Multicenter Italian Trials in Ovarian Cancer (MITO-7) randomized trial [62]. In this study, over 800 women with stage Ic to IV EOC were treated with a total of six cycles using carboplatin and paclitaxel on either a standard (every 3 weeks) or on a weekly schedule, with both agents administered on days 1, 8, and 15 every 21 days. At a median follow-up of 22 months, similar PFS (18 versus 17 months; HR, 0.96; 95 % CI, 0.80–1.16) was found in the experimental arm compared with standard treatment, with no statistically overall survival differences between two arms (77 versus 79 % of probability of survival at 24 months, respectively, of HR 1.20 and 95 % CI 0.90–1.61), but a better tolerability profile and quality of life founded in the weekly arm. The MITO-7 trial differs from JGOG 3016 in several aspects. In contrast to the Japanese one, the European trial the total dose of the drugs is similar between the arms, but both carboplatin and paclitaxel are administrated weekly. The most interesting advice that at least emerged from these trials concerns the race of the enrolled population (Asian versus Caucasian), which may explain the discrepancy of results probably related to distinct profiles of response and tolerability, often imputed to genetic polymorphisms involved in drug metabolism and chemosensitivity.

Another smaller European trial did not find a benefit from a regimen including induction therapy with three cycles of dose-dense weekly paclitaxel and weekly platinum over a standard three-weekly regimen [76]. The JGOG 3016 dose-dense regimen was also evaluated in the USA through the GOG 262 phase III trial, where a similar schedule was analyzed but with the optional addition of bevacizumab (at physician choice) [15]. The use of bevacizumab in most patients enrolled (85 %) and in both arms prevents a strict comparison between GOG 262 and JGOG 3016, except in the small subset of patients (15 %) where bevacizumab was not added to chemotherapy. No significant difference in efficacy was found between both arms, with a difference in favor of the dose-dense weekly regimen observed only in patients who did not receive bevacizumab. The limited series of patients in this trial precludes any definitive conclusion. There is currently no data suggesting that the weekly dose-dense regimen is beneficial to non-Japanese women. Thus, the three-weekly carboplatin/paclitaxel regimen remains the standard in Caucasian populations, although we await further data; the ICON8 (https://clinicaltrials.gov/ct2/show/NCT01654146), which is ongoing, is a phase III trial, comparing three possible schedules of paclitaxel/carboplatin combination (three-weekly carboplatin and paclitaxel, three-weekly carboplatin plus weekly paclitaxel, weekly carboplatin and paclitaxel), and might help to definitively clarify the role of dose-dense chemotherapy.

As the majority of clinical recurrences are generally confined to the peritoneal cavity, there is a strong rationale for administering cytotoxic drugs directly into the abdomen (intraperitoneal chemotherapy), thus increasing the dose intensity delivered to any residual tumor while avoiding additional systemic toxicity. Intraperitoneal chemotherapy (IP) is unable to penetrate deeply into tissues so it is only likely to be suitable for patients who have undergone optimal cytoreductive surgery with minimal residual disease.

There have been three large phase III trials comparing intraperitoneal (IP) chemotherapy with IV chemotherapy. In the first study, 654 patients were randomly assigned to receive six cycles of IV cyclophosphamide in combination with either IV or IP cisplatin. The median OS was significantly longer in the IP arm (49 versus 41 months; $p=0.02$; HR, 0.76) [2]. This questionable trial was carried out before the introduction of taxanes; however, it formed the basis for further trials of IP chemotherapy. The second study, GOG 114, incorporated IV paclitaxel in each arm. Patients were randomly assigned to receive either IV paclitaxel 135 mg/m^2 over 24 h followed by IV cisplatin 75 mg/m^2 every 3 weeks for six courses or IV carboplatin (AUC 9) every 28 days for two courses, then IV paclitaxel 135 mg/m^2 over 24 h followed by intraperitoneal cisplatin 100 mg/m^2 every 3 weeks for six courses. In the 462 assessable patients, a substantial improvement in PFS was observed but the difference in OS was not significant ($p=0.05$). Again toxic effects were higher in the experimental arm and 18 % of patients received <2 courses of IP treatment [48]. The use of IP chemotherapy as a viable alternative to intravenous (IV) treatment is supported by European and American guidelines on the basis of a large phase III randomized trial (the GOG172) that randomized 415 among the 429 women with stage III EOC treated with optimal debulking surgery (residual disease ≤1 cm) [3] to receive IV paclitaxel and cisplatin or IV paclitaxel followed by IP cisplatin (d 1) and paclitaxel (d 8). In the experimental arm, the patients received IP cisplatin (100 mg/m^2) on day 1 and IP paclitaxel (60 mg/m^2) on day 8; in the control arm, both cisplatin (75 mg/m^2) and paclitaxel (135 mg/m^2) were administered intravenously on days 1 and 2, respectively, every 3 weeks. The experimental arm showed a significant benefit compared with the control arm in PFS (23.8 versus 18.3 months, $p=0.05$). A significant improvement in OS was also demonstrated, 65.6 vs. 49.7 months, respectively, in the IP arm compared to IV arm ($p=0.03$). It is worth to be mentioned that only 42 % of patients was able to complete six cycles of IP chemotherapy. Grade 3–4 toxicity was greater and quality-of-life scores were significantly worse in the IP arm. The three trials described above all recorded favorable PFS or OS results for the IP arms. Data from the GOG 114 and 172 trials were recently retrospectively analyzed by Tewari and colleagues [74] to determine 10-year long-term survival and prognostic factors linked to IP therapy. After a median follow-up of 10.7 years, the survival benefit for IP chemotherapy was confirmed, with a median survival with IP therapy of 61.8 months (95 % CI, 55.5–69.5), compared with 51.4 months (95 % CI, 46.0–58.2) for intravenous therapy. Factors associated with poorer survival included: clear, mucinous versus serous histology (AHR, 2.79; 95 % CI, 1.83–4.24; $p<.001$), gross residual versus no visible disease (AHR, 1.89; 95 % CI, 1.48–2.43; $p<.001$), and fewer versus more cycles of IP chemotherapy (AHR, 0.88; 95 % CI, 0.83–0.94; $p<.001$). In this setting, also, an interesting field of study is related to tumor genomic alterations. Recently, an analysis of somatic loss of BRCA1 in patients participating in GOG-172 demonstrated a profound effect on overall survival [40]. In this analysis of 393 patients (94 % of GOG-172 participants), somatic loss of BRCA1 was observed in 48 %, and the median overall survival for IP vs. IV therapy was 84 vs. 47 months ($p=.0002$), amounting to a 33 % reduction in the hazard for death.

Despite such encouraging and undoubted findings on the impact of overall survival, IP chemotherapy still raises many concerns among oncologists and has been adopted only in a few countries [10]. The additional toxicity (grade 3–4 pain, fatigue, and hematologic toxicities were significantly more common in the IP cohort), lack of familiarity with placement and use of peritoneal catheters, the worse quality-of-life scores observed in the experimental arms, and concern over the design of trials have hindered its widespread use. In the last months conflicting results from two important phase II [59] and phase III trials (PERTROC-OV21 and the GOG 252 trial) [26] on adjuvant IP treatment in OC patients have been presented at the 2016 Annual Meeting of the Society of Gynecologic Oncology and at the 2016 ASCO Annual Meeting. To further elucidate the role of IP in the treatment of ovarian cancer and better define which patients will truly benefit from this approach, other studies [31] are ongoing, the researchers are also conducting correlative studies on collected tissue samples to determine whether certain biologic characteristics may be associated with improved outcomes using IP versus IV chemotherapy.

Since the majority of patients with EOC achieve a complete clinical remission after surgery and frontline chemotherapy, but ultimately recur the idea of delaying recurrence through a maintenance, the therapy has been investigated. No randomized phase III maintenance or consolidation study has shown a statistically significant improvement in outcome with maintenance chemotherapy. Data from a meta-analysis of six randomized trials ($n = 902$) concluded for the absence of significant improvement in 5-year overall survival for the administration of maintenance chemotherapy (relative risk, 1.07; 95 % CI, 0.91–1.27) [49]. An ongoing study, GOG 212, is further investigating the role of maintenance taxanes. In addition, randomized trials evaluating some therapeutic monoclonal antibodies that directed mucin Ca125 as a maintenance strategy have shown no benefit in either relapse-free or overall survival compared with placebo [7, 67].

Molecular-Targeted Therapies

The addition of biological agents to standard frontline chemotherapy is currently the main topic of research. Angiogenesis represents one of the most promising targets in ovarian cancer [37]. One of the key mediators of angiogenesis is vascular endothelial growth factor (VEGF), a heparin-binding growth factor that selectively promotes proliferation and survival of vascular endothelial cells [41]. VEGF also induces vascular permeability and angiogenesis in a variety of in vivo models [22]. EOC is characterized by high levels of intra-tumoral VEGF [18] that has been shown to significantly affect prognosis compared to tumors with lower VEGF expression [11]. In parallel with these results, there are several studies which report poor survival to be associated with high serum VEGF levels in patients with advanced disease [50, 71].

Bevacizumab is a recombinant humanized monoclonal antibody (IgG1) targeting VEGF-A [65]. Its effects include a direct antiangiogenic activity and additional effects on tumor vasculature, interstitial pressure, and blood vessel permeability, leading to enhanced chemotherapy delivery to tumor cells [32]. Prompted by the encouraging phase II results, two prospective randomized phase III trials, GOG-0218 and ICON7, were initiated to investigate the role of bevacizumab administered in combination with frontline chemotherapy and continued as single-agent maintenance therapy. Both trials have reported that the addition of bevacizumab to carboplatin and paclitaxel, followed by maintenance therapy with the anti-VEGF, significantly prolongs PFS. The double-blind, placebo-controlled randomized phase III GOG-0218 trial included 1873 patients with stage III (incompletely resected) or stage IV (any surgical outcome) epithelial ovarian, primary peritoneal, or fallopian tube cancer [12]. Patients were randomized to receive carboplatin plus paclitaxel for six cycles (arm 1/control), or the same regimen for six cycles plus bevacizumab (15 mg/kg q3w) for five cycles (i.e., concomitantly with chemotherapy, arm 2), or the same chemotherapy for six cycles and bevacizumab (15 mg/kg q3w) for 22 cycles (i.e., concomitant with chemotherapy followed by maintenance, arm 3). The two bevacizumab-containing arms were both compared with the control arm. PFS was the primary endpoint. As expected, at a median follow-up of 17.4 months, a statistically significant improvement in PFS was seen from the addition of bevacizumab concurrently and as maintenance therapy up to overall 15 months of therapy, when compared to chemotherapy alone (10.3 vs. 14.1 months; HR, 0.72; 95 % CI, 0.63–0.83; p <0.001). It is worth of mentioning that the maximum convergence between PFS survival curves was at 15 months, which is the protocol-defined point where bevacizumab therapy was stopped. Subgroup analyses showed that the PFS benefit was maintained in all subgroups evaluated (disease stage, residual disease, histological subtype, tumor grade, age, and performance status). The median OS was 40.6, 38.8, and 43.8 months, respectively, for the control group, the concomitant-only bevacizumab group, and the concomitant and maintenance bevacizumab group [66]. A possible confounding factor, affecting overall survival analysis, is the higher crossover to bevacizumab in subsequent lines (28 % in the control arm vs. 15 % in arm 3). Of note, in the subgroup of patients with stage IV disease, who have a poorer prognosis and thus shorter post-progression survival, an exploratory analysis showed an HR for OS of 0.72 (95 % CI, 0.53–0.97), favoring bevacizumab. The ICON7 trial was a randomized phase III trial that recruited 1528 patients with high-risk early-stage disease or advanced-stage EOC. Patients received conventional carboplatin plus paclitaxel for six cycles or the same treatment plus bevacizumab (7.5 mg/kg q3w) during chemotherapy, with bevacizumab monotherapy continuing for an additional 36 weeks. The results of this open-label trial are consistent with those of GOG 0218, showing an improvement of PFS [58]. At a median follow-up of 28 months, there was only a 1.7 months of difference in the bevacizumab group (HR, 0.81; 95 % CI, 0.70–0.94), PFS was 17.3 months in the control arm and 19.8 months in the bevacizumab arm, with clear evidence of non-proportional hazards ($p<0.001$). Interestingly, once again the maximum separation of the PFS curves occurred at around 12 months, corresponding with the time where bevacizumab was discontinued, but the curves finally converged at 22 months. At the final OS analysis, there was no difference in OS between treatment arms. The HR was 0.99 (95 % CI 0.85–1.14), with median OS of 58.6 months in the chemotherapy-alone group and 58.0 months in the bevacizumab arm [56]. The overall benefit seen in ICON7 was less marked than in the GOG 0218 study due to the inclusion of a large proportion of patients with earlier-stage and lower-risk disease. As the ICON7 trial included patients with early-stage ovarian cancer (18 % of the population stages I and II), a subgroup analysis of PFS was undertaken focusing on patients considered to be at high risk of progression, predefined in this study as FIGO stage III with residual disease >1 cm or stage IV with any surgical debulking. In patients subcategorized as high risk for disease progression, median PFS improved from 10.5 to 15.9 months with addition of bevacizumab (HR, 0.68; 95 % CI, 0.55–0.85; $p < 0.001$) [58]. On the basis of these results, the European Medicines Agency (EMA) in December 2011 approved bevacizumab use in first-line treatment of advanced ovarian cancer (FIGO IIIb–IV) in concomitance with carboplatin/paclitaxel for six cycles followed by bevacizumab at a dose of 15 mg/kg in a three-weekly maintenance schedule for a total of 15 months. This approval was independent of the outcome of initial surgery in terms of residual disease, except that patients with FIGO stage IIIa were excluded from the label. Additionally a recently published final analysis of the ICON7 data revealed 4.8 months of survival advantage (34.5–39.3 months, $p = 0.03$) with bevacizumab compared to standard treatment arm in patients with high-risk features, while no survival improvement was evident in the general study population [56].

In the ICON7, the subgroup analysis was not planned at the time of trial design, but the "high-" and "low-risk" subgroups were subsequently identified, after the presentation of the GOG218 primary analysis. This analysis was a post hoc subgroup analysis and requires prospective validation before being accepted as a definitive result. It is worth to be noted that a relevant proportion (about one third) of patients enrolled in the GOG218 trial had a residual disease after surgery not greater than 1 cm. According to the global result of the GOG218, also these patients can benefit from the addition of bevacizumab to standard chemotherapy, and there was no suggestion of a differential effect in terms of PFS according to residual disease. These findings have been confirmed during the last ASCO meeting [13], where a recent update of the post hoc exploratory analysis of subgroups defined by stage and extent of residual disease at diagnosis was performed for the ICON 7 trial. At a prolonged follow-up, the PFS benefit from bevacizumab observed in the ITT population was seen consistently in all subgroups explored with an HR (95 % CI) of 0.77 (0.59–0.99). These results were obtained irrespective of stage and residual tumor and, therefore, also in patients categorized as having "low-risk" tumor with the absence of any residual disease at the time of primary surgery.

Despite these results, there are still many open questions regarding the use of bevacizumab in EOC. It remains unclear whether patients would benefit from its use as a first-line treatment or whether the maintenance with bevacizumab should be prolonged beyond 15 months. The BOOST trial (ClinicalTrials.gov identifier: NCT01462890) will hopefully address these questions. Several proposals have been done to identify molecular biomarkers able to guide the choice of treatment with bevacizumab in the different diseases where it is approved; to date, none of those proposed have been accepted in clinical practice. At ASCO 2014, Gourley et al. [27] presented the results of a 63-gene expression signature, which was applied to samples from the ICON7. Three major subgroups were identified: two with angiogenic gene upregulation and one with angiogenic gene repression and immune gene upregulation. The assay showed that for patients in the immune molecular subgroup (41 % of cases), the addition of bevacizumab resulted in worse PFS (HR: 1.73; 95 % CI: 1.12–2.68) and OS (HR: 2.0:95 % CI: 1.11–3.61) compared to chemotherapy alone. The hypothesis is that this subgroup having repressed angiogenesis-related gene expression may benefit less from bevacizumab. These results should be validated in additional datasets and laboratories.

Interesting biomarkers are currently under development as predictive factors of response to bevacizumab (e.g., circulating levels of Ang1 and Tie2) [5] and immune versus proangiogenic tumor molecular subgroups [27]. Several ongoing trials, including the MITO16/MANGO-2, are focused on these aspects, which aim to identify which patients could benefit from treatment based on such molecular features.

Over the last decade, a number of new agents have shown evidence of antitumor activity in patients with ovarian carcinoma. Phase III trials have been conducted with oral tyrosine kinase inhibitors with antiangiogenic properties that target VEGF receptors 1, 2, and 3, platelet-derived growth factor receptors (PDGFR), and fibroblast growth factor receptor (FGFR) [8, 24, 38, 44, 45]. Some of those target agents have been evaluated in first-line studies.

Pazopanib is an oral, multikinase inhibitor of VEGFR-1, VEGFR-2, and VEGFR-3, PDGFR-α and PDGFR-ß, and c-Kit. The effectiveness of pazopanib as switch maintenance in ovarian cancer patients was studied in the AGO-OVAR 16, a phase III randomized study [20]. This trial addressed for the first time a solely antiangiogenic maintenance therapy. Patients with stage II–IV disease who had not progressed after first-line chemotherapy were randomized to receive pazopanib (800 mg p.o. once daily or placebo) subsequent to standard for first-line chemotherapy with carboplatin and paclitaxel for up to 24 months. This study met its primary endpoint. A significant improvement in PFS of 5.6 months for patients in the experimental arm was noted (median, 17.9 vs. 12.3 months; HR, 0.77; 95 % CI, 0.64–0.91; $p=0.002$). There were no significant differences between two groups in terms of OS in the second preplanned interim analysis (HR = 1.076, $p=0.4985$). Due to a higher rate of grade 3 and 4 adverse events, mainly hypertension (30.8 %), neutropenia (9.9 %), liver-related toxicity (9.4 %), and diarrhea (8.2 %) reported in the pazopanib arm, about 30 % of patients discontinued treatment. Of note, it seems that pazopanib was more beneficial in terms of PFS in non-Asian patients (HR = 0.69; median PFS benefit, 5.9 months), in which pazopanib exerted a detrimental effect on OS (HR, 1.16).

Encouraging data come from another phase III trial, AGO-OVAR 12/LUME-OVAR-1, that tested the activity as first-line maintenance therapy of another multitarget antiangiogenic agent nintedanib (BIBF 1120). It is an oral intracellular inhibitor that targets multiple receptor tyrosine kinases, including the VEGF, FGFR, and PDGFR. In this randomized phase III trial, a total of 1366 stage IIb–IV ovarian cancer patients were randomized after primary surgery to standard chemotherapy (carboplatin–paclitaxel) with placebo or nintedanib for six cycles and then followed by maintenance therapy with placebo or nintedanib for up to 120 weeks. The primary end point was median PFS that was higher in experimental arm with 16.6 compared to 17.3 months (HR, 0.84; 95 % CI, 0.72–0.98; $p=0.024$), and a greater benefit was observed in the subgroup of "low-risk" patients (stages II–III and optimally debulked) with a median PFS of 20.8 versus 27.1 months (HR = 0.75, 95 % CI = 0.61–0.92, $p=0.005$). Of note, treatment-related toxicity was significantly increased in the nintedanib arm with predominantly hematologic and gastrointestinal AEs (Grad ≥3 22 vs. 2 %) [19]. Although approval of this multikinase inhibitor is currently not expected, AGO-OVAR 12 trial highlighted the importance of tolerability in these phase III trials and of patient selection in structuring clinical trials. Also agents targeting the angiopoietin axis have been developed as antiangiogenic therapy in first-line treatment of EOC. AMG 386 (trebananib), a peptibody inhibiting the interaction of angiopoietin-1 and angiopoietin-2 to the Tie2 receptor, obtained promising results in phase II trials in relapsed setting (TRINOVA 1 trial) that have led to further exploration in the upfront treatment of EOC within the TRINOVA 3 trial. This phase III, double-blind study compares carboplatin/paclitaxel to trebananib in combination with standard chemotherapy followed by a subsequent weekly trebananib maintenance therapy vs. placebo (AGO-OVAR 18, TRINOVA 3). The TRINOVA 3 trial has completed recruitment and is currently under follow-up.

Perspectives

Among the potential "druggable" molecular pathways related to ovarian cancer, one of the most promising is that of homologous recombination repair mechanism (HRD). The rationale for testing agents affecting these pathways in ovarian tumor is the observation that HRD deficiency is present in almost 50 % of high-grade serous EOC, including 20 % of genetic disorders (17 % germline, 3 % somatic) linked to BRCA1 and BRCA2 genes [73]. HRD-deficient tumors are particularly sensitive to platinum-based treatments. PARP family proteins are involved in single-strand DNA break (SSB) repair and indirectly also in DSBs caused by the persistence of SSBs. Therefore, in tumors with HRD-defective pathway, the inactivation of PARP1 enzyme causes cell death. This phenomenon is called "synthetic lethality" [42]. Given their demonstrated activity as single agents in the recurrent setting and based on the toxicity profiles that prevent the combination with chemotherapy, trials are investigating PARP inhibitors as maintenance treatment after chemotherapy rather than in combinations with antineoplastic drugs. Olaparib is the first compound of the anti-PARP class and in 2014 obtained approval for ovarian cancer in relapse both by the EMA and FDA. A phase III registration trial (SOLO 1) is ongoing (ClinicalTrials.gov identifier: NCT01844986) with olaparib as maintenance treatment after first-line chemotherapy in HGSOC with known BRCA germline mutation. Other PARP inhibitors are also under development, namely, niraparib (ClinicalTrials.gov identifier: NCT01847274) and rucaparib (ClinicalTrials.gov identifier: NCT01891344), both of which are currently being tested in platinum-sensitive recurrence and first line. The efficacy of PARP1 in patients with "BRCA-like" or "BRCaness" genetic profiling is also a matter of future research. Encouraging data regarding the synergistic activity of the combination of antiangiogenic drugs and PARP inhibitors in the reccurrent setting prompted the PAOLA1 trial. This is a European Network of Gynaecological Oncology Trial (ENGOT) trial testing in first line the combination of bevacizumab and olaparib in maintenance in patients having responded or with no evidence of disease after a first-line treatment combining chemotherapy and bevacizumab [21].

Future Perspectives

The treatment of ovarian cancer remains challenging despite many advances in therapeutic options. There is still place for investigating better ways of scheduling known drugs and the results of ongoing trials over the next few years will further increase our knowledge about the optimal use of chemotherapy.

Molecular-targeted therapy is moving into earlier phases of treatment. There is need of a greater focus on identifying predictive markers of response to new biological agents.

More tailored therapies based on individual histological and biological characteristics are expected to be developed in the years to come.

References

1. AIOM Linee guida Tumori dell'ovaio. 2015. Available at: http://www.aiom.it.
2. Alberts DS, Liu PY, Hannigan EV, et al. Intraperitoneal cisplatin plus intravenous cyclophosphamide versus intravenous cisplatin plus intravenous cyclophosphamide for stage III ovarian cancer. N Engl J Med. 1996;335:1950–5.
3. Armstrong D, Bundy B, Wenzel L, et al. Intraperitoneal cisplatin and paclitaxel in ovarian cancer. N Engl J Med. 2006;354:34–43. J Clin Oncol. 2006 1;24(28):4531–3.
4. Armstrong DK, Brady MF. Intraperitoneal therapy for ovarian cancer: a treatment ready for prime time. J Clin Oncol. 2006;24(28):4531–3.
5. Backen A, Renehan AG, Clamp AR, et al. The combination of circulating Ang1 and Tie2 levels predicts progression-free survival advantage in bevacizumab-treated patients with ovarian cancer. Clin Cancer Res. 2014;20:4549–58.
6. Bell J, Brady MF, Young RC, et al. Randomized phase III trial of three versus six cycles of adjuvant carboplatin and paclitaxel in early stage epithelial ovarian carcinoma: a gynecologic oncology group study. Gynecol Oncol. 2006;102:432–9.
7. Berek J, Taylor P, McGuire W, et al. Oregovomab maintenance mono immunotherapy does not improve outcomes in advanced ovarian cancer. J Clin Oncol. 2009;27(3):418.
8. Biagi JJ, Oza AM, Chalchal HI, et al. A phase II study of sunitinib in patients with recurrent epithelial ovarian and primary peritoneal carcinoma: an NCIC clinical trials group study. Ann Oncol. 2011;22:335–40.
9. Bookman MA, Brady MF, McGuire WP, et al. Evaluation of new platinum-based treatment regimens in advanced-stage ovarian cancer: a phase III trial of the Gynecologic Cancer Intergroup. J Clin Oncol. 2009;27:1419–25.
10. Bookman MA, Brady MF. Intraperitoneal chemotherapy: long-term outcomes revive a long-running debate. J Clin Oncol. 2015;33:1424–6.
11. Byrne AT, Ross L, Holash J, Nakanishi M, et al. Vascular endothelial growth factor-trap decreases tumor burden, inhibits ascites, and causes dramatic vascular remodeling in an ovarian cancer model. Clin Cancer Res. 2003;9(15):5721–8.
12. Burger RA, Brady MF, Bookman MA, et al. Incorporation of bevacizumab in the primary treatment of ovarian cancer. N Engl J Med. 2011;365:2473–83.
13. Burger IA, Goldman DA, Vargas HA, et al. Incorporation of postoperative CT data into clinical models to predict 5-year overall and recurrence free survival after primary. Cytoreductive surgery for advanced ovarian cancer. Gynecol Oncol. 2015;138:554–910.

14. Chan JK, Tian C, Fleming GF, et al. The potential benefit of 6 vs. 3 cycles of chemotherapy in subsets of women with early-stage high-risk epithelial ovarian cancer: an exploratory analysis of a gynecologic oncology group study. Gynecol Oncol. 2010;116:301.
15. Chan J, Brady MF, Penson R, et al. Phase III trial of every-3-week paclitaxel vs. dose dense weekly paclitaxel with carboplatin +/–bevacizumab in epithelial ovarian, peritoneal, fallopian tube cancer: GOG 262 (NCT01167712). Int J Gynecol Cancer. 2013;23 Suppl 1:9–10.
16. Chiara S, Conte P, Franzone P, et al. High-risk early-stage ovarian cancer. Randomized clinical trial comparing cisplatin plus cyclophosphamide versus whole abdominal radiotherapy. Am J Clin Oncol. 1994;17(1):72.
17. Cho KR, Shih Ie M. Ovarian cancer. Annu Rev Pathol. 2009;4:287–313.53.
18. Cooper BC, Ritchie JM, Broghammer CL, et al. Preoperative serum vascular endothelial growth factor levels: significance in ovarian cancer. Clin Cancer Res. 2002;8(10):3193–7.
19. du Bois A, Kristensen G, Ray-Coquard I, et al. AGO-OVAR 12: a randomized placebo-controlled GCIG/ENGOT-Intergroup phase III trial of standard frontline chemotherapy +/– nintedanib for advanced ovarian cancer. Abstracts from the 18th international meeting of the European Society of Gynaecological Oncology (ESGO), 2013, Liverpool, UK. Int J Gynecol Cancer. 2013;23(8 Suppl 1).
20. du Bois A, Floquet A, Kim JW, et al. Incorporation of pazopanib in maintenance therapy of ovarian cancer. J ClinOncol. 2014;32(30):3374–82. pii: JCO.2014.55.7348.
21. ENGOT ov-25, EudraCT 2014-004027-52.
22. Ferrara N. Vascular endothelial growth factor: basic science and clinical progress. Endocr Rev. 2004;25:581–611.
23. Ferlay J, Soerjomataram I, Ervik M, et al. GLOBOCAN 2012 v1.0, Cancer Incidence and Mortality Worldwide: IARC CancerBase No. 11 [Internet]. Lyon: International Agency for Research on Cancer; 2013.
24. Friedlander M, Hancock KC, Rischin D, et al. A phase II, open-label study evaluating pazopanib in patients with recurrent ovarian cancer. Gynecol Oncol. 2010;119:32–7.
25. Frumovitz M, Schmeler KM, Malpica A, et al. Unmasking the complexities of mucinous ovarian carcinoma. Gynecol Oncol. 2010;117(3):491–6.
26. Walker JL, Brady MF, DiSilvestro PA, et al. A phase III clinical trial of bevacizumab with IV versus IP chemotherapy in ovarian, fallopian tube and primary peritoneal carcinoma NCI-supplied agent(s): bevacizumab (NSC #704865, IND #7921) NCT01167712 a GOG/NRG trial (GOG 252). Presented at: 2016 SGO Annual Meeting. March 19-22, 2016. San Diego, CA. Late-breaking abstract.
27. Gourley C, McCavigan A, Perren T, et al. Molecular subgroup of high-grade serous ovarian cancer (HGSOC) as a predictor of outcome following bevacizumab. J Clin Oncol. 2014;(32 Suppl):abstr 5502.
28. Hoskins PJ. Triple cytotoxic therapy for advanced ovarian cancer: a failed application, not a failed strategy. J Clin Oncol. 2009;27:1355–8.
29. Hreshchyshyn MM, Park RC, Blessing JA, et al. The role of adjuvant therapy in stage I ovarian cancer. Am J Obstet Gynecol. 1980;138(2):139–45.
30. ICON8, ClinicalTrials.gov Identifier: NCT01654146.
31. iPOC, ClinicalTrials. gov identifier: NCT01506856.
32. Jain RK. Normalizing tumor vasculature with anti-angiogenic therapy: a new paradigm for combination therapy. Nat Med. 2001;7(9):987–9.
33. Katsumata N, Yasuda M, Isonishi S, et al. Long-term results of dose-dense paclitaxel and carboplatin versus conventional paclitaxel and carboplatin for treatment of advanced epithelial ovarian, fallopian tube, or primary peritoneal cancer (JGOG 3016): a randomized, controlled, open-label trial. Lancet Oncol. 2013;14:1020–6.
34. Kurman RJ, Shih Ie M. The origin and pathogenesis of epithelial ovarian cancer: a proposed unifying theory. Am J Surg Pathol. 2010;34(3):433–43.
35. Kurman RJ, Shih Ie M. Molecular pathogenesis and extraovarian origin of epithelial ovarian cancer–shifting the paradigm. Hum Pathol. 2011;42(7):918–31.
36. Lawrie TA, Winter-Roach BA, Heus P, Kitchener HC. Adjuvant (post-surgery) chemotherapy for early stage epithelial ovarian cancer. Cochrane Database Syst Rev. 2015;(12):CD004706.

37. Ledermann JA, Marth C, Carey, et al. Gynecologic Cancer InterGroup. Role of molecular agents and targeted therapy in clinical trials for women with ovarian cancer. Int J Gynecol Cancer. 2011;21:763–70.
38. Ledermann JA, Hackshaw A, Kaye S, et al. Randomized phase II placebo controlled trial of maintenance therapy using the oral triple angiokinase inhibitor BIBF 1120 after chemotherapy for relapsed ovarian cancer. J Clin Oncol. 2011;29:3798–804.
39. Ledermann JA, Raja FA ,Fotopoulou C, et al. On behalf of the ESMO guidelines working group. Newly diagnosed and relapsed epithelial ovarian carcinoma: ESMO clinical practice guidelines for diagnosis, treatment and follow-up. Ann Oncol. 2013;24(Suppl 6):vi24–32.
40. Lesnock JL, Darcy KM, Tian C, et al. BRCA1 expression and improved survival in ovarian cancer patients treated with intraperitoneal cisplatin and paclitaxel: a Gynecologic Oncology Group Study. Br J Cancer. 2013;108:1231–7.
41. Leung DW, Cachianes G, Kuang WJ, et al. Vascular endothelial growth factor is a secreted angiogenic mitogen. Science. 1989;246:1306–9.
42. Liu JF, Konstantinopoulos PA, Matulonis UA. Olaparib maintenance therapy in platinum-sensitive relapsed ovarian cancer. Gynecol Oncol. 2014;133(2):362–9.
43. Lopes NM, Adams EG, Pitts TW, Bhuyan BK. Cell kill kinetics and cell cycle effects of taxol on human and hamster ovarian cell lines. Cancer Chemother Pharmacol. 1993;32: 235–42.
44. Matei D, Sill MW, Lankes HA, et al. Activity of sorafenib in recurrent ovarian cancer and primary peritoneal carcinomatosis: a gynecologic oncology group trial. J Clin Oncol. 2011;29:69–75.
45. Matulonis UA, Berlin S, Ivy P, et al. Cediranib, an oral inhibitor of vascular endothelial growth factor receptor kinases, is an active drug in recurrent epithelial ovarian, fallopian tube, and peritoneal cancer. J Clin Oncol. 2009;27:5601–6.
46. McCluggage WG. Morphological subtypes of ovarian carcinoma: a review with emphasis on new developments and pathogenesis. Pathology. 2011;43(5):420–32.
47. McGuire WP, Hoskins WJ, Brady MF, et al. Cyclophosphamide and cisplatin compared with paclitaxel and cisplatin in patients with stage III and stage IV ovarian cancer. N Engl J Med. 1996;334:1–6.
48. McGuire WP. Intraperitoneal therapy for ovarian cancer. J Clin Oncol. 2001;19:921–3.
49. Mei L, Chen H, Wei DM, et al. Maintenance chemotherapy for ovarian cancer. Cochrane Database Syst Rev. 2010;(9):CD007414.
50. Mesiano S, Ferrara N, Jaffe RB, et al. Role of vascular endothelial growth factor in ovarian cancer: inhibition of ascites formation by immunoneutralization. Am J Pathol. 1998;153(4): 1249–56.
51. NCIC-OV21 trial ClinicalTrials.gov Identifier: NCT00993655.
52. Neijit JP, Engelholm SA, Tuxen MK, et al. Exploratory phase III study of paclitaxel and cisplatin versus paclitaxel and carboplatin in advanced ovarian cancer. J Clin Oncol. 2000;18:3084–92. 7.
53. NICE clinical guideline. Ovarian cancer – the recognition and initial management of ovarian cancer. 2011. Available online: http://nice.org.uk/guidance.
54. Ovarian cancer including fallopian tube cancer and primary peritoneal cancer. NCCN clinical practice guidelines in oncology (v.2.2015) . Available online at: http://www.nccn.com.
55. Ozols RF, Bundy BN, Greer BE, Fowler JM, et al. Phase III trial of carboplatin and paclitaxel compared with cisplatin and paclitaxel in patients with optimally resected stage III ovarian cancer: a Gynecologic Oncology Group study. J Clin Oncol. 2003;21(17): 3194–200.
56. Oza AM, Cook AD, Pfisterer J, Embleton A, et al. Standard chemotherapy with or without bevacizumab for women with newly diagnosed ovarian cancer (ICON7): overall survival results of a phase 3 randomised trial. Lancet Oncol. 2015;16(8):928–36.
57. Pectasides D, Pectasides E, Psyrri A, et al. Treatment issues in clear cell carcinoma of the ovary: a different entity? Oncologist. 2006;11:1089–94.

58. Perren TJ, Swart AM, Pfisterer J, Ledermann JA, Pujade-Lauraine E, Kristensen G, et al. ICON7 Investigators, 2011. A phase 3 trial of bevacizumab in ovarian cancer. N Engl J Med. 2011;365:2484–96.
59. Mackay H, Gallagher CJ,Parulekar W R,et al. OV21/PETROC: A randomized Gynecologic Cancer Intergroup (GCIG) phase II study of intraperitoneal (IP) versus intravenous (IV) chemotherapy following neoadjuvant chemotherapy and optimal debulking surgery in epithelial ovarian cancer (EOC). J Clin Oncol 34, 2016 (suppl; abstr LBA5503).
60. Piccart MJ, Bertelsen K, James K, et al. Randomized Intergroup Trial of cisplatin-paclitaxel versus cisplatin-cyclophosphamide in women with advanced epithelial ovarian cancer: three-year results. J Natl Cancer Inst. 2000;92:699–708.6.
61. Pignata S, Scambia G, Ferrandina G, et al. Carboplatin plus paclitaxel versus carboplatin plus pegylated liposomal doxorubicin as first-line treatment for patients with ovarian cancer: the MITO-2 randomized phase III trial. J Clin Oncol. 2011;29:3628–35.
62. Pignata S, Scambia G, Katsaros D, et al. Carboplatin plus paclitaxel once a week versus every 3 weeks in patients with advanced ovarian cancer (MITO-7): a randomised, multicentre, open-label, phase 3 trial. Lancet Oncol. 2014;15:396–405.
63. Prat J. New insight into ovarian cancer pathology. Ann Oncol. 2012;23(10):111–7.
64. Prat J for the FIGO committee on gynecologic oncology. Staging classification for the cancer of the ovary, fallopian tube, and peritoneum. Int J Gynaecol Obstet. 2014;124(1):1–5.
65. Presta LG, Chen H, O'Connor SJ, et al. Humanization of an anti-vascular endothelial growth factor monoclonal antibody for the therapy of solid tumors and other disorders. Cancer Res. 1997;57(20):4593–9.
66. Randall L, Burger R, Nguyen H, et al. Outcome differences in patients with advanced epithelial ovarian, primary peritoneal and fallopian tube cancers treated with and without bevacizumab. Gynecol Oncol. 2013;130:e33 (abstract 80).
67. Sabbatini P, Harter P, Scambia G, et al. Abagovomab as maintenance therapy in patients with epithelial ovarian cancer: a phase III trial of the AGO OVAR, COGI, GINECO, and GEICO-the MIMOSA study. J Clin Oncol. 2013;31(12):1554.
68. Schmeler KM, Gershenson DM. Low-grade serous ovarian cancer: a unique disease. Curr Oncol Rep. 2008;10:519–23.
69. Shih Ie M, Kurman RJ. Ovarian tumorigenesis: a proposed model based on morphological and molecular genetic analysis. Am J Pathol. 2004;164(5):1511–8.
70. Sigurdsson K, Johnsson JE, Tropé C. Carcinoma of the ovary, stages I and II. A prospective randomized study of the effects of postoperative chemotherapy and radiotherapy. Ann Chir Gynaecol. 1982;71(6):321–9.
71. Spannuth WA, Sood AK, Coleman RL. Angiogenesis as a strategic target for ovarian cancer therapy. Nat Clin Pract Oncol. 2008;5(4):194–204.
72. Swart AC, on behalf of ICON collaborators. Long-term follow-up of women enrolled in a randomized trial of adjuvant chemotherapy for early stage ovarian cancer (ICON1). J Clin Oncol. 2007;25 abstr 5509.
73. The cancer genome atlas research network. Integrated genomic analysis of ovarian carcinoma. Nature. 2011;474(7353):609–15.
74. Tewari D, Java JJ, Salani R, et al. Long-term survival advantage and prognostic factors associated with intraperitoneal chemotherapy treatment in advanced ovarian cancer. J Clin Oncol. 2015;33:1460–6.
75. Trimbos JB, Parmar M, Vergote I, et al. International Collaborative Ovarian Neoplasm trial 1 and Adjuvant ChemoTherapy In Ovarian Neoplasm trial: two parallel randomized phase III trials of adjuvant chemotherapy in patients with early-stage ovarian carcinoma. J Natl Cancer Inst. 2003;95(2):105–12.
76. Van Der Burg ME, Onstenk W, Boere IA, et al. Long-term results of a randomized phase III trial of weekly versus three-weekly paclitaxel/platinum induction therapy followed by standard or extended three-weekly paclitaxel/platinum in European patients with advanced epithelial ovarian cancer. Eur J Cancer. 2014;50:2592–601.

77. Vasey PA, Jayson GC, Gordon A, et al. Phase III randomized trial of docetaxel-carboplatin versus paclitaxel-carboplatin as first-line chemotherapy for ovarian carcinoma. J Natl Cancer Inst. 2004;96(22):1682–91.
78. Vergote I, De Brabanter J, Fyles A, et al. Prognostic importance of degree of differentiation and cyst rupture in stage I invasive epithelial ovarian carcinoma. Lancet. 2001;357(9251): 176–82.
79. Winter-Roach BA, Kitchener HC, Lawrie TA, et al. Adjuvant (post-surgery) chemotherapy for early stage epithelial ovarian cancer. Cochrane Database Syst Rev. 2001;357(9251):176–82.

Ovarian Cancer in the Elderly

9

C. Falandry

Abstract

Elderly patients represent an increasing proportion of ovarian cancer patients. While prognosis has improved in younger patients with treatment standardisation and new treatment strategies, age stays a strong predictor of poor survival in elderly patients and major heterogeneity in practices. This review summarises current evidence, proposed treatment guidelines and future challenges for elderly ovarian cancer patients. It highlights the need for prospective specific data integrating assessment of geriatric covariates and patient-centred outcomes.

Introduction

Management of advanced ovarian cancer has been progressively standardised during last decades, as the association of an extensive debulking surgical step and adjuvant chemotherapy allowed overall survival rates to improve, with the median survival exceeding 35 months [1]. Nevertheless the reported overall survival of elderly patients, in population-based studies or even in randomised trials, is largely worse. These differences may be sometimes explained simply by a suboptimal management but also by excessive toxicities, leading to dose limitations or treatment stoppage. In this context, standard treatment feasibility needed to be explored in elderly-specific populations and specific conclusions to be

C. Falandry
Geriatrics Unit, Lyon University Hospital, Lyon University,
Pierre Benite, Lyon, France
e-mail: Claire.falandry@chu-lyon.fr

E. Pujade-Lauraine et al. (eds.), *Ovarian Cancers*,
DOI 10.1007/978-3-319-32110-3_9

drawn. An extensive effort has already been made, in order to explore both surgical and chemotherapic management in elderly populations. Nevertheless, highly variable populations have been depicted, starting with age definition (from over 60 to over 75 and even 80).

Tumour Characteristics

Demographics

Ovarian cancer is the leading cause of death from gynaecological cancer in the Western world [2]. Incidence and mortality increase with age, with incidence peaking between 75 and 79 and mortality between 80 and 84. About half of the cases appear in women over the age of 65 years [3]. Age has been long recognised as an independent prognostic factor for ovarian cancer [4, 5], and differences in survival rates have increased with treatment and management improvements [6–8].

Histopathologic Features

Advanced stages, i.e. FIGO stages III or IV, represent the majority of the cases of ovarian cancer and even more in the elderly population [9, 10]. This can be explained by an asymptomatic disease at early stages and a delay in clinic examinations. Histo-prognostic features of ovarian cancer in the elderly subject are generally worse than in their younger counterparts: more advanced stages, mixed histology, and less differentiated tumours. High-grade serous carcinomas (HGSC) account for 70 % of them. On the contrary, low-grade serous carcinomas are rare in the elderly, frequently associated with a serous borderline tumour or corresponding to a recurrent lesion after a diagnosis of borderline tumour. Clear cell carcinomas usually occur at a younger age than HGSC but may be seen in 10 % of the cases in elderly patients. Their prognosis at an advanced stage is worst than HGSC.

As ovarian cancer diagnosis is based on a histopathological examination, the question may frequently rise in the elderly, of whether a surgical exploration is needed, in order to provide sufficient material. In vulnerable patients for whom a laparoscopic exploration is contraindicated, a percutaneous peritoneal fine-needle biopsy or even cytology of ascites may help in making the diagnosis of malignancy with a good accuracy (60 % sensitivity, 100 % specificity). An association of a radiologic pelvic mass, a compatible cytology and a CA125/CEA ratio (cancer antigen 125/carcinoembryonic antigen) over 25 is usually accepted for the diagnosis of an epithelial ovarian cancer [11]. However, cytology alone is not able to distinguish between different subtypes of carcinomas.

A Worse Outcome with Different Origins

Age is an independent pejorative prognostic factor for survival [4, 5], and this difference has tended to worsen with time and technique improvement [6–8], which highlights the impact of age on treatment decisions, often considered as suboptimal.

The main improvements in the last five decades in ovarian cancer management can be summarised as a surgical step – seeking to achieve the smallest tumour residue – and development of platinum-based poly-chemotherapy. The current accepted standard of care for patients newly diagnosed with advanced stage ovarian cancer is optimal surgical debulking (i.e. no macroscopic residual disease) performed either upfront or in a delayed fashion by a trained gynaecologic oncologist [12, 13] and six cycles of platinum-taxane-based chemotherapy given either in adjuvant or neoadjuvant setting. Both surgery and chemotherapy outcomes have been studied in an elderly population. In both cases, some contradictions arise when comparing trial results – usually promoting standard treatments – and real-time practice, as it has been analysed from the SEER (Surveillance, Epidemiology and End Results) programme data and a study from the German AGO (Arbeitsgemeinschaft Gynaekologische Onkologie) collaborative group on "non-enrolled" patients.

This contradiction between theoretical standards, considered as feasible in selected elderly patients and real practice, illustrates the necessity, commonly accepted in geriatric oncology, to adapt the treatment plan based on a geriatric assessment. However, this necessity encounters three major difficulties:

First, and as in many oncogeriatric fields, elderly patients are either excluded from trials or selected within restrictive inclusion criteria favouring biased results and conclusions and also justifying some hesitations in applying standard treatments to vulnerable cancer patients. Indeed, in a SWOG (Southwest Oncology Group) retrospective analysis of 16,396 patients enrolled in 164 trials during the 1990s, increasing age appeared to be a limitation to trial enrolment [14]. In ovarian cancer, patients older than 65 years accounted for 30 % of trial-included patients while representing more than 48 % of the overall population of patients. In a survey from the US Food and Drug Administration comparing patients enrolled into registration trials for new drugs to SEER cancer demographics, only 9 % of cancer patients older than 75 years were included in clinical trials, while representing 31 % of the overall ovarian cancer patients [15].

Second, clinical trial including elderly patients rarely integrates a geriatric assessment, leading to a restriction of inclusions due to either restrictive inclusion criteria or self-restriction upon the "clinical look" of the investigators. Factors interfering with elderly patients' inclusion into clinical trials have been extensively reviewed and include physician's perceptions, fear of time consumption, restrictive inclusion criteria notably on comorbid conditions or functional status or lack of social support [16, 17]. The "unenrolled" cohort of ovarian cancer patients of AGO were older than their "enrolled" counterparts (mean age 66.7

versus 57.2 years), and cancer management differed mainly on surgical debulking [18].

Lastly, specific trials on elderly patients are often small and non-comparative phase II trials and suffer from the heterogeneity of the geriatric covariates explored. In this context, results are often noncomparable, and guidelines may be difficult to elaborate.

Should Ovarian Cancer in the Elderly Be Considered a Specific Entity?

A Topic Gaining an Increasing Interest

The Research Area

Historically, first elderly-specific data in ovarian cancer have been retrospective cohorts on surgical or chemotherapeutic management, subgroup analyses of randomised trials or epidemiologic data. Since the end of last century, collaborative groups have developed prospective trials: the GINECO (Groupe d'investigateurs Nationaux pour l'Etude des Cancers de l'Ovaire et du sein) with the EWOT (Elderly Woman with Ovarian cancer Trials) programme and the MITO (Multicentre Italian Trial in Ovarian cancer) with MITO-5 study. During the plenary session of the 4th Ovarian Cancer Consensus Conference of the GCIG in 2011, the delegates reached the consensus that additional research involving elderly patients with ovarian cancer was imperative [19]. Recommendations for the design of future clinical trials were proposed:

1. Collaborative groups should promote the inclusion of elderly patients in prospective trials by suppressing the upper age limit in the eligibility criteria, thus avoiding excessive exclusion and reducing selection bias.
2. In randomised trials, elderly patients should be better identified and evaluated, using parameters from the geriatric assessment and a priori planned predictive/prognostic analyses after stratification by age.
3. Specific trials devoted to elderly patients are important because patients excluded from randomised trials have different characteristics and a poorer prognosis from those who are included, despite frequently receiving the same treatment (control arm). In addition, the so-called standard treatments recommended in younger counterparts should be specifically evaluated in elderly patients presenting with criteria of vulnerability (significant comorbidity, lack of autonomy, malnutrition or cognitive disorder). In this context, comprehensive geriatric assessment parameters would help investigators discriminate patients at higher risk of toxicity and/or lower clinical benefit due to a reduced life expectancy. Pharmacokinetic and other biological studies should be encouraged because specificities of elderly subjects regarding these parameters are still unknown.

Clinical Guidelines

In 2012, the Nice/Saint Paul de Vence 2012 clinical guidelines on ovarian cancer proposed specific recommendations for elderly patients [22]. These French national guidelines are translated in this review (paragraphs 4.3 for surgery and 6.4 for chemotherapy). In 2015, NCCN (National Comprehensive Cancer Network) included in its version 2.2015 the following updates for the clinical practice guidelines for ovarian cancer [23]:

"For the 2015 update, the NCCN panel added the weekly carboplatin/paclitaxel regimen and suggests considering the weekly regimen for elderly patients or those with poor PS based on the phase III MITO-7 trial. Note the carboplatin may also be used for neoadjuvant chemotherapy".

"OV-B3 of 3 – the following intravenous regimen and footnote were added":

- Paclitaxel 60 mg/m^2 IV over 1 h plus carboplatin AUC2 IV over 30 min weekly for 18 weeks (category 1).
- Footnote "5": "This regimen may be considered for elderly patients or those with poor performance status".

In addition, the following general assumption was added:

"For elderly patients (>age 65) and/or those with comorbidities:

Elderly patients and those with comorbidities may be intolerant to the combination chemotherapy regimens recommended in these NCCN Guidelines. Single-agent platinum agents may be appropriate in selected patients. Algorithms have been developed for predicting chemotherapy toxicity (seen NCCN Guidelines for Older Adult Oncology)".

To our knowledge, neither British NICE guidelines [20], German AGO (Arbeitsgemeinschaft Gynaekologische Onkologie) [21] nor other learned society mentioned specific recommendations for elderly patients.

Is a Geriatric Assessment Needed? For Which Purpose?

A comprehensive geriatric assessment has been for long recommended in elderly patients (more than 70) when considering any cancer treatment [24], as such a procedure increases global knowledge on the patient [25]. More recently, a screening procedure has been proposed, in order to exclude "fit" patients, with a weak risk of geriatric problems, from an automatic geriatric assessment. The tools used for such a screening are diverse, G8 being currently considered as the best compromise for its sensitivity and specificity thresholds ([26], Table 9.1). A G8 $\leq$ 14/17 implies the necessity for a comprehensive geriatric assessment and a geriatric intervention plan [27]. In the context of surgery, a specific assessment tool was developed (PACE = Preoperative Assessment of Cancer in the Elderly) which combines a pre-anaesthesia assessment tool (ASA), a comprehensive geriatric assessment, a screening of comorbidities (Satariano index) and a Brief Fatigue Inventory (BFI). This tool was able to identify a subgroup of patients with a high risk of 30 days morbi-mortality and long hospitalisation stay (see Sect. 4.2).

Table 9.1 The G8 questionnaire

	Items	Possible responses (score)
A	Has food intake declined over the past 3 months due to loss of appetite, digestive problems, chewing or swallowing difficulties?	0 = severe decrease in food intake
		1 = moderate decrease in food intake
		2 = no decrease in food intake
B	Weight loss during the last 3 months?	0 = weight loss >3 kg
		1 = does not know
		2 = weight loss between 1 and 3 kg
		3 = no weight loss
C	Mobility?	0 = bed or chair bound
		1 = able to get out of bed/chair but does not go out
		2 = goes out
E	Neuropsychological problems?	0 = severe dementia or depression
		1 = mild dementia
		2 = no psychological problems
F	BMI? (weight in kg)/(height in m^2)	0 = BMI <19
		1 = BMI 19 to <21
		2 = BMI 21 to <23
		3 = BMI ≥23
H	Takes more than three prescription drugs per day?	0 = yes
		1 = no
P	In comparison with other people of the same age, how does the patient consider his/her health status?	0.0 = not as good
		0.5 = does not know
		1.0 = as good
		2.0 = better
	Age	0: >85
		1: 80–85
		2: <80
	Total Score	**0–17**

Adapted from Bellera et al. *Ann Oncol* 2012

Surgical Strategies

Historical Controversies

Elderly ovarian cancer patients often undergo less radical surgery than their younger counterparts, even with equivalent comorbidities [29]. While maximum debulking surgery remains, during the platinum era, one of the most powerful determinants of survival in advanced ovarian cancer [30], the rate of complete surgery decreases with age [31]. In addition to age itself, reduced debulking contributes to the poorer outcome in elderly patients [31].

Nevertheless, according to many published series, age itself should not interfere with optimal surgical management. For some authors, in optimal surgical conditions, maximal debulking rates are not decreased with age [29, 32–34]. In a retrospective cohort published by Bruchim et al. comparing management of 46 patients 70 years or older to 143 younger patients, only 54.3 % of elderly patients had primary debulking surgical interventions compared to 84.5 % of the younger group ($p=0.001$), but age was not a limiting factor for optimal debulking in patients who underwent surgery (53 % vs. 54 % in old versus young groups) [33]. The same conclusions were drawn by Uyar et al. in a multi-institutional review of ovarian cancer management (131 elderly patients ≥70 years) and Wright et al. in a retrospective series (129 younger patients <70 and 46 ≥ 70) [29, 32]. In both studies, age had no impact on postoperative complication rates, and Wright found that younger and older groups had the same duration of hospital stay and survival [32]. For both Bruchim and Uyar studies, age had a significant impact on platinum-based chemotherapy with higher rates of treatment-related toxicities (mainly haematological), dose reductions and treatment delays in the older group [29, 33]. Such non-significant differences between elderly and non-elderly patients' outcomes after surgery can be explained by significant improvements in surgical techniques and perioperative intensive care during the 1980s that yielded to a decrease in perioperative mortality from 8.9 % to 3.2 % in pre-planned surgical conditions [35].

However, other series suggest a pejorative impact of age on both postoperative outcomes and quality of resection. As suggested by a GOG (Gynecologic Oncology Group) retrospective analysis of six clinical trials, even in standardised surgical procedures and on relatively selected patients, advancing age is associated with larger volumes of residual disease [5]. In a retrospective study on patients older than 80 years, debulking surgery induced a 38 % risk of major postoperative morbidity and 11 % of death or prolonged hospitalisation, but most of them were discharged to home and were able to receive postoperative chemotherapy [36]. Moreover, optimal debulking of less than 1 cm had a major impact on overall survival (32.5 months versus 3.5 months) but was achieved in only 25 % of the patients despite aggressive surgical effort. In another retrospective study (2001–2006) on 85 octogenarians patients, 86 % presented with advanced disease, 80 % had cytoreductive surgery and 74 % were left with <1 cm residual disease. But death prior to hospital discharge and within 60 days of surgery occurred in, respectively, 13 % and 20 % of patients. Among patients who underwent surgery, 13 % were unable to receive planned adjuvant therapy, 22 % were treated with single-agent platinum and 37 % completed less than three cycles of chemotherapy. This led the authors to conclude that patients over 80 years may not tolerate combination surgery and chemotherapy and that the high proportion of postoperative complications and deaths argues for a more prudent approach to management in this group of patients [37]. Similar conclusions can be driven from a population-based cohort performed during the 1990–2000 time period. Short-term outcomes of 168 octogenarians were compared to those of 2249 younger patients. Octogenarian patients were significantly more likely to have a longer hospital stay (median 10 days vs. 7 days, $p<0.0001$) and a 2.3-fold higher 30-day mortality rate (5.4 % vs. 2.4 %, $p=0.036$) [38].

More globally and according to the SEER cancer statistic reviews, age remains the most predictive factor for suboptimal surgical management. Optimal surgical procedures were performed in 43.7 % of patients <60, 29.5 % between 60 and 79 years and 21.7 % ≥80 years between 1973 and 1999 [3]. Similar rates (21 % and 40 %, respectively) have been observed in two successive phase II trials from the French GINECO group, designed for analysing the feasibility of two chemotherapy regimens, the first from 1998 to 2000 and the second from 2000 to 2003 [39, 40]. Reasons for this suboptimal surgical treatment include fear of more advanced cancers at time of diagnosis, presence of comorbidities and some nonmedical factors such as socio-economic or racial origins [41, 42]. Elderly people also are more often cared for by nononcologists such as general surgeons and obstetricians/gynaecologists [43] or in emergency conditions [38] for cancer complications (occlusion, perforation, infection) and are less likely to undergo surgery at a university hospital [38].

According to 1995–2005 SEER database, among the 5475 women aged 65 and older who had primary debulking surgery for stage III or IV epithelial ovarian cancer, the overall 30-day mortality was 8.2 %, 5.6 % for those admitted electively and 20.1 % for those admitted emergently. Risk factors among patients admitted electively were advancing age, increasing stage and comorbidities. A subgroup of patients at high risk of 30-day mortality (12.7 % [95 % CI 10.7–14.9 %]) was identified and included patients aged 75 or older with either a stage IV disease or a stage III disease and a comorbidity score of 1 or more [44].

Finally, Jorgensen published in 2012 the results of a vast nationwide database evaluating the clinicians' behaviours when facing ovarian cancer in the elderly in Denmark. During the 2005–2006 time period, patients aged 70 and older were 348 and represented 36.2 % of the whole population of patients. Age ≥ 70 was independently predictive of not receiving surgery (OR 0.2 [95 % CI 0.1–0.5]), not receiving a carboplatin–paclitaxel standard treatment (OR 0.03 [95 % CI 0.01–0.1]) and poorer PFS and OS. However, this unfavourable impact of age on outcomes ceased after 16 months. In addition, comorbidity was also independently predictive of both not receiving surgery (OR 0.2 [95 % CI 0.1–0.5]) and not receiving standard chemotherapy (OR 0.03 [95 % CI 0.01–0.1]).

These controversial results after surgery and the surgeons' frequent reluctance to undertake maximal cytoreductive surgery in vulnerable elderly patients led some teams to consider other management strategies, including secondary surgery (see Chap. 6).

Impact of Geriatric Parameters on Surgical Outcomes

In the context of high perioperative morbidity and mortality risks, another challenging question is the place of preoperative assessment. The elderly population should not be considered as a uniform but as a highly heterogeneous population, in which medical and functional assessments play a central role.

In the large field of surgical management of elderly patients, because of higher risks of postoperative morbi-mortality and longer hospital stays, some authors have considered the need for specific preoperative geriatric assessment tools. Some retrospective analyses have identified some covariates of interest, and low serum albumin levels before surgery are significantly associated with suboptimal cytoreduction in univariate and with death in multivariate analyses, along with increasing age [45]. Comorbidities also impact on perioperative morbidity and mortality, as well as the specialty of the surgeon who undertakes the surgery [38].

Since usually used preoperative assessments are not validated in geriatric cancer populations [46], Audisio et al. developed PACE (Preoperative Assessment of Cancer in the Elderly), a specific screening assessment [47] combining indices from geriatric and anaesthesia fields (a screening tool called CGA for "Comprehensive Geriatric Assessment", the BFI or Brief Fatigue Index and ASA and Satariano indices). Its validation included 389 older patients, although inclusion was restricted to patients having a MMS score ≥ 18 for ethical reasons, rendering it difficult to extend to mild to moderate cognition deficits. Some components of this mixed screening tool were predictive of 30-day morbidity and mortality and length of hospital postoperative stay – IADL (instrumental activities of daily living) score < 8, PS (performance status) > 1 and moderate to severe fatigue (BFI) score (>3) – yielding the authors to conclude that this screening tool should be used for future studies.

More recently, two articles explored the correlation between frailty screening tools and gynaecological cancer surgery outcomes in the elderly. Frailty is considered as a major topic in geriatrics, defined consensually as "a state of increased vulnerability to poor resolution of homeostasis after a stressor event, which increases the risk of adverse outcomes", but a matter of debate considering its outlines. A first theory interprets frailty as a multidomain phenotype due to the accumulation of deficits and/or comorbidities. This view favours an extensive comprehensive geriatric assessment and was evaluated using the modified Frailty Index (mFI) developed by George et al. The mFI correlates with morbi-mortality after a gynaecological cancer surgery [48]. A second theory – called the phenotypic theory – interprets frailty as a special entity, closely linked to sarcopenia and denutrition [49]. According to this theory, some functional markers as the gait speed, fatigue and weight loss are more significant markers. Such a view was favoured by Cesari et al., who demonstrated that Short Physical Performance Battery (SPPB), usual gait speed (UGS) and instrumental activities of daily living (IADL) score are the best predictors of elderly patients operated for gynaecological cancers [50].

What Is it Recommended by Clinical Guidelines?

In their 2012 session, Nice/Saint Paul de Vence practical guidelines on ovarian cancer have proposed the following recommendations:

- Whatever the patient's age, the quality of cytoreductive surgery is a major prognostic factor *Level 1, Grade A.*
- Its objective should be radical (R0).
- The surgical environment is fundamental. Its impact on perioperative morbidity and mortality increases with age *Level 2, Grade B.*
- It should imply:
  - A trained surgeon
  - A reference centre
  - A scheduled surgery
- Nevertheless surgery should be used with caution:
  - Age has a major impact on perioperative morbi-mortality.
  - The likelihood of R0 resection decreases with age.
  - It can jeopardise the execution of subsequent chemotherapy *Level 2.*
- Preoperative rehabilitation (prehabilitation) comprises:
  - Preoperative geriatric assessment
  - Preoperative nutrition (ESPEN guidelines)
  - Preoperative immunonutrition in all cases
  - Enteral nutrition 10–14 days before the procedure if severe malnutrition *Level 1, Grade A.*
- The intraoperative assessment is an important aid for decision and prognostic evaluation.
  - First laparoscopic *Professional agreement*
- The objective of the FA of the support is to adapt the sequence surgery/chemotherapy to the patient, avoiding the overtreatment but especially the under-treatment. *Professional agreement*
- Some surgical procedures are to avoid:
  - Simple exploratory laparotomy
  - Extended resections
  - Digestive stomias

The Neoadjuvant Era

Controversial results on surgery patients and frequent reluctance of surgeons to perform cytoreductive surgery in vulnerable patients led some teams to discuss, specifically in the elderly population, the neoadjuvant approach. Non-elderly-specific trials evaluated the place of a secondary cytoreduction after either a non-maximal primary surgery (EORTC 55865 trial, [51]) or after a maximal primary debulking effort [52]. According to the EORTC 55971-NCIC trial, interval debulking surgery does not seem to worsen prognosis compared to primary debulking surgery and yields lower complications rates [53]. Although elderly people represented only a minority of those included in these trials, it is tempting to consider this treatment as an alternative for vulnerable elderly patients with high initial tumour burden [54, 55]. According to retrospective data, neoadjuvant chemotherapy is more systematic after 70 years (43.3 % versus 13.4 %, $p<0.001$) [33]. It allows a decrease in postoperative complications but also chemo-induced toxicities [56].

Chemotherapic Strategies

Historical Controversies

As with surgical management, some differences appear in the literature between dogma and real practice. During the first randomised trials of the platinum era, elderly people were either excluded or selected on restrictive inclusion criteria. Nevertheless, some subgroup analyses were published, concluding that the chemotherapy protocols have similar risk benefit ratios [57], with perhaps slightly increased hematotoxicity but decreased gastrointestinal secondary events, better quality of life during chemotherapy [58] and the same efficacy [59, 60]. In a subgroup analysis of the AGO-OVAR3 trial which recruited 103 patients over 70 years (median age: 73), there was no difference between elderly and younger patients in terms of paclitaxel, carboplatin or cisplatin dose intensity as well as chemotherapy tolerance and patient's quality of life. Febrile neutropenia was more common in older subjects (5 % vs. 1 %, $p=0.005$), and treatment was more often prematurely stopped [61]. Despite these increased limiting toxicities, in Eisenhaurer's analysis of 108 patients older than 65 years, compared to 184 younger ones, treated between 1998 and 2004 at the Memorial Sloan Kettering Cancer Centre, elderly patients demonstrated similar rates of initial response, platinum resistance, PFS and OS to younger patients [60]. Hershman et al. also concluded, from a population-based analysis of the SEER programme database, that even if only half of the patients over age 65 years were treated with platinum-based therapy, survival should improve by 38 % in this group, with similar benefit rates as described among younger patients, justifying an increasing effort to treat elderly patients in a similar way to younger ones [59].

Some controversies appeared from series of older and frailer patients. In Uyar's analysis of treatment patterns by decades in elderly patients at a multi-institutional level, 36 % of patients of 70–79 years and 41 % of patients over 80 treated with platinum-based chemotherapy required dose reductions or termination of therapy [29]. In Bruchim's retrospective cohort comparing cancer management of 46 patients over age 70 years to 143 younger ones, elderly patients had significantly more haematological toxicities (75 % vs. 36.3 %; $p=0.001$) and were more likely to have dose reductions and treatment delays (60 % vs. 22.4 %; $p<0.001$, and 46.6 % vs. 19.1 %; $p=0.004$, respectively) [33]. In Ceccaroni's retrospective analysis of 148 patients over 70 years treated between 1990 and 2000 (median age: 73) in Italian cancer centres, treatment delays over 7 days were often required (16.9 % of the cases) [62]. Villella drew the same conclusion while comparing treatment delays of 31 patients over 70 years to 44 under 55 treated between 1996 and 2001 at the Columbia University College of Physicians and Surgeons [63].

In 2008, Pignata et al. reported the MITO-5 (Multicentre Italian Trial in Ovarian cancer) study, a phase II trial of 26 stage IC–IV ovarian cancer patients. It assessed the tolerance of a weekly carboplatin + paclitaxel schedule: carboplatin AUC 2 + paclitaxel 60 mg/m^2 d1, d8, and d15 every 4 weeks. They included elderly patients, with a median age of 77, a significant proportion of them having some ADL and/or IADL dependencies, although most were *PS* 0 or 1 [64]. Only three limiting toxicities were observed (heart rhythm, prolonged haematological toxicity, liver transaminase increase), and four individuals developed grade 1 peripheral neuropathy. Thus this weekly schedule appears currently to be an alternative to the usual carboplatin–paclitaxel standard regimen.

More recently, Pignata published a strictly weekly regimen of carboplatin AUC 2 and paclitaxel 60 mg/m^2 during 18 weeks, in a nonspecifically geriatric population [65]. Despite the absence of demonstrated benefit of the weekly arm, and perhaps an opposite trend in the older population (151 pts over 70), this regimen was considered in the last NCCN guidelines as an option in the elderly and/or patients with comorbid conditions [23].

Considering the treatment of platinum-sensitive, cancer relapse, CALYPSO randomised clinical trial which compared a carboplatin + pegylated liposomal doxorubicin to a carboplatin + paclitaxel standard in platinum-sensitive relapse. In a subgroup analysis of patients older than 70 (median age: 73) who represented 16 % of the whole populations of patients, an excess in grade 2 and over neuropathies was demonstrated in the carboplatin–paclitaxel treatment arm [66].

To summarise, the real geriatric population is frequently excluded from large prospective studies due to either selective inclusion criteria or investigators' reluctance to include elderly people in clinical trials. Chronological age, rather than distinct geriatric syndromes which may be reversible, seems the main selection factor. While standard adjuvant chemotherapy with six cycles of carboplatin–paclitaxel [67, 68], is well described, real practice is different. Population-based studies, mainly from the SEER programme, showed a higher rate of monotherapies or even abstention from therapy in elderly people. According to the analysis of Sundarajan et al., using 1992–1996 SEER programme data, abstention reached 17 % of patients over 65 years. Compared to the 65–69 age group, the odds ratio by age group for receiving therapy within 4 months of diagnosis was 0.96 for patients 70–74 years, 0.65 for patients 75–79 years, 0.24 for patients 80–84 years and 0.12 for patients over 85 years of age, showing a dramatic decrease of chemotherapy after 80 years. Reasons for suboptimal treatment include age itself [69], fear of comorbidities but also some nonmedical factors such as socio-economic or racial origin [70]. As previously explained, extensive surgical management itself seems to compromise chemotherapy feasibility in vulnerable elderly people [29, 33], yielding some authors to consider either delayed surgical treatment or even surgical abstention [37].

Impact of Geriatric Parameters on Chemotherapy Completion

Since the subgroup analyses of large randomised trials frequently reflect only a partial and biased picture of the real treatment tolerance in elderly people, since 1997 the GINECO dedicated a specific programme to elderly ovarian cancer patients. Its first purpose was to analyse the feasibility of some "standard" chemotherapies in the light of geriatric assessment, with as large inclusion criteria as possible ($PS \leq 3$, absence of severe disease limitation, no cognitive exclusion criteria except patient's inability to understand and accept treatment procedures). According to EWOT1 (1997–2000), which evaluated the feasibility of carboplatin cyclophosphamide, three factors were associated with decreased overall survival: depression ($p = 0.03$), a FIGO stage IV disease ($p = 0.043$) and having six or more co-medications per day ($p = 0.043$). Three factors were predictive of a high toxicity risk: depression ($p = 0.006$), ADL and IADL dependency ($p = 0.048$) and a $PS \geq 2$ [40]. According to EWOT2 (2001–2004), which evaluated the treatment completion of six courses of standard carboplatin–paclitaxel, overall survival was correlated with a HADS score (Hospital Anxiety and Depression Scale) ≥ 15. In a combined analysis of both studies, four cofactors associated with a decrease in the prognosis were the existence of depressive disorders (HR = 5.11; $p < 0.001$), a FIGO stage IV, an initial lymphopenia and the use of paclitaxel [39]. With the limit of a cautious interpretation of a retrospective analysis of a relatively small population, those data raised the (debated [71]) question of the usefulness of combining paclitaxel to platinum in elderly patients with advanced ovarian carcinoma, leading to EWOT3 (2007–2010), which evaluated the impact of psychogeriatric covariates on the outcomes of first-line elderly ovarian cancer patients. This study led to the development of a geriatric vulnerability score (GVS), including ADL score < 6, IADL score < 25, a serum albumin < 35 g/L, lymphopenia < 1G/L, a HADS score > 14. GVS is highly predictive of both decreased overall survival (median 11.5 months versus 21.7 months; HR 2.94 [95 % CI 1.79–4.84], $p < 0.0001$) and treatment completion rates (65.5 % versus 82.1 %; OR of 0.41 [95 % CI 0.17–0.99], $p = 0.044$).

Currently, two prospective studies are being recruiting:

- GOG273 observational study was designed to evaluate the impact of a geriatric assessment on elderly patients' quality of life study. In this three parallel arms study, the investigators were free to propose, depending on their own decision, either a 3-week carboplatin AUC5 paclitaxel 135 mg/m^2 association (regimen 1), a carboplatin monotherapy (regimen 2) or a 3-week carboplatin regimen associated with weekly 60 mg/m^2 paclitaxel (regimen 3) [72].

Preliminary data on regimen 1 and 2 cohorts have been presented and concluded that the population included in regimen 2 cohort was more vulnerable and more prone to premature treatment stopping. However and even when prematurely stopped, chemotherapy tended to ameliorate patients' quality of life [73].

- EWOC-1 [74]: Carboplatin ± Paclitaxel in Vulnerable Elderly Patients With Stage III-IV Advanced Ovarian Cancer. This international multicentre randomised phase II trial will compare the success rate of delivering six courses of chemotherapy with evidence of efficacy and without premature termination for progression, death or unacceptable toxicity of three different chemotherapy regimens in a selected population of vulnerable elderly patients, defined as those with a GVS ≥ 3:
  - Arm A: Paclitaxel 175 mg/m^2/3 h IV and carboplatin AUC 5 IV every 3 weeks
  - Arm B: Carboplatin monotherapy AUC 5 or 6 every 3 weeks
  - Arm C: Weekly paclitaxel 60 mg/m^2/1 h and weekly carboplatin AUC 2 (d1, d8, and d15 every 4 weeks)

How to Deal with Targeted Therapies

There is currently no specific test for elderly patients, examining the effectiveness and safety of anti-angiogenic drugs. Neither ICON7 and GOG218 trials included upper age limit in terms of inclusion criteria; the median age of patients included was 57 and 60, with a maximum of 82 and 89 years in ICON7 and study of GOG, respectively. However, no specific analysis was reported for the subgroup of older patients and the impact of comorbidities, particularly cardiovascular, on their tolerability. Provided a careful assessment of comorbidities, its use seems possible, however, by analogy to other settings. Indeed, a study on 623 patients with lung cancer reported no additional bevacizumab-related toxicity after 65 [75]. Similar results were obtained in a pooled analysis of four randomised studies on colorectal cancer, which showed no significant increase of adverse events after 75 [76]. However, a recent-population-based analysis showed that bevacizumab was used commonly in breast, colon and lung cancer patients despite presenting contraindications to the drug, such circumstances concerning one third of the patients and leading to a high increase of complications rates compared to clinical trials [77]. Consequently, a careful benefit/risk evaluation is recommended, as well as a systemic monitoring for potential adverse events (hypertension, proteinuria, arterial and venous thromboembolic events) [78]. Subgroup analysis of elderly patients' outcomes when treated with other antiangiogenics (pazopanib, nintedanib, cediranib) is awaited.

What Is it Recommended by Clinical Guidelines?

Nice/Saint Paul de Vence 2012 clinical guidelines on ovarian cancer in the elderly have proposed the following recommendations:

First-line chemotherapy

- Real-life data in elderly women:
  - Increased abstention and monochemotherapies
  - Increased premature treatment stops
  - When performed, same efficacy of chemotherapy
- Theoretical data (subgroup analyses):
  - Paclitaxel carboplatin feasible in a selected population
  - Excess toxicities but even better quality of life and digestive tolerance
- Specific data (vulnerable populations)
- Good rates of treatment completion with:
  - Carboplatin and cyclophosphamide
  - Carboplatin–paclitaxel AUC5 standard
  - AUC5 carboplatin
  - A protocol adapted from AUC2 carboplatin–paclitaxel 60 mg/m2 3w/4 (MITO-5)
- In the absence of comparison, these protocols are treatment options

Level 2, Grade B

Targeted therapies in the adjuvant setting

- The available data are insufficient to make recommendations.
- Bevacizumab: no elderly-specific study (ICON7, GOG218)
- Necessary assessment of:
  - Comorbidities (hypertension, cardiomyopathy, etc.)
  - Associated risk factors (history of arterial event, digestive anastomoses)

Chemotherapy after relapse

- No standardised attitude.
- Same recommendations as in the younger patients according to her condition and her personal wishes.
- The decision depends on platinum-free interval:
  - Platinum-sensitive disease: the carboplatin–pegylated liposomal doxycyclin association provides the same benefit as in the younger patient (subgroup analysis).
  - Early relapse: no specific data
  - Prioritise support and supportive care.

Elderly Specific Research: Current Directions

According to a recent review on how to design clinical trials in elderly patients with ovarian cancer, Pignata et al. proposed the following outline:

1. Limit retrospective – consequently biased – studies.
2. In large prospective randomised trials, integrate a (limited) geriatric assessment of elderly patients to evaluate the impact of both age and geriatric covariates on treatment outcomes.

3. Integrate both a functional evaluation of the patients and QoL assessment.
4. Consider assessment of each grade of toxicity, provided that even a grade 2 toxicity can induce decompensation in the elderly.
5. Stratify patients by ages, comorbid conditions and functional status.
6. Determine fit, vulnerable and frail populations in order to evaluate in each group the feasibility of treatments.

Considering judgement criteria, overall survival but also disease-specific survival, QoL and functionality are the main end points to include, either as primary, co-primary or composite end points.

Finally, the authors highlighted the need for an enhanced multidisciplinary cooperation between geriatricians, medical oncologists and gynaecologic/oncologic surgeons [28].

Conclusions

Despite demographics showing a higher incidence and mortality rates over the age of 70 years, ovarian cancer clinical trials have long restricted elderly patients' inclusion either on inclusion criteria or even age limit. This led to a paradox: currently accepted standards have been established on included patients with a median age between 50 and 55, when median age is actually over 65 years in the Western world. In addition, many contradictions appear while analysing published trials on ovarian cancer in elderly individuals, since populations of interest have been highly heterogeneous and rarely characterised by geriatric parameters. A considerable work has been made during the last 20 years, in order to develop elderly-specific prospective trials. The challenge for oncologists is to explore this heterogeneity and to disentangle it on the basis of oncogeriatric assessment. This may reduce current barriers to elderly patients entering into clinical trials, lead to different treatment strategies based on patients' vulnerability and globally improve patients' outcomes. A specific work has to be done, in order to adapt clinical end points to patients' wills and goals.

References

1. Spriggs DR. Ovarian cancer as a chronic disease: a new treatment paradigm. Highlights of a roundtable discussion. Cancer Control. 2001;8(6 Suppl 1):5–7; discussion 8–18.
2. Jemal A, Murray T, Ward E, Samuels A, Tiwari RC, Ghafoor A, Feuer EJ, Thun MJ. Cancer statistics, 2005. CA Cancer J Clin. 2005;55(1):10–30.
3. Ries LA. Ovarian cancer. Survival and treatment differences by age. Cancer. 1993;71(2 Suppl):524–9.
4. Alberts DS, Dahlberg S, Green SJ, Garcia D, Hannigan EV, O'Toole R, Stock-Novack D, Surwit EA, Malviya VK, Jolles CJ. Analysis of patient age as an independent prognostic factor for survival in a phase III study of cisplatin-cyclophosphamide versus carboplatin-cyclophosphamide in stages III (suboptimal) and IV ovarian cancer. A Southwest Oncology Group study. Cancer. 1993;71(2 Suppl):618–27.

5. Thigpen T, Brady MF, Omura GA, Creasman WT, McGuire WP, Hoskins WJ, Williams S. Age as a prognostic factor in ovarian carcinoma. The Gynecologic Oncology Group experience. Cancer. 1993;71(2 Suppl):606–14.
6. Chan JK, Urban R, Cheung MK, Osann K, Shin JY, Husain A, Teng NN, Kapp DS, Berek JS, Leiserowitz GS. Ovarian cancer in younger vs older women: a population-based analysis. Br J Cancer. 2006;95(10):1314–20. Epub 2006 Oct 1331.
7. Barnholtz-Sloan JS, Schwartz AG, Qureshi F, Jacques S, Malone J, Munkarah AR. Ovarian cancer: changes in patterns at diagnosis and relative survival over the last three decades. Am J Obstet Gynecol. 2003;189(4):1120–7.
8. Chan JK, Loizzi V, Lin YG, Osann K, Brewster WR, DiSaia PJ. Stages III and IV invasive epithelial ovarian carcinoma in younger versus older women: what prognostic factors are important? Obstet Gynecol. 2003;102(1):156–61.
9. Young R, Fuks Z, Hoskins W. Cancer of the ovary. In: De Vita VT Jr, Hellman S, Rosenberg SA, editors. Cancer principles in practice of oncology. 1989. P. 1162–96.
10. Yancik R. Ovarian cancer. Age contrasts in incidence, histology, disease stage at diagnosis, and mortality. Cancer. 1993;71(2 Suppl):517–23.
11. Yedema CA, Kenemans P, Wobbes T, Thomas CM, Bon GG, Mulder C, Voorhorst FJ, Verstraeten AA, van Kamp GJ, Hilgers J. Use of serum tumor markers in the differential diagnosis between ovarian and colorectal adenocarcinomas. Tumour Biol. 1992;13(1–2):18–26.
12. Delgado G, Oram DH, Petrilli ES. Stage III epithelial ovarian cancer: the role of maximal surgical reduction. Gynecol Oncol. 1984;18(3):293–8.
13. Venesmaa P, Ylikorkala O. Morbidity and mortality associated with primary and repeat operations for ovarian cancer. Obstet Gynecol. 1992;79(2):168–72.
14. Hutchins LF, Unger JM, Crowley JJ, Coltman Jr CA, Albain KS. Underrepresentation of patients 65 years of age or older in cancer-treatment trials. N Engl J Med. 1999;341(27): 2061–7.
15. Talarico L, Chen G, Pazdur R. Enrollment of elderly patients in clinical trials for cancer drug registration: a 7-year experience by the US Food and Drug Administration. J Clin Oncol. 2004;22(22):4626–31.
16. Townsley CA, Selby R, Siu LL. Systematic review of barriers to the recruitment of older patients with cancer onto clinical trials. J Clin Oncol. 2005;23(13):3112–24.
17. Villella J, Chalas E. Optimising treatment of elderly patients with ovarian cancer: improving their enrollment in clinical trials. Drugs Aging. 2005;22(2):95–100.
18. Harter P, du Bois A, Schade-Brittinger C, Burges A, Wollschlaeger K, Gropp M, Schmalfeldt B, Huober J, Staehle A, Pfisterer J. Non-enrolment of ovarian cancer patients in clinical trials: reasons and background. Ann Oncol. 2005;16(11):1801–5. Epub 2005 Aug 1809.
19. Freyer G, Tinker AV. Clinical trials and treatment of the elderly diagnosed with ovarian cancer. Int J Gynecol Cancer. 2011;21(4):776–81.
20. Ovarian cancer: recognition and initial management; 2011. http://nice.org.uk/guidance/cg122.
21. Wagner U, Harter P, Hilpert F, Mahner S, Reuss A, du Bois A, Petru E, Meier W, Ortner P, Konig K, et al. S3-guideline on diagnostics, therapy and follow-up of malignant ovarian tumours: short version 1.0 – AWMF registration number: 032/035OL, June 2013. Geburtshilfe. 2013;73(9):874–89.
22. Falandry C, Fabbro M, Lesoin A, Guérin O, Kurtz JE. Cancer de l'ovaire de la patiente âgée. Onko+. 2013;41(5);suppl 2:14–23.
23. NCCN clinical practice guidelines in oncology: ovarian cancer (including fallopian tube cancer and primary peritoneal cancer)- Version 2.2015. www.nccn.org/professionals/physician_gls/f_guidelines.asp#ovarian.
24. Extermann M, Aapro M, Bernabei R, Cohen HJ, Droz JP, Lichtman S, Mor V, Monfardini S, Repetto L, Sorbye L, et al. Use of comprehensive geriatric assessment in older cancer patients: recommendations from the task force on CGA of the International Society of Geriatric Oncology (SIOG). Crit Rev Oncol Hematol. 2005;55(3):241–52.
25. Repetto L, Fratino L, Audisio RA, Venturino A, Gianni W, Vercelli M, Parodi S, Dal Lago D, Gioia F, Monfardini S, et al. Comprehensive geriatric assessment adds information to Eastern

Cooperative Oncology Group performance status in elderly cancer patients: an Italian Group for Geriatric Oncology Study. J Clin Oncol. 2002;20(2):494–502.
26. Hamaker ME, Jonker JM, de Rooij SE, Vos AG, Smorenburg CH, van Munster BC. Frailty screening methods for predicting outcome of a comprehensive geriatric assessment in elderly patients with cancer: a systematic review. Lancet Oncol. 2012;13(10):70259.
27. Soubeyran P, Bellera C, Goyard J, Heitz D, Cure H, Rousselot H, Albrand G, Servent V, Jean OS, van Praagh I, et al. Screening for vulnerability in older cancer patients: the ONCODAGE Prospective Multicenter Cohort Study. PLoS One. 2014;9(12):2014.
28. Pignata S, Cecere SC, Tambaro R. How to design clinical trials? In: Freyer G, editor. Ovarian cancer in elderly patients. Switzerland: Springer International Publishing, Switzerland; 2016. P. 79–93.
29. Uyar D, Frasure HE, Markman M, von Gruenigen VE. Treatment patterns by decade of life in elderly women (> or =70 years of age) with ovarian cancer. Gynecol Oncol. 2005;98(3):403–8.
30. Bristow RE, Tomacruz RS, Armstrong DK, Trimble EL, Montz FJ. Survival effect of maximal cytoreductive surgery for advanced ovarian carcinoma during the platinum era: a meta-analysis. J Clin Oncol. 2002;20(5):1248–59.
31. Wimberger P, Lehmann N, Kimmig R, Burges A, Meier W, Hoppenau B, du Bois A. Impact of age on outcome in patients with advanced ovarian cancer treated within a prospectively randomized phase III study of the Arbeitsgemeinschaft Gynaekologische Onkologie Ovarian Cancer Study Group (AGO-OVAR). Gynecol Oncol. 2006;100(2):300–7.
32. Wright JD, Herzog TJ, Powell MA. Morbidity of cytoreductive surgery in the elderly. Am J Obstet Gynecol. 2004;190(5):1398–400.
33. Bruchim I, Altaras M, Fishman A. Age contrasts in clinical characteristics and pattern of care in patients with epithelial ovarian cancer. Gynecol Oncol. 2002;86(3):274–8.
34. Ben-Ami I, Vaknin Z, Schneider D, Halperin R. Perioperative morbidity and mortality of gynecological oncologic surgery in elderly women. Int J Gynecol Cancer. 2006;16(1):452–7.
35. Lichtinger M, Averette H, Penalver M, Sevin BU. Major surgical procedures for gynecologic malignancy in elderly women. South Med J. 1986;79(12):1506–10.
36. Cloven NG, Manetta A, Berman ML, Kohler MF, DiSaia PJ. Management of ovarian cancer in patients older than 80 years of Age. Gynecol Oncol. 1999;73(1):137–9.
37. Moore KN, Reid MS, Fong DN, Myers TK, Landrum LM, Moxley KM, Walker JL, McMeekin DS, Mannel RS. Ovarian cancer in the octogenarian: does the paradigm of aggressive cytoreductive surgery and chemotherapy still apply? Gynecol Oncol. 2008;110(2):133–9. Epub 2008 May 2020.
38. Diaz-Montes TP, Zahurak ML, Giuntoli 2nd RL, Gardner GJ, Gordon TA, Armstrong DK, Bristow RE. Surgical care of elderly women with ovarian cancer: a population-based perspective. Gynecol Oncol. 2005;99(2):352–7. Epub 2005 Aug 2001.
39. Trédan O, Geay JF, Touzet S, Delva R, Weber B, Cretin J, Provencal J, Martin J, Pujade-Lauraine E, Freyer G. Carboplatin Cyclophosphamide or Carboplatin Paclitaxel in elderly with advanced ovarian cancer? Analysis of two consecutive trials from the GINECO. Ann Oncol. 2007;18(2):256–62.
40. Freyer G, Geay JF, Touzet S, Provencal J, Weber B, Jacquin JP, Ganem G, Tubiana-Mathieu N, Gisserot O, Pujade-Lauraine E. Comprehensive geriatric assessment predicts tolerance to chemotherapy and survival in elderly patients with advanced ovarian carcinoma: a GINECO study. Ann Oncol. 2005;16(11):1795–800.
41. Chan JK, Zhang M, Hu JM, Shin JY, Osann K, Kapp DS. Racial disparities in surgical treatment and survival of epithelial ovarian cancer in United States. J Surg Oncol. 2008;97(2):103–7.
42. Vercelli M, Capocaccia R, Quaglia A, Casella C, Puppo A, Coebergh JW. Relative survival in elderly European cancer patients: evidence for health care inequalities. The EUROCARE Working Group. Crit Rev Oncol Hematol. 2000;35(3):161–79.
43. Hightower RD, Nguyen HN, Averette HE, Hoskins W, Harrison T, Steren A. National survey of ovarian carcinoma. IV: patterns of care and related survival for older patients. Cancer. 1994;73(2):377–83.

44. Thrall MM, Goff BA, Symons RG, Flum DR, Gray HJ. Thirty-day mortality after primary cytoreductive surgery for advanced ovarian cancer in the elderly. Obstet Gynecol. 2011; 118(3):537–47.
45. Alphs HH, Zahurak ML, Bristow RE, Diaz-Montes TP. Predictors of surgical outcome and survival among elderly women diagnosed with ovarian and primary peritoneal cancer. Gynecol Oncol. 2006;103(3):1048–53. Epub 2006 Jul 1027.
46. Audisio RA, Bozzetti F, Gennari R, Jaklitsch MT, Koperna T, Longo WE, Wiggers T, Zbar AP. The surgical management of elderly cancer patients; recommendations of the SIOG surgical task force. Eur J Cancer. 2004;40(7):926–38.
47. Audisio RA, Pope D, Ramesh HS, Gennari R, van Leeuwen BL, West C, Corsini G, Maffezzini M, Hoekstra HJ, Mobarak D, et al. Shall we operate? Preoperative assessment in elderly cancer patients (PACE) can help. A SIOG surgical task force prospective study. Crit Rev Oncol Hematol. 2008;65(2):156–63.
48. George EM, Burke WM, Hou JY, Tergas AI, Chen L, Neugut AI, Ananth CV, Hershman DL, Wright JD. Measurement and validation of frailty as a predictor of outcomes in women undergoing major gynaecological surgery. BJOG. 2015;2015(23):1471–528.
49. Fried LP, Tangen CM, Walston J, Newman AB, Hirsch C, Gottdiener J, Seeman T, Tracy R, Kop WJ, Burke G, et al. Frailty in older adults: evidence for a phenotype. J Gerontol A Biol Sci Med Sci. 2001;56(3):M146–56.
50. Cesari M, Cerullo F, Zamboni V, Di Palma R, Scambia G, Balducci L, Antonelli Incalzi R, Vellas B, Gambassi G. Functional status and mortality in older women with gynecological cancer. J Gerontol A Biol Sci Med Sci. 2013;68(9):1129–33.
51. van der Burg ME, van Lent M, Buyse M, Kobierska A, Colombo N, Favalli G, Lacave AJ, Nardi M, Renard J, Pecorelli S. The effect of debulking surgery after induction chemotherapy on the prognosis in advanced epithelial ovarian cancer. Gynecological Cancer Cooperative Group of the European Organization for Research and Treatment of Cancer. N Engl J Med. 1995;332(10):629–34.
52. Rose PG, Nerenstone S, Brady MF, Clarke-Pearson D, Olt G, Rubin SC, Moore DH, Small JM. Secondary surgical cytoreduction for advanced ovarian carcinoma. N Engl J Med. 2004;351(24):2489–97.
53. Vergote I, Trope CG, Amant F, Kristensen GB, Ehlen T, Johnson N, Verheijen RH, van der Burg ME, Lacave AJ, Panici PB, et al. Neoadjuvant chemotherapy or primary surgery in stage IIIC or IV ovarian cancer. N Engl J Med. 2010;363(10):943–53.
54. Chi DS, Bristow RE, Armstrong DK, Karlan BY. Is the easier way ever the better way? J Clin Oncol. 2011;29(31):4073–5.
55. Vergote I, Trope CG, Amant F, Ehlen T, Reed NS, Casado A. Neoadjuvant chemotherapy is the better treatment option in some patients with stage IIIc to IV ovarian cancer. J Clin Oncol. 2011;29(31):4076–8.
56. McLean KA, Shah CA, Thompson SA, Gray HJ, Swensen RE, Goff BA. Ovarian cancer in the elderly: outcomes with neoadjuvant chemotherapy or primary cytoreduction. Gynecol Oncol. 2010;118(1):43–6.
57. Giovanazzi-Bannon S, Rademaker A, Lai G, Benson 3rd AB. Treatment tolerance of elderly cancer patients entered onto phase II clinical trials: an Illinois Cancer Center study. J Clin Oncol. 1994;12(11):2447–52.
58. Le T, Leis A, Pahwa P, Wright K, Ali K, Reeder B, Hopkins L, Fung MF. Quality of life evaluations in patients with ovarian cancer during chemotherapy treatment. Gynecol Oncol. 2004;92(3):839–44.
59. Hershman D, Jacobson JS, McBride R, Mitra N, Sundararajan V, Grann VR, Neugut AI. Effectiveness of platinum-based chemotherapy among elderly patients with advanced ovarian cancer. Gynecol Oncol. 2004;94(2):540–9.
60. Eisenhauer EL, Tew WP, Levine DA, Lichtman SM, Brown CL, Aghajanian C, Huh J, Barakat RR, Chi DS. Response and outcomes in elderly patients with stages IIIC-IV ovarian cancer receiving platinum-taxane chemotherapy. Gynecol Oncol. 2007;106(2):381–7.

61. Hilpert F, du Bois A, Greimel ER, Hedderich J, Krause G, Venhoff L, Loibl S, Pfisterer J. Feasibility, toxicity and quality of life of first-line chemotherapy with platinum/paclitaxel in elderly patients aged>=70 years with advanced ovarian cancer – a study by the AGO OVAR Germany. Ann Oncol. 2006;18(2):282–7.
62. Ceccaroni M, D'Agostino G, Ferrandina G, Gadducci A, Di Vagno G, Pignata S, Poerio A, Salerno MG, Fanucchi A, Lapresa MT, et al. Gynecological malignancies in elderly patients: is age 70 a limit to standard-dose chemotherapy? An Italian retrospective toxicity multicentric study. Gynecol Oncol. 2002;85(3):445–50.
63. Villella JA, Chaudhry T, Pearl ML, Valea F, DiSilvestro PA, Pollack S, Chalas E. Comparison of tolerance of combination carboplatin and paclitaxel chemotherapy by age in women with ovarian cancer. Gynecol Oncol. 2002;86(3):316–22.
64. Pignata S, Breda E, Scambia G, Pisano C, Zagonel V, Lorusso D, Greggi S, De Vivo R, Ferrandina G, Gallo C, et al. A phase II study of weekly carboplatin and paclitaxel as first-line treatment of elderly patients with advanced ovarian cancer. A Multicentre Italian Trial in Ovarian cancer (MITO-5) study. Crit Rev Oncol Hematol. 2008;66(3):229–36. Epub 2008 Feb 2001.
65. Pignata S, Scambia G, Katsaros D, Gallo C, Pujade-Lauraine E, De Placido S, Bologna A, Weber B, Raspagliesi F, Panici PB, et al. Carboplatin plus paclitaxel once a week versus every 3 weeks in patients with advanced ovarian cancer (MITO-7): a randomised, multicentre, open-label, phase 3 trial. Lancet Oncol. 2014;15(4):396–405.
66. Kurtz JE, Hilpert F, Dorum A, Veillard A, Elit L, Buck M, Petru E, Reed N, Scambia G, Varsellona N. Can elderly patients with recurrent ovarian cancer (ROC) be treated with a platinum-based doublet? Results from the CALYPSO trial. J Clin Oncol. 2010;28(15s):Suppl; abstr 5031.
67. Begg CB, Carbone PP. Clinical trials and drug toxicity in the elderly. The experience of the Eastern Cooperative Oncology Group. Cancer. 1983;52(11):1986–92.
68. Higgins RV, Naumann RW, Gardner J, Hall JB. Is age a barrier to the aggressive treatment of ovarian cancer with paclitaxel and carboplatin? Gynecol Oncol. 1999;75(3):464–7.
69. Maas HA, Kruitwagen RF, Lemmens VE, Goey SH, Janssen-Heijnen ML. The influence of age and co-morbidity on treatment and prognosis of ovarian cancer: a population-based study. Gynecol Oncol. 2005;97(1):104–9.
70. Sundararajan V, Hershman D, Grann VR, Jacobson JS, Neugut AI. Variations in the use of chemotherapy for elderly patients with advanced ovarian cancer: a population-based study. J Clin Oncol. 2002;20(1):173–8.
71. Zola P, Ferrero A. Is carboplatin-paclitaxel combination the standard treatment of elderly ovarian cancer patients? Ann Oncol. 2007;18(2):213–4.
72. Chemotherapy toxicity on quality of life in older patients with stage I, stage II, stage III, or stage IV ovarian epithelial, primary peritoneal cavity, or fallopian tube cancer; 2016. https://www.clinicaltrials.gov/ct2/show/NCT01366183.
73. von Gruenigen VE, Huang H, Tew WP. Geriatric assessment and tolerance to chemotherapy in elderly women with ovarian, primary peritoneal or fallopian tube cancer: a Gynecology Oncology Group study. Gynecol Oncol. 2014;133:abstr 439.
74. http://www.clinicaltrials.gov/ct2/show/NCT02001272; 2016.
75. Laskin J, Crino L, Felip E, Franke F, Gorbunova V, Groen H, Jiang GL, Reck M, Schneider CP. Safety and efficacy of first-line bevacizumab plus chemotherapy in elderly patients with advanced or recurrent nonsquamous non-small cell lung cancer: safety of avastin in lung trial (MO19390). J Thorac Oncol. 2012;7(1):203–11.
76. Cassidy J, Saltz LB, Giantonio BJ, Kabbinavar FF, Hurwitz HI, Rohr UP. Effect of bevacizumab in older patients with metastatic colorectal cancer: pooled analysis of four randomized studies. J Cancer Res Clin Oncol. 2010;136(5):737–43.
77. Hershman DL, Wright JD, Lim E, Buono DL, Tsai WY, Neugut AI. Contraindicated use of bevacizumab and toxicity in elderly patients with cancer. J Clin Oncol. 2013;31(28):3592–9.
78. Tredan O, Ray-Coquard I. Management of antiangiogenic agents. In: Freyer G, editor. Ovarian cancer in elderly patients. Switzerland: Springer International Publishing Switzerland; 2016. P. 69–77.

Treatment at Relapse (Surgery and Systemic Treatments)

10

Anne Floquet and Jacobus Pfisterer

Abstract

Relapses are an important part of epithelial ovarian cancer history due to the natural course of disease and due to inadequate primary treatment. Presently, first relapse means an evolution towards a chronic disease. However, treatments at relapse as chemotherapy, targeted therapy and potentially surgery have substantially prolonged life. So, it is of particular interest to give the patient the best strategy for a better life despite recurrences. Decision making is now mainly based on the expected chemosensitivity of the disease, which was reflected until now by platinum-free interval. This has recently changed. It illustrates biological features of the tumour and host's profile such as immune and genetics characteristics. Quality of life remains the cornerstone of treatment choice, and benefit-risk balance evaluation should be the main goal for decision.

Introduction

Despite better well-defined first-line treatment combining radical surgery [1] and chemotherapy with platinum and taxanes ± bevacizumab [2, 3], relapses of epithelial ovarian carcinoma (EOC) are still a matter of concern. Approximately 70 % of patients treated for advanced EOC are facing relapses with a median progression-free survival around 18 months. Unfortunately, a patient who recurs from EOC

A. Floquet, MD
GINECO Group, Institut Bergonié, Bordeaux, France
e-mail: a.floquet@bordeaux.unicancer.fr

J. Pfisterer, MD, PhD (✉)
AGO Study Group, Gynecologic Oncology Center, Kiel, Germany
e-mail: jacobus.pfisterer@googlemail.com

E. Pujade-Lauraine et al. (eds.), *Ovarian Cancers*,
DOI 10.1007/978-3-319-32110-3_10

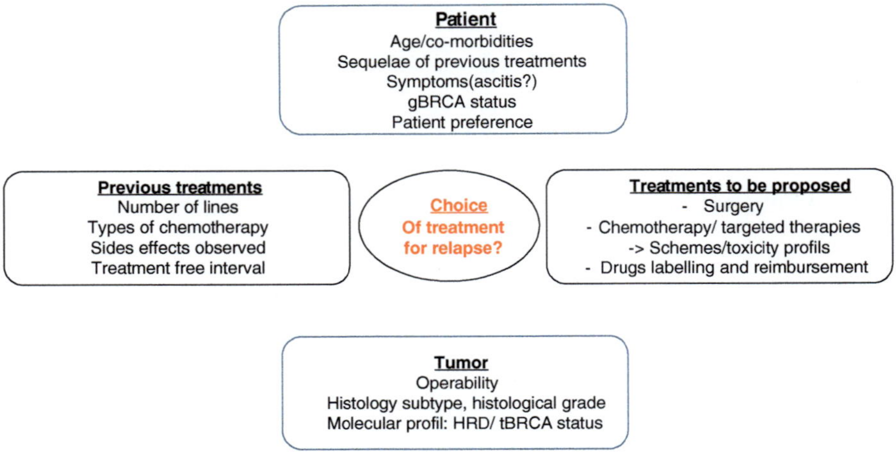

Fig. 10.1 Criteria for decision making

remains today incurable, making the situation as a chronic disease [4]. Nonetheless, different chemotherapy regimens have contributed to substantially prolong survival as shown by the AGO-GINECO analysis from their three randomised phase III studies which concluded that a maximum of three lines of subsequent relapse treatments may be beneficial in case of recurrent ovarian carcinoma [5]. The place of surgery for selected cases is still to be proven. Prognosis at relapse is mainly dominated by chemosensitivity of the tumour which is a reflection of biological features of the tumour and of its environment. The delay of recurrence from the end of first-line platinum-based treatment is the major prognostic factor. The choice of chemotherapy modalities depends on several factors such as platinum-free interval (PFI), persistent side effects of prior treatments, schedules, and toxicity profiles of next therapies and patient preferences [6]. Figure 10.1 highlights the main decision criteria. The results showed by recent trials with new targeted therapies such as anti-angiogenic agents or PARP inhibitors (which will not be discussed here) have redefined the landscape of new strategies for dealing with relapses. However, these trials are most of the time designed for first, second and eventually third relapses, and very few evidence-based data are available beyond.

When Should the Relapse Be Treated?

In most of cases, CA 125 elevation is the first signal of recurrence; it can be observed some months before clinical symptoms or radiological signs. It remains difficult in routine practice to know if a treatment has to be immediately initiated. The MRC OV05/EORTC 55955 addressed this question in a randomised trial comparing early versus delayed treatments in case of asymptomatic rising of CA125. No difference was observed in overall survival (OS) in the delayed treatment group (median delayed time: 4.8 months) in comparison with the earlier treated one; furthermore, the quality of life in the delayed group was better [7]. Since the results of that study, there have been a lot of debates on the needs to better document the recurrence (particularly with PET CT), to explore the role of surgery and to evaluate the role of alternative treatments to chemotherapy in such a situation. However, it is commonly assumed that raised CA125 alone is not sufficient to systematically recommend treatment.

Platinum-Free Interval

Until now, mainly for clinical trial design, relapses have been defined according to time spent between end of the last platinum-based chemotherapy and detection of recurrence, which is called "platinum-free interval (PFI)". Then relapses are named as platinum refractory (0–3 months), platinum resistant (<6 months), platinum partially sensitive (6–12 months) and platinum sensitive (>12 months) [8]. These definitions are meant to move on with better knowledge on biological behaviour of each tumour. The introduction of non-platinum chemo regimens and targeted therapies may also jeopardise these predefined intervals. They are currently being discussed (5th Ovarian Carcinoma Consensus Conference, Tokyo, November 2015) and are awaiting publication. It seems that we may consider only early and delayed relapses as a reflection of tumour ability to respond to subsequent medical treatments. The delay of relapse is also an important criterion to select patient amenable to surgery.

Surgery at Relapse

Surgery at relapse is commonly performed in routine practice based on some retrospective data [9, 10]. It usually concerns first relapses with low volume, accessible anatomical sites and long treatment-free interval. Disease-free interval is the most important prognostic factor at relapse; more than 6 months is generally mandatory to consider secondary cytoreductive surgery (SCS) [11]. The later the relapse, the better the benefit of surgery seems to be; however, the best disease-free interval to indicate surgery was not well established. A meta-analysis with heterogeneous and retrospective studies has shown correlation between residual disease after surgery and overall survival [12, 13]. There are no evidence-based phase III results to validate this routine practice, and the place of SCS remains to be defined yet. The Fourth Ovarian Cancer Consensus Meeting recommendations were that a complete resection must be the main objective of a trial designed to access surgery at relapse [14]. Two prospective trials have addressed this issue, the DESKTOP III trial and GOG 0213, at first relapse beyond 6 months. These two trials compare platinum-based chemotherapy with or without SCS with the aim of no residual disease. Their principal objective is overall survival. Selection criteria for SCS were studied by the Arbeitsgemeinschaft Gynakologische Onkologie (AGO) group in two consecutive studies. The DESKTOP I trial validated a score to identify patients who can benefit from the surgical approach [15]. This score has three items: it is positive if the primary surgery was complete, patient performance status is good and there is no ascites. In every other situation, the score is negative. The DESKTOP II trial prospectively validated the impact of a positive AGO score to obtain a complete resection at relapse [16]. Finally, the DESTKTOP III randomised trial was designed to compare, in case of relapse beyond 6 months and positive AGO score, surgery followed by platinum-based chemotherapy versus platinum-based chemotherapy alone. GOG 0213 trial shared the same main selection criteria. These two prospective trials are closed, and results are awaited in the next years.

Early Relapse

They are defined by relapses during first-line treatment or in the few following months. They are called refractory (0–3 months after) or resistant (3–6 months after). But platinum resistance is the final event of all relapses of EOC. As such, they represent a very heterogeneous group of various biological tumour behaviours. They are difficult to treat due to the lack of response to chemotherapy, and for the more previously treated patients, persistence of side effects can be limiting. In these bad prognosis situations, the main objective of treatment is to give the best efficacy, and, as it is uncertain, attention must be focused on toxicity profile. The recommendation in this situation is not to reintroduce platinum especially for refractory relapses. However, in case of platinum-resistant disease, some reports mentioned responses to platinum-based chemotherapy [17, 18]; it is for sure a way to investigate further. Combinations of chemotherapy are not superior to monotherapy and responsible of more side effects. The main available drugs are represented by weekly paclitaxel, liposomal doxorubicin, topotecan and gemcitabine [19–23]. These four drugs offer similar objective responses rates (10–20 %), median progression-free survival (PFS) (3–4 months) and OS (around 12 months) with different toxicity profiles. The AURELIA trial evaluated in a phase III randomised trial the addition of bevacizumab to chemotherapy versus chemotherapy alone in first or second relapses of EOC. Chemotherapy was according to investigator's choice weekly paclitaxel, topotecan or pegylated liposomal doxorubicin. After completion of chemotherapy, bevacizumab was given in maintenance until progression or toxicity. Better responses (27.3 versus 11.8 %, $p=0.001$) and PFS (HR 0.48; 95 % CI 0.38–0.60; $p<0.001$) were observed with chemotherapy associated with bevacizumab [24]. Median PFS was 6.7 months with chemotherapy plus bevacizumab versus 3.4 months with chemotherapy alone. Responses were of particular interest in cases of ascites with a significant impact in reductions of paracentesis needs. Combination of chemotherapy and bevacizumab was associated with improvement of symptoms as evaluated by patient-reported outcomes [25]. No benefit was observed in OS. Bevacizumab (Avastin™) was licensed in this setting.

Other anti-angiogenic agents (trebananib, pazopanib, nintedanib, cediranib) showed some efficacy in phase II or III studies but none has been licensed yet [26–29]. The phase III trial TRINOVA 1 [26] compared weekly paclitaxel + trebananib (P + T) or placebo (P) in recurrent EOC with PFI <12 months and less than three previous lines of chemotherapy. The results showed a better PFS with weekly paclitaxel associated with trebananib (HR 0.66; 95 % CI 0.57–0.77; p <0.001) 7.2 months versus 5.4 months. They also interestingly displayed a benefit in OS in the subgroup with ascites. In this case, with a median follow-up of 17.7 m, the median OS was 14.5 m (P+T) versus 12.3 m with P alone (HR=0.72, 95 % CI 0.55–0.93; p=0.011) [30]. No benefit was observed in OS in the intent to treat population as in previous studies with bevacizumab. The mechanism of action of trebananib is very different from monoclonal vascular endothelial growth factor antibody bevacizumab. It is a peptibody (Fc-peptide fusion molecule) blocking binding of angiopoietins Ang1/2 to the Tie 2 receptor. The toxicity profile is also different with mainly oedema, ascites and pleural effusion and less cardiovascular and renal effects.

Relapses After 6 Months

They are called platinum sensitive [31, 32] and generally more responsive to chemotherapy. Chemosensitivity is supposed to increase with the widening of the interval. For first relapse, platinum-based chemotherapy is still the most active agents with comparable efficacy of cisplatin and carboplatin [33, 34] but with a toxicity profile in favour of carboplatin. Combination of carboplatin with a second drug (paclitaxel, gemcitabine, pegylated liposomal doxorubicin) has shown better efficacy than platinum monotherapy; it also gives more manageable side effects [32, 35, 36] depending on the second associated drug. A meta-analysis published in 2013, using individual patient data, demonstrated with inclusion of four randomised trials (exploring platinum monotherapy versus platinum combination) and 1300 patients, the superiority of the platinum combination in terms of PFS (HR=0.68; 95 % CI 0.57–0.81; p<0.001) and OS (HR=0.80; 95 % CI 0.64–1.00; p=0.05) [37]. As patients will be exposed to subsequent lines of chemotherapy, the issue of tolerance must be kept in mind in order to avoid excessive or cumulative toxicities. The CALYPSO trial [36] compared carboplatin plus 3 weekly paclitaxel and carboplatin plus pegylated liposomal doxorubicin. It was designed as a non-inferiority trial. The results showed a better PFS for platinum-pegylated liposomal doxorubicin (HR 0.82, 95 % CI 0.72–0.94) with better toxicity profile and less discontinuing of treatment.

Some have explored an artificial extension of PFI by delivering a non-platinum-based chemotherapy. The OVA 301 trial compared a population of relapsing EOC regardless of PFI in a phase III randomised study pegylated liposomal doxorubicin alone or in combination with a new drug named trabectedin [38]. Trabectedin is a new compound with original antineoplastic properties, the best known being the possibility to bind DNA minor groove. The results showed for platinum-sensitive patients an improved PFS with the combination (HR 0.73; CI 95 % 0.56–0.95; p=0.0170) and better objective response rate 35.3 % versus 22.6 %. Observed toxicities with the combination were mainly neutropenia, grade ¾ transaminase transient elevations. Meaningful results were observed in the partially platinum-sensitive population (PFI between 6 and 12 months) in which rechallenging with platinum-based chemotherapy could be difficult or not wished. PFS was improved in the combination arm (HR = 0.65 CI 95 % 0.45–0.92) as well as OS (HR = 0.59; CI 95 % 0.43–0.82) [39]. To definitively confirm this concept, a prospective trial was designed, INOVATYON trial, in the partially platinum-sensitive population, comparing platinum-based chemotherapy with PLD-carboplatin with crossover at progression. This study is still ongoing.

More recently, the place of bevacizumab was evaluated in a phase III randomised trial (OCEANS) comparing the doublet carboplatin-gemcitabine with (experimental arm) or without bevacizumab (standard arm) for patients bevacizumab naive [40]. Bevacizumab was given during chemotherapy then in maintenance until progression or unacceptable toxicity. The study met its primary objective, PFS increased in the chemo-bevacizumab arm with 12.4 months versus 8.4 months (HR 0.484; 95 % CI 0.388–0.605; $p < 0.0001$). The objective response rate was also significantly improved: 78.5 versus 57.4 % ($p < 0.0001$). However, no benefit was seen in OS. Treatment was well tolerated with no new signal. No gastrointestinal perforation was observed. The main grade 3 or more toxicities were hypertension (17.4 versus 0.4 %) and proteinuria (8.5 versus 0.9 %). In Europe, these results led the license of bevacizumab (Avastin™) in association with carboplatin-gemcitabine in this setting. However, bevacizumab was already indicated in primary treatment in association with carboplatin-paclitaxel combination in advanced EOC. There is no data concerning benefit of bevacizumab rechallenging in relapsed EOC. That hypothesis is tested in an ongoing Italian phase III trial (MITO 16 study) comparing platinum-based chemotherapy (carbo-paclitaxel, carbo-gemcitabine or carbo-pegylated liposomal doxorubicin) with or without bevacizumab.

Another anti-angiogenic compound has been evaluated in late recurrences. The ICON 6 trial compared in a randomised phase III, cediranib during platinum-based chemotherapy followed by cediranib in maintenance for 18 months versus cediranib during platinum-based chemotherapy followed by placebo in maintenance during the same duration versus platinum-based chemotherapy with placebo. The results demonstrated a better PFS (HR 0.56; 95 % CI 0.44–0.72; $p < 0.0001$), OS data are immature yet (HR 0.77; 95 % CI 0.55–1.07; $p = 0.11$) in arm with cediranib during chemotherapy and in maintenance in comparison to the standard arm with chemotherapy alone [41]. The main side effects were hypertension, fatigue, nausea and diarrhoea.

Cediranib is a small oral molecule VEGF receptor tyrosine kinase inhibitor, which also inhibits both platelet-derived and fibroblast growth factor receptors, explaining the different toxicity profile.

This new compound was recently assessed in a randomised phase II in association with olaparib versus olaparib alone in 86 patients with a platinum-sensitive ovarian cancer relapse. This "all oral no-chemo doublet" showed impressive results in term of efficacy: PFS was extended by 8.7 m (9 m with olaparib alone versus 17.7 m with the combination). The improvement was observed regardless of germinal BRCA status. Toxicity was significant with mainly grade 3/4 hypertension, fatigue and diarrhoea [42]. The place of such combination remains to be evaluated on larger population. Olaparib belongs to PARP inhibitors family and is so far the most evaluated agent. Olaparib (Lynparza™) was licensed in Europe, in platinum-sensitive relapse of m BRCA serous ovarian cancer, in case of response to platinum-based chemotherapy, following the results of Study 19 [43]. This phase II randomised study compared, after good response to platinum-based chemotherapy, treatment by olaparib 400 mg twice a day (introduced after the chemotherapy) versus placebo in 265 women with platinum-sensitive relapse: adding olaparib showed a benefit. In that study, 51 % of patients had germinal or somatic BRCA mutations. The benefit of olaparib was greater in the mBRCA group with a reduced risk of progression of 82 % (HR 0.18; 95 % CI 0.11–0.31, $p < 0.00001$). The median PFS was 11.2 m in the mBRCA group versus 4.3 m for the others. However, data for OS are not mature yet.

Conclusion

Besides old classic drugs, the availability of new-targeted ones such as anti-angiogenic agents expands the perspective of treatments in relapsed epithelial ovarian carcinoma. Many other compounds are currently being assessed, especially PARP inhibitors. Actually, the identification of homologous recombination repair pathway defects and the implication of BRCA genes in ovarian carcinoma have offered new perspectives for prevention and treatment in these last 10 years. Surgery may be another chance for selected patients. The challenge in the near future is to find selection criteria to avoid undue side effects and then offer the patients longer and better quality of life. For the moment, we are lacking routine tests to evaluate chemo-sensibility or resistance of tumours, and the more used criterion remains platinum-free interval. This is susceptible to move on with the idea of continuum in the biological history of the tumour, the introduction of non-platinum chemo regimens and targeted therapies especially if they are given in maintenance setting.

References

Introduction

1. Harter P, Hilpert F, Mahner S, et al. Prognostic factors for complete debulking in first and second line ovarian cancer. Int J Gynecol Cancer. 2009;19:14–7.
2. Burger RA, Brady MF, Bookman, MA, et al.; Gynecologic Oncology Group. Incorporation of bevacizumab in the primary treatment of ovarian cancer. N Engl J Med. 2011;365(26): 2473–83.
3. Perren TJ, Swart AM, Pfisterer J, et al.; ICON 7 Investigators. A phase 3 trial of bevacizumab in ovarian cancer. N Eng J Med. 2011;365(26):2484–96.
4. Markman M. Viewing ovarian cancer as a "chronic disease": what exactly does this mean? Gynecol Oncol. 2006;100:229–30.
5. Hanker L, Loibl S, Buchardi N, et al. The impact of second to sixth line therapy on survival of relapsed ovarian cancer after primary taxane/platinum based therapy. Ann Oncol. 2012; 23:2605–12.

6. Baumann KH, Wagner U, du Bois A. The changing landscape of the therapeutic strategies for recurrent ovarian cancer. Future Oncol. 2012;8:1135–47.
7. Rustin GJ, van der Burg ME, Griffin CL, et al. Early versus delayed treatment of relapsed ovarian cancer (MRC OV05/EORTC 55955): a randomised trial. Lancet. 2010;376:1155–63.

Platinum Free Interval

8. Stuart G, Kitchener H, Bacon M, et al. 2010 Gynecologic Cancer Intergroup (GCIG) consensus statement on clinicals trials in ovarian cancer: report from the Fourth Ovarian Cancer Consensus Conference. Int J Gynecol Cancer. 2011;21:750–5.

Surgery

9. Eisenkop SM, Friedman RL, Spirtos NM. The role of secondary cytoreductive surgery in the treatment of patients with recurrent epithelial ovarian carcinoma. Cancer. 2000;88:144–53.
10. Chi DS, McCaughty K, Diaz JP, et al. Guidelines and selection criteria for secondary cytoreductive surgery in patients with recurrent, platinum-sensitive epithelial ovarian carcinoma. Cancer. 2006;106:1933–9.
11. Shih KK, Chi DS. Maximal cytoreductive effort in epithelial ovarian cancer surgery. J Gynecol Oncol. 2010;21:75–80.
12. Bristow RE, Puri I, Chi DS. Cytoreductive surgery for recurrent ovarian cancer: a meta-analysis. Gynecol Oncol. 2009;112:265–74.
13. Zang RY, Harter P, Chi DS, et al. Predictors of survival in patients with recurrent ovarian cancer undergoing secondary cytoreductive surgery based on the pooled analysis of an international collaborative cohort. Br J Cancer. 2011;105:890–6.
14. Friedlander M, Trimble E, Tinker A, et al. Clinical trials in recurrent ovarian cancer. Int J Gynecol Cancer. 2011;21:771–5.
15. Harter P, du Bois A, Hahmann M, et al. Surgery in recurrent ovarian cancer: the Arbeitsgemeinschaft Gynaekologische Onkologie (AGO) DESKTOP OVAR trial. Ann Surg Oncol. 2006;12:1702–10.
16. Harter P, Sehouli J, Reuss A, et al. Prospective validation study of a predictive score for operability of recurrent ovarian cancer: the Multicenter Intergroup Study DESKTOP II. A project of the AGO Kommission OVAR, AGO study group, NOGGO, AGO- Austria, and MITO. Int J Gynecol Cancer. 2011;21:289–95.

Early Relapse

17. Rose P, Mossbruger K, Fusco N, et al. Gemcitabine reverses cisplatin resistance :demonstration of activity in platinum and multidrug resistant ovarian and peritoneal carcinoma. Gynecol Oncol. 2003;88:17–21.
18. Sharma R, Graham J, Mitchell H, et al. Extended weekly dose-dense paclitaxel/carboplatin is feasible and active in heavily pre-treated platinum-resistant recurrent ovarian cancer. Br J Cancer. 2009;100:707–12.
19. Buda A, Floriani I, Rossi R, et al. Randomised controlled trial comparing single agent paclitaxel vs epidoxorubicin plus paclitaxel in patients with advanced ovarian cancer in early progression after platinum-based chemotherapy: an Italian Collaborative Study from the "Mario Negri" Institute, Milan, G.O.N.O. (Gruppo Oncologico Nord Ovest) group and I.O.R (Istituto Oncologica Romagnolo) group. Br J Cancer. 2004; 90:2112–7.

20. Gordon A, Fleagle J, Guthrie D, et al. Recurrent epithelial ovarian carcinoma: a randomized phase III study of pegylated liposomal doxorubicin versus topotecan. J Clin Oncol. 2001; 19:3312–22.
21. Ten Bokkel Huinink W, Gore M, Carmichael J, et al. Topotecan versus paclitaxel for the treatment of recurrent epithelial ovarian cancer. J Clin Oncol. 1997;15:2183–93.
22. Mutch D, Orlando M, Goss T, et al. Randomized phase III trial of gemcitabine compared with pegylated liposomal doxorubicin in patients with platinum-resistant ovarian cancer. J Clin Oncol. 2007;25:2811–8.
23. Cottu P, Floquet A, Weber B, et al. RPC Saint Paul de Vence: Chimiothérapies (à l'exclusion des thérapies ciblées) et cancer de l'ovaire en rechute. Onko +. 2013;5:33–8.
24. Pujade Lauraine E, Hilpert F, Weber B, et al. Bevacizumab combined with chemotherapy for platinum-resistant recurrent ovarian cancer: the AURELIA open-label randomized phase III trial. J Clin Oncol. 2014;32:1–8.
25. Stockler M, Hilpert F, Friedlander M, et al. Patient reported outcome results from the open label phase III AURELIA trial evaluating bevacizumab containing therapy for platinum resistant ovarian cancer. J Clin Oncol. 2014;32:1309–16.
26. Monk BJ, Poveda A, Vergote I, et al. Anti-angiopoietin therapy with trebananib for recurrent ovarian cancer (TRINOVA-1): a randomised, multicentre, double blind, placebo-controlled phase 3 study. Lancet Oncol. 2014;15:799–808.
27. Pignata S, Lorusso D, Scambia G, et al. Pazopanib plus weekly paclitaxel versus weekly paclitaxel alone for platinum-resistant or platinum-refractory advanced ovarian cancer (MITO 11); a randomised, open label, phase 2 trial. Lancet Oncol. 2015;16:561–8.
28. Ledermann JA, Hackshaw A, Kaye S, et al. Randomized phase II placebo-controlled trial of maintenance therapy using the oral triple angiokinase inhibitor BIBF 1120 after chemotherapy for relapsed ovarian cancer. J Clin Oncol. 2011;29:3798–804.
29. Matulonis UA, Berlin S, Ivy P, et al. Cediranib, an oral inhibitor of vascular endothelial growth factor receptor kinases, is an active drug in recurrent epithelial ovarian, fallopian tube, and peritoneal cancer. J Clin Oncol. 2009;27:5601–6.
30. Monk BJ, Poveda A, Vergote I, et al. Impact of trebananib plus weekly paclitaxel on overall survival (OS) in patients (pts) with recurrent ovarian cancer and ascites: results from the phase III TRINOVA-1 study. J Clin Oncol. 2015;33(Suppl; abstr 5503).

Late Relapse

31. Fung-Kee-Fung M, Oliver T, Elit L, et al. Optimal chemotherapy treatment for women with recurrent ovarian cancer. Curr Oncol. 2007;14:195–208.
32. Parmar MK, Ledermann JA, Colombo N, et al. Paclitaxel plus platinum-based chemotherapy versus conventional platinum-based chemotherapy in women with relapsed ovarian cancer: the ICON4/AGO 2.2 trial. Lancet. 2003;361:2099–106.
33. Ozols RF, Bundy BN, Greer BE, et al. Phase III trial of carboplatin and paclitaxel compared with cisplatin and paclitaxel in patients with optimally resected stage III ovarian cancer; A Gynecologic Oncology Group Study. J Clin Oncol. 2003;21:3194–200.
34. du Bois A, Luck HJ, Meier W, et al. A randomized clinical trial of cisplatin/paclitaxel versus carboplatin/paclitaxel as first line treatment of ovarian cancer. J Natl Cancer Inst. 2003;95: 1320–9.
35. Pfisterer J, Plante M, Vergote I, et al. Gemcitabine plus carboplatin compared with carboplatin in patients with platinum-sensitive recurrent ovarian cancer: an intergroup trial of AGO-OVAR, the NCIC-CTG, and the EORTC GCG. J Clin Oncol. 2006;24:4699–707.
36. Pujade-Lauraine E, Wagner U, Aavall-Lundqvist E, et al. Pegylated liposomal doxorubicin and carboplatin compared with paclitaxel and carboplatin for patients with platinum sensitive ovarian cancer in late relapse. J Clin Oncol. 2010;28:3323–9.

37. Raja FA, Cousell N, Colombo N, et al. Platinum versus platinum combination chemotherapy in platinum-sensitive recurrent ovarian cancer: a meta-analysis using individual patient data. Ann Oncol. 2013;24:3028–34.
38. Monk BJ, Herzog TJ, Kaye SB, et al. Trabectedin plus pegylated liposomal Doxorubicin in recurrent ovarian cancer. J Clin Oncol. 2010;28:3107–14.
39. Poveda A, Vergote I, Tjulandin S, et al. Trabectedin plus pegylated liposomal doxorubicin in relapsed ovarian cancer: outcomes in the partially platinum-sensitive (platinum-free interval 6–12 months) subpopulation of OVA-301 phase III randomized trial. Ann Oncol. 2011;22: 39–48.
40. Aghajanian C, Blank SV, Goff BA, et al. OCEANS: A randomized double-blind, placebo-controlled phase III trial of chemotherapy with or without bevacizumab in patients with platinum-sensitive recurrent epithelial ovarian, primary peritoneal, or fallopian tube cancer. J Clin Oncol. 2012;30(17):2039–45.
41. Ledermann JA, Embleton AC, Raja F, et al. Cediranib in patients with relapsed platinum-sensitive ovarian cancer (ICON6): a randomised, double blind, placebo-controlled phase 3 trial. Lancet. 2016;387:1066–74.
42. Liu JF, Barry WT, Birrer M, et al. A randomized phase 2 study of combination cediranib and olaparib versus olaparib alone as recurrence therapy in platinum-sensitive ovarian cancer. Lancet Oncol. 2014;15:1207–14.
43. Ledermann J, Harter P, Gourley C, et al. Olaparib maintenance therapy in patients with platinum-sensitive relapsed serous ovarian cancer: a preplanned retrospective analysis of outcomes by BRCA status in a randomised phase 2 trial. Lancet Oncol. 2014;15:852–61.

The Future in Ovarian Cancer: Advances in Immunotherapies

11

Amani Makkouk, Cariad Chester, and Holbrook E. Kohrt

Abstract

Recent advances in understanding the role of the immune system in ovarian cancer have culminated in the introduction of multiple promising immunotherapeutic treatment strategies. These include the adoptive transfer of immune effectors such as monoclonal antibodies and T cells, vaccination, and immunomodulatory therapy. In this chapter, we discuss the various therapeutic strategies, their mechanisms of action, and their key clinical trials in ovarian cancer. We also highlight promising combinatorial treatment regimens and present the challenges that are being critically addressed by clinicians and researchers to enhance the efficacy of immunotherapy.

Introduction

Recent advances in understanding the role of the immune system in ovarian cancer have culminated in the introduction of multiple promising immunotherapeutic treatment strategies. Mounting clinical evidence suggested that ovarian cancers are immunogenic, with the early observation that patients with tumor-infiltrating $CD3^+$

A. Makkouk • H.E. Kohrt (✉)
Division of Oncology, Department of Medicine, Stanford University, Stanford, CA 94305, USA
e-mail: amakkouk@stanford.edu; kohrt@stanford.edu

C. Chester
Division of Oncology, Department of Medicine, Stanford University, Stanford, CA 94305, USA

Institute for Immunity, Transplantation and Infection, Stanford University School of Medicine, Stanford, CA 94305, USA

E. Pujade-Lauraine et al. (eds.), *Ovarian Cancers*,
DOI 10.1007/978-3-319-32110-3_11

T cells had improved responses to chemotherapy and increased overall survival [1]. Other studies subsequently confirmed tumor-infiltrating lymphocytes (TILs), specifically CD8 T cells, as predictors of favorable clinical outcome [2–4]. On the other hand, the presence of immunosuppressive $CD4^{+}CD25^{+}Foxp3^{+}$ regulatory T cells (Tregs) in tumors correlated with poor outcome [5]. Furthermore, several tumor-associated antigens (TAAs) recognized by peripheral blood T cells or TILs have been identified, including mutated cell cycle regulatory proteins (p53), cancer-testis antigens (NY-ESO-1), cancer antigens (CA-125), growth-activating receptors (EGFR and HER2/neu), and folate receptors (folate receptor alpha, FRα) [6–9]. These TAAs serve not only as markers of disease progression but also as potential therapeutic targets for several immunotherapies. Lastly, the expression of immune inhibitory receptors such as programmed death 1 (PD-1) on TILs and its ligand (PD-L1) on tumor cells has created opportunities for combination therapies with checkpoint inhibitors [10–12].

This book chapter will review various immunotherapeutic approaches, their mechanisms of action, and their key clinical trials in ovarian cancer. Therapeutic strategies are divided into three categories: adoptive transfer of immune effectors, vaccination, and immunomodulatory therapy.

Immunotherapies for Ovarian Cancer

Adoptive Transfer of Immune Effectors

Immune effectors employed in adoptive transfer include monoclonal antibodies (mAbs) against antigenic targets expressed by tumor cells or within the tumor microenvironment, as well as autologous or allogeneic antitumor T cells (also known as adoptive T-cell therapy or ACT). Both of these approaches bypass the need for in vivo antigen presentation and immune effector proliferation [13].

Monoclonal Antibodies (mAbs)

With the US Food and Drug Administration (FDA) approval of rituximab (anti-CD20) in 1997 for chemotherapy-resistant non-Hodgkin lymphoma, a new era of cancer therapy dawned. The FDA has since approved more than 20 mAbs for clinical use in oncologic care. Based on their antigenic target, mAbs can be classified into mAbs that target tumor cells (direct tumor cell killers), mAbs that target the tumor microenvironment (TME) (TME modifiers), and mAbs that target immune checkpoints (checkpoint inhibitors), among others [14, 15]. mAbs have shown promise in ovarian cancer and are increasingly being examined in clinical trials. The latter category of mAbs (checkpoint inhibitors) will be discussed in section "Depleting Tregs".

In addition to neutralizing the function of their antigenic targets by inhibiting their signaling pathways (such as tumor growth and angiogenesis), mAbs can modulate the immune response against tumor cells, such as increasing dendritic cell (DC) maturation, priming effector cells (T cells and natural killer "NK" cells), and activating complement-dependent cytotoxicity (CDC) and antibody-dependent cell-mediated cytotoxicity (ADCC) pathways. Conjugation to antineoplastic toxins in antibody-drug conjugates (ADCs) bestows additional cytotoxic activity to mAbs and allows more precise delivery of chemotherapy following their binding to target antigen and subsequent internalization into tumor cells [16, 17].

mAbs Targeting Tumor Cells

Anti-EGFR (Cetuximab and Panitumumab)

The epidermal growth factor receptor (EGFR) is overexpressed by 9–62 % of ovarian cancers and has been associated with high tumor grade and poor patient outcome [18]. Cetuximab (Erbitux®, BMS and Eli Lilly) is an FDA-approved chimeric IgG1 mAb that binds to the extracellular domain of EGFR, preventing EGFR signaling and promoting receptor internalization and ubiquitin-mediated degradation [19, 20]. Single-agent studies of cetuximab reported minimal activity. In a phase II trial of weekly cetuximab monotherapy in patients with persistent/recurrent ovarian or primary peritoneal carcinoma, none of the 25 patients achieved complete response (CR), 9 patients had stable disease (SD), and only one patient achieved a partial response (PR) [21]. On the other hand, cetuximab in combination with chemotherapy showed only modest activity. In a phase II trial of cetuximab and carboplatin in patients with relapsed, platinum-sensitive ovarian cancer, 9 of the 26 patients with EGFR-positive tumors developed an objective response (OR) and eight had SD. Additionally, response to this treatment regimen did not correlate with tumor EGFR expression and was associated with dermatologic toxicity in the majority of patients [22]. These observations highlight the need for developing effective combination therapies with chemotherapy and for determining more robust predictors for patient responsiveness in order to improve responses to anti-EGFR therapy and patient outcomes [18].

Panitumumab (Vectibix®, Amgen) is another FDA-approved anti-EGFR mAb of the IgG2 isotype that has shown encouraging results in a recent phase II clinical trial. In patients with platinum-resistant ovarian cancer, the combination of panitumumab and the chemotherapeutic pegylated liposomal doxorubicin (PLD) demonstrated 9 % PR and 19 % SD [23]. It should be mentioned that in the intent-to-treat population, the overall response rate (18.7 %) was similar to that reported in other phase II clinical trials of monotherapy with PLD in patients with platinum-refractory/platinum-resistant disease (19.7 %) [24].

Anti-mesothelin (Amatuximab) and Anti-CA-125 (Abagovomab and Oregovomab)

The high frequency of expression of the TAAs mesothelin and CA-125 in ovarian cancer has made them potential targets for mAb therapy. Mesothelin is a glycosylphosphatidylinositol (GPI)-anchored cell surface protein that is involved in tumor resistance to several chemotherapeutic drugs and in promoting tumor metastasis through its interaction with the mucin CA-125 [25]. CA-125 (also known as MUC16) is a TAA that is also overexpressed in ovarian cancer. CA-125 can be proteolytically cleaved from the tumor cell surface and has been employed as a serum biomarker to screen for ovarian cancer as well as to monitor responses to therapy. In addition to promoting tumor invasion and metastasis, CA-125 exerts immunosuppressive activity through protecting tumor cells from NK cell attack [26]. Attempts at targeting the mesothelin-MUC16 interaction using mAbs have met limited success. In a phase I trial in patients with mesothelin-expressing tumors (including four with ovarian cancer) receiving amatuximab (anti-mesothelin chimeric IgG1 mAb, MORAb-009, Morphotek), no CR or PR was seen [27]. Amatuximab is currently in a phase II trial for mesothelioma patients. Abagovomab (anti-idiotypic CA-125 murine IgG1 mAb) and oregovomab (anti-CA-125 murine IgG1 mAb, OvaRex®, AltaRex) failed to show a survival benefit in large clinical trials [28–30]. Oregovomab is currently in a phase II trial in combination with chemotherapy for patients with advanced epithelial ovarian cancer (NCT01616303). ADCs may prove a more promising strategy and are being explored in preclinical studies and ongoing clinical trials, as will be discussed.

Anti-FRα (Farletuzumab)

FRα is widely expressed on epithelial ovarian cancers, especially in platinum-resistant patients, but not on normal ovarian tissues [31, 32]. Farletuzumab (Morphotek) is an investigational humanized IgG1 anti-FRα mAb that mediates tumor cell cytotoxicity via CDC and ADCC rather than blocking folate transport [32]. In a phase II trial in platinum-sensitive ovarian cancer patients experiencing a first relapse, farletuzumab alone was poorly effective but when combined with chemotherapy (carboplatin and taxanes) improved objective response rates (ORR) to 75 %. Additionally, 80.9 % of patients normalized CA-125 [33]. However, a recent phase III trial was discontinued after farletuzumab in combination with paclitaxel failed to meet its end point of improving progression-free survival (PFS) in platinum-resistant ovarian cancer patients. Since a trend toward improved PFS was observed, additional analyses will be required to determine whether farletuzumab may improve outcome for patients [34]. In 2015, a phase II trial was launched to assess the combination of farletuzumab with carboplatin and paclitaxel or PLD in patients with low CA-125 platinum-sensitive ovarian cancer (NCT02289950).

mAbs Targeting Tumor Microenvironment

Anti-VEGF (Bevacizumab)

The vascular endothelial growth factor (VEGF) binds to its receptors on endothelial cells and activates signaling pathways that regulate normal development of the vasculature as well as pathologic angiogenesis in cancer [35]. In ovarian cancer, tumor VEGF gene expression correlates with a poor prognosis [36]. Bevacizumab (Avastin®, Roche) is a humanized IgG1 anti-VEGF mAb that can neutralize all isoforms of VEGF. In addition to its antiangiogenic activity, bevacizumab can also modulate the immune response by increasing DC maturation and priming of T cells, as demonstrated in multiple myeloma and melanoma [37, 38]. Bevacizumab is active in platinum-resistant ovarian cancer, both as monotherapy and in combination with chemotherapy [39–42]. In the phase III AURELIA trial in platinum-resistant ovarian cancer, combining bevacizumab with chemotherapy improved PFS (increased from 3.4 to 6.7 months) and ORR (increased from 11 to 27 %) [43].

Anti-TAMs (Anti-CSF-1R, Anti-CCL22, and Anti-B7-H4)

Similar to DCs, macrophages are phagocytic innate immune cells that can, to a lesser extent, induce T-cell activation. Macrophages are broadly classified into classical (M1-polarized) and alternative (M2-polarized) phenotypes. M1 macrophages are involved in Th1 responses through antigen presentation and secretion of immunostimulatory cytokines such as interleukins 6 and 12 (IL-6 and IL-12), while M2 macrophages are involved in Th2 responses through secretion of immunosuppressive cytokines such as IL-10 and transforming growth factor β (TGF-β). Tumor-associated macrophages (TAMs) are a major component of the TME and, in agreement with the M2 signature, have been associated with enhanced tumor progression, angiogenesis, and immunosuppression [44]. M2 TAMs are abundantly present in ovarian cancers and malignant ascites, and their numbers correlate with malignancy, while elevated M1 to M2 TAM ratios correlate with improved 5-year prognosis [45–47].

The macrophage colony-stimulating factor-1 receptor (CSF-1R) binds CSF-1 (also known as macrophage CSF or M-CSF) and is involved in regulating macrophage migration, proliferation, survival, and function [48]. Inhibiting CSF-1R activation using an antagonistic mAb has been shown in preclinical murine tumor models of high TAM infiltration to strongly reduce TAMs and enhance the CD8/CD4 T-cell ratio [49]. RG7155 (by Roche) is an investigational humanized anti-CSF-1R mAb that has recently entered clinical trials. In an ongoing phase Ia/Ib trial in patients with tenosynovial giant cell tumor (NCT01494688), RG7155 markedly reduced TAMs and was well tolerated [50]. CSF-1R blockade may thus be a promising strategy for depleting TAMs in ovarian cancer.

Another promising strategy is to modulate TAM-T-cell interactions in the TME. TAMs can recruit Tregs to the TME through the chemokine CCL22, which in turn suppresses tumor-specific T-cell immunity. In xenograft models of primary human ovarian tumors, neutralizing CCL22 using anti-CCL22 mAb inhibited Treg migration to tumors [5]. Tregs can also secrete IL-10, which can stimulate the expression of the checkpoint B7-H4 on macrophages. B7-H4 is expressed by >70 % of freshly isolated TAMs and negatively regulates T-cell responses [51, 52]. It is also expressed by ovarian cancer tumor cells, but only B7-$H4^+$ macrophages suppress T-cell immunity and are negatively associated with patient outcome [52, 53]. Blocking B7-H4 interactions with single-chain fragments of antibody variable regions (scFvs) rescued tumor antigen-specific T-cell activation in vitro and delayed the growth of established tumors in mice [54]. The use of mAbs to reverse TAM-mediated immunosuppression represents a promising therapeutic approach to enhance T-cell tumor immunity in ovarian cancer.

Bispecific Antibodies

Anti-EpCAM × Anti-CD3 (Catumaxomab)

The epithelial cell adhesion molecule (EpCAM) is a transmembrane glycoprotein mediating calcium-independent cell-cell adhesion in the epithelium. It is overexpressed in primary, metastatic, and recurrent epithelial ovarian cancers across subtypes and has been associated with poor prognosis [55–58]. In ovarian cancer-associated malignant ascites, EpCAM is expressed by tumor cells in 70–100 % of cases [59]. Catumaxomab (Removab®, Fresenius Biotech GmbH) is a chimeric, bispecific, trifunctional antibody that binds to epithelial tumor cells via EpCAM and to T cells via CD3, facilitating the localization of T cells to the tumor tissue. Additionally, catumaxomab has a functional Fc domain (composed of mouse IgG2a and rat IgG2b) that can activate Fc receptor-expressing NK cells and mediate tumor cell cytotoxicity via ADCC [60, 61]. In a randomized phase II/III trial in patients with malignant ascites (including 129 ovarian cancer patients), catumaxomab prolonged puncture-free survival (PuFI: time to first need for paracentesis after treatment or time to death, whichever occurred first) [59] and received market approval by the European Medicines Agency (EMA) for this indication. In a recent phase II trial in chemotherapy-refractory ovarian cancer patients with malignant ascites, catumaxomab prolonged both the PuFI and the time to first therapeutic puncture (TTPu) and had a beneficial effect on the quality of life through improving ascites symptoms [62].

ADCs

Anti-mesothelin Conjugated to DM4 (Anetumab Ravtansine) and Anti-CA-125 Conjugated to MMAE (Sofituzumab Vedotin)

Anetumab ravtansine (BAY 94–9343, Bayer) is an ADC that consists of a human anti-mesothelin IgG1 mAb conjugated to the microtubule-targeting drug DM4 via a reducible disulfide linker. Following binding and internalization by tumor cells, degradation of the linker releases a cytotoxic DM4 metabolite. Anetumab ravtansine was superior to standard-of-care treatments in patient-derived xenograft models of ovarian cancer and led to complete eradication. Furthermore, its efficacy correlated with the expression level of mesothelin [63, 64]. Currently, anetumab ravtansine is being evaluated in a phase I clinical trial (NCT01439152).

Sofituzumab vedotin (RG7458 or DMUC5754A, Roche/Genentech) consists of a humanized anti-CA-125 IgG1 mAb conjugated to the microtubule-targeting drug monomethyl auristatin E (MMAE) via a protease-cleavable peptide linker. In a phase I trial in 44 patients with platinum-resistant ovarian cancer (NCT01335958), sofituzumab vedotin demonstrated a toxicity profile that was comparable to other current therapeutics and led to 1 CR and 4 PR. Similar to anetumab ravtansine, its efficacy correlated with the TAA expression level [65].

Anti-FRα Conjugated to DM4 (Mirvetuximab Soravtansine)

Mirvetuximab soravtansine (IMGN853, ImmunoGen) consists of a chimeric anti-FRα IgG1 mAb conjugated to DM4 via a reducible disulfide linker. Preclinical studies in xenograft models showed that the ADC efficiently targeted FRα⁺ tumors and was also cytotoxic to adjacent FRα⁻ tumor cells (bystander effect), reflecting an ability to eradicate tumors with heterogeneous expression of FRα [66]. In an ongoing phase I trial in patients with platinum-resistant epithelial ovarian cancer (NCT01609556), mirvetuximab soravtansine as a single agent demonstrated promising preliminary clinical activity with an ORR of 53 % in the overall cohort and 80 % in the high FRα expression subset. Preliminary analysis suggested that FRα expression correlates well with ADC activity [67, 68]. Other ongoing trials are comparing the efficacy of mirvetuximab soravtansine to chemotherapy in patients with FRα⁺ advanced epithelial ovarian cancer (NCT02631876) or combining it with chemotherapy (NCT02606305).

Adoptive T-Cell Therapy (ACT)

Adoptive T-cell therapy (ACT) involves using ex vivo activated tumor-specific T cells that are either derived from tumors (TILs) and enriched for particular antigen specificity or are genetically engineered to express either tumor-specific T-cell receptors (TCRs) or chimeric antigen receptors (CARs). Prior to reinfusion into the cancer patient, cells are expanded with IL-2, and lymphodepleting chemotherapy and/or radiotherapy is administered to promote the in vivo survival and expansion of adoptively transferred T cells by increasing cytokines and antigen-presenting cell (APC) activity and eliminating immunosuppressive cells [69, 70]. Ongoing intensive research aims to improve this attractive (albeit labor-intensive and expensive) approach by improving T-cell constructs, automating T-cell generation, and optimizing toxicity management [13].

TILs

The use of TILs for ACT benefits from the natural selection of patient TMEs to polyclonal, tumor-specific T cells which have escaped thymic deletion and homed to tumors [71]. In the 1990s, the adoptive transfer of TILs expanded ex vivo with IL-2 was examined in ovarian cancer [72–74]. Aoki et al. reported that in 17 patients with advanced or recurrent ovarian cancer, ACT alone administered to seven patients led to 1 CR and 4 PR, while ACT administered to ten patients in conjunction with cisplatin led to 7 CR and 2 PR [73]. In a pivotal trial, Fujita et al. reported that in patients with advanced-stage epithelial ovarian cancer, ACT after optimal debulking surgery and cisplatin chemotherapy improved the 3-year overall survival rates to 100 % versus 67.5 % for patients not receiving ACT [74]. The drawbacks of ACT using TILs are numerous, including tolerance to self-antigens and the low yield of tumor-specific lymphocytes for ex vivo expansion [75]. Attempts to overcome these drawbacks have led to the use of genetically engineered T cells from peripheral blood for ACT.

Genetically Engineered T Cells

To redirect the T-cell specificity of normal peripheral blood lymphocytes (PBLs), T cells are genetically modified to recognize TAA using viral vectors encoding for either TCRs (which are MHC-restricted) or CARs. In CARs, TCR intracellular signaling domains are coupled with surface variable regions of antibodies; CARs can thus recognize TAA in an MHC-unrestricted fashion and their activation is enhanced upon TAA contact [70]. A phase I/IIa trial is currently ongoing for ACT with TCRs recognizing the TAA NY-ESO-1 in patients with recurrent or treatment-refractory ovarian cancer carrying the HLA-A201 allele (NCT01567891). In addition, several CAR trials are under way. The first trial was conducted in 2006 in 14 patients with advanced FRα$^+$ ovarian cancer using FRα-specific CARs. However, transferred CARs were undetectable at 1 month, and no clinical benefit was observed [76]. The addition of costimulatory signaling capabilities to the intracytoplasmic domain of CARs (such as CD137) has improved in vivo CAR persistence and activity [77, 78]. Mesothelin-specific CARs are also being pursued in ovarian cancer. In an ongoing phase I trial in patients with mesothelin-expressing tumors (including two with ovarian cancer), CARs were adoptively transferred without lymphodepletion and were found to traffic to tumor sites and to persist in the blood for 3–4 weeks post infusion [79]. Other trials are also ongoing (NCT02159716 and NCT01583686).

Vaccination

Therapeutic cancer vaccines aim to "teach" the immune system to recognize tumor cells through supplying whole tumor cells or tumor-derived peptides. These are provided together with immune adjuvants, including pattern recognition receptor ligands (such as poly-ICLC and the incomplete Freund's adjuvant Montanide) and granulocyte-macrophage colony-stimulating factor (GM-CSF), to promote DC activity. Unlike passive immunotherapy with adoptively transferred mAbs or T cells, vaccines are an active immunotherapy strategy that can generate long-lasting immunological memory. The convenience and low toxicity have made vaccines an attractive approach in ovarian cancer as in other types of cancer. Nonetheless, limited efficacy has been observed [6, 80]. Efforts to improve performance include optimizing target antigens, improving vaccine platforms by using DCs and oncolytic viruses, and developing combinatorial approaches with immunomodulatory therapy (the latter will be discussed in section "Combination Therapies").

Vaccination Based on Tumor Peptides or Tumor Cells

Peptide Vaccines

Peptide vaccines employ short peptides from TAAs that can directly bind to exact HLA class I molecules on DCs, bypassing the need for antigen processing and generating CD8 T-cell responses (albeit short-lived). In addition to using adjuvants to increase peptide immunogenicity, recent advances in improving the efficacy of peptide vaccines include the use of synthetic or overlapping long peptides, which require antigen processing by DCs but are efficiently presented to both CD4 and CD8 T cells [81].

NY-ESO-1

NY-ESO-1 is an immunogenic TAA that is expressed by 40 % of epithelial ovarian cancers and generates antibody and cellular immune responses in multiple cancer patients [82, 83]. In a pilot study of patients with advanced ovarian cancer and minimal disease burden, administration of NY-ESO-1 peptide of HLA class I/II specificities with Montanide induced both NY-ESO-1-specific CD4 and CD8 T-cell responses in the majority of patients and improved PFS. Importantly, a patient who experienced complete regression had a recurrence later with an NY-ESO-1-negative tumor, highlighting the drawback of immune escape tumor variants with peptide (single target) vaccines [84]. In a phase I trial in high-risk ovarian cancer patients in their first remission, NY-ESO-1 peptide with Montanide led to NY-ESO-1-specific CD8 T-cell responses in both NY-ESO-1-positive and NY-ESO-1-negative tumors and CR in 33 % of patients [85]. A phase I trial in 28 patients with advanced ovarian cancer in second or third remission examined overlapping long peptides (OLPs) from NY-ESO-1 either alone or in combination with Montanide or Montanide and poly-ICLC. Antibody and CD8 T-cell responses specific to NY-ESO-1 were undetectable with OLP alone but were detected in 91 % of patients receiving OLP and both adjuvants, where each had a distinct effect for the induction of NY-ESO-1-specific Th1 cells [86, 87]. Recently, a phase I trial in 12 patients with relapsed ovarian cancer examined the effect of adding decitabine (a DNA methyltransferase inhibitor) as an epigenetic modifier to NY-ESO-1 peptide vaccine administered with the adjuvants Montanide and GM-CSF and the chemotherapeutic liposomal doxorubicin. Increased NY-ESO-1 serum antibodies and T-cell responses were observed in the majority of patients, while SD or PR was noted in six out of ten evaluable patients [88].

p53

p53 is a protein that is encoded by the tumor suppressor gene *TP53* and regulates the fate of cells upon DNA damage [89]. p53 is overexpressed in 50–60 % of ovarian cancers, and the presence of p53 antibodies has been identified as a positive prognostic factor in ovarian cancer patients [90, 91]. In addition, circulating and tumor-infiltrating p53-specific memory T cells were detected in patients with ovarian cancer [92]. In a phase II trial in patients with advanced-stage ovarian cancer, a p53 peptide vaccine administered with IL-2, GM-CSF, and Montanide as adjuvants led to immune responses (as measured by interferon γ (IFN-γ) production and tetramer assays). However, IL-2 administration increased toxicity and induced Treg expansion, leading the authors to suggest the removal of IL-2 from this vaccine regimen. Importantly, the trial found that the subcutaneous p53 peptide vaccine had a similar efficacy to an intravenous vaccine of DCs pulsed with p53 peptides, suggesting that the peptide vaccine is a superior choice given its simpler approach in preparation and administration [93]. Another phase II trial examined p53 synthetic long peptides (p53-SLP) with Montanide in patients with recurrent ovarian cancer. While IFN-γ-producing p53-specific CD4 T cells were induced, Th2 cytokines dominated the p53-specific response, and no improvement in clinical outcome was observed [94, 95].

HER-2/neu

A phase I trial in 19 patients with breast or ovarian cancer showed that vaccination with HER-2/neu-derived MHC class II "helper" peptides, which contain MHC class I epitopes, administered with GM-CSF as adjuvant induced potent and long-lasting HER-2-specific IFN-γ-producing CD8 T cells. A larger, phase I trial examined HER-2/neu peptides with GM-CSF in patients with advanced HER-2/neu$^+$ cancers (including five patients with ovarian cancer). The vaccine induced HER-2/neu-specific T-cell responses in 92 % of patients. Importantly, the responses were long-lived, and epitope spreading to additional HER-2/neu epitopes and to p53, was observed in some patients [96, 97].

Tumor Cell Vaccines

Personalized vaccines based on whole tumor cells represent an alternative to peptide vaccines that allow the generation of a diverse immune response directed at multiple TAAs. Because they incorporate both MHC class I and class II epitopes, tumor cell vaccines can limit tumor escape variants. On the other hand, using whole tumor cells carries the risk of stimulating tolerogenic or autoimmune, rather than immunogenic, responses due to the significant presence of self-antigens [98]. The FANG vaccine represents an elegant approach to enhance the immunogenicity of whole tumor cells. It is composed of autologous tumor cells genetically modified to encode GM-CSF (as an adjuvant) and a bifunctional short hairpin RNAi that inhibits TGF-β by targeting furin transferase. In a phase I trial that included five patients with ovarian cancer, the vaccine was safe and elicited an immune response correlating with prolonged survival [99]. A follow-up phase II/III trial is currently ongoing in patients with advanced ovarian cancer achieving CR following primary surgical debulking and chemotherapy (NCT02346747). Preliminary results show that 92 % of vaccinated patients developed immunity (as measured by IFN-γ production), and the median regression-free survival (RFS) was 399 days versus 94 days for control patients [99, 100].

Vaccination Based on DCs

DC-based vaccines were developed to overcome the low number and/or defective ability of DCs in cancer patients to process and present tumor antigens. Autologous DCs are generated ex vivo from peripheral blood monocytes in the presence of cytokine and growth factor cocktails that induce DC expansion and maturation. DCs are then loaded with TAAs or whole tumor lysates prior to reinfusion into patients [101].

A promising TAA for DC-based vaccines is mucin 1 (MUC-1), a heavily glycosylated surface protein that is overexpressed and aberrantly glycosylated in a large number of cancers including ovarian cancer [102]. In a phase I trial in advanced-stage ovarian cancer patients, DCs pulsed with MUC-1 peptides generated tumor-specific CD8 T cells [103]. A phase II study examined the CVac® vaccine (Prima BioMed) of MUC-1-loaded DCs in 63 patients with epithelial ovarian cancer in complete remission. In patients who had achieved a remission after second-line therapy, PFS and OS were improved with the CVac vaccine as compared to patients receiving standard-of-care therapy [104]. Another potential TAA is HER-2/neu. A phase I trial involving four ovarian cancer patients evaluated lapuleucel-T (Neuvenge®, Dendreon), a DC-based vaccine composed of autologous peripheral blood mononuclear cells (including APCs) cultured ex vivo with HER-2/neu peptides linked to GM-CSF. The vaccine generated HER-2-specific T-cell responses and led to short-term SD in two of the four patients [105].

DCs loaded with whole tumor lysates have also shown promise in ovarian cancer. In a phase I trial in six patients with recurrent advanced ovarian cancer, patients received DCs pulsed with whole tumor lysates and keyhole limpet hemocyanin (KLH) as an adjuvant. The treatment was well tolerated, and three of the six patients showed PFS of 25–45 weeks [106]. A phase II trial further examined the tumor lysate-pulsed DCs and KLH that was administered with low-dose IL-2 as an adjuvant in ten ovarian cancer patients with minimal residual disease. The vaccine resulted in 3 CR for 38–83 months and induced tumor-related immunity in responders, including NK cell activity and IFN-γ-producing T cells [107]. In another pilot study in five patients with recurrent ovarian cancer, DCs pulsed with tumor lysates oxidized with hypochlorous acid (which enhances immunogenicity), two patients had a PFS of 24 months or more [108].

Vaccination Based on Viruses

Recombinant viral vaccines are attractive TAA delivery systems due to their inherent immunogenicity and ability to exploit DC trafficking to the injection site for enhanced TAA uptake and presentation. Commonly employed viral vectors are members of the *Poxviridae* family and include vaccinia and fowlpox viruses. The vaccinia vector induces strong cellular and humoral immune responses to the transgene it encodes but is limited by the development of host-induced neutralizing antibodies to the vector itself and by the exclusion of use in immunocompromised patients. On the other hand, fowlpox viruses can be administered in booster doses due to absence of neutralizing antibody development but are less efficient than vaccinia vectors in inducing immune responses [109].

In a pilot study involving three ovarian cancer patients, the PANVAC vaccine regimen was evaluated. It consisted of the transgenes for the TAAs carcinoembryonic antigen (CEA) and MUC-1 along with the transgenes for the TRICOM adjuvant (the costimulatory molecule CD80, intercellular adhesion molecule-1 (ICAM-1), and leukocyte function-associated antigen-3 (LFA-3)) engineered into vaccinia (PANVAC-V) as a prime and fowlpox (PANVAC-F) as booster vaccinations. Immune responses to MUC-1 and/or CEA were observed post vaccination [110]. In a follow-up study involving 14 patients with ovarian cancer, median OS was 15 months in patients receiving the PANVAC vaccine, and those with limited tumor burden and minimal prior chemotherapy seemed to derive the most benefit [111]. Another heterologous prime-boost vaccine regimen was recently examined in a phase II trial in 22 patients with advanced ovarian cancer in clinical remission. Patients received NY-ESO-1-vaccinia as a prime and NY-ESO-1-fowlpox as booster vaccinations. CD4 and CD8 T-cell responses were induced and found to correlate with improved OS. Ovarian cancer patients showed a median PFS and OS of 21 and 48 months, respectively [112].

Immunomodulatory Therapy

Immunomodulatory therapy aims to tip the balance in the immunosuppressive TME from immune tolerance to immune reactivity. The traditional use of cytokines, including IL-2, IL-12, type I and II IFNs, and tumor necrosis factor α (TNF-α), as immunotherapeutic agents that broadly activate T cells has proven challenging due to systemic toxicity and has met with limited success in ovarian cancer [6, 113]. T-cell activation is regulated not only by costimulatory receptors (including CD28 and CD137) but also by inhibitory receptors or checkpoints, which are induced following TCR stimulation (Fig. 11.1). Therapeutic approaches that block the suppressive signals of checkpoints (checkpoint blockade) or selectively target

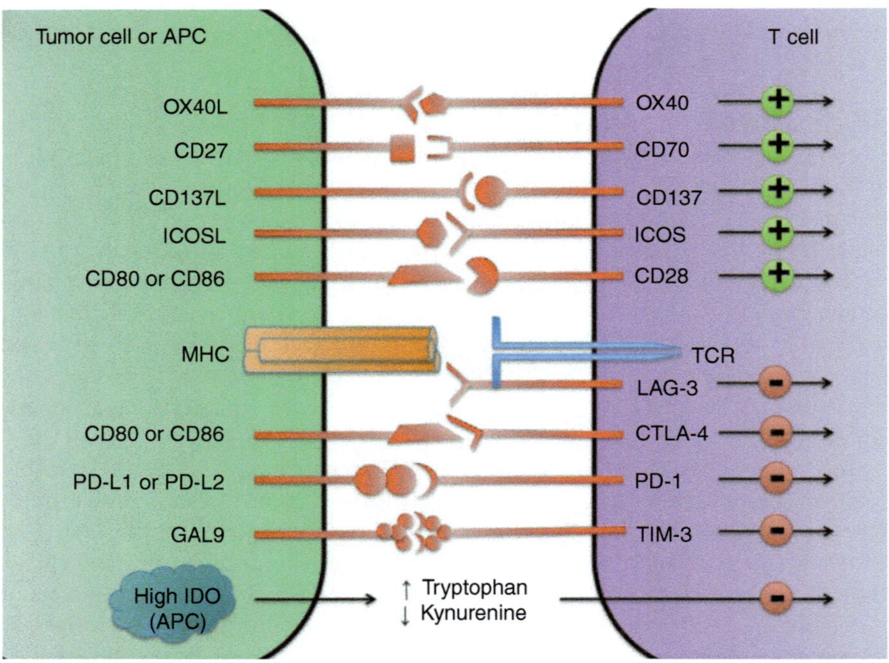

Fig. 11.1 The major T cell-based immunotherapeutic targets and their tumor or antigen-presenting cell ligands. The activation of T cells and their conversion to a cytotoxic phenotype is governed by a network of activating and inhibitory receptors. Using immunotherapeutic agents to increase activation and decrease inhibitory signaling has the potential to generate T cells with enhanced tumor lytic capacity. *APC* antigen-presenting cell, *GAL* galectin-9, *IDO* indoleamine 2,3-dioxygenase, *ICOS* inducible T-cell costimulator, *MHC* major histocompatibility complex, *PD-1* programmed death 1, *PD-L* PD-1 ligand, *TCR* T-cell receptor, *TIM-3* T-cell immunoglobulin and mucin domain 3

immunosuppressive cells in the TME (such as Tregs) can sustain the activation and proliferation of tumor-specific T cells and represent one of the most rapidly moving and exciting areas in clinical oncology.

Depleting Tregs

Targeting CD25: Anti-CD25 (Daclizumab) and Denileukin Diftitox

Tregs constitutively express the IL-2 receptor α chain (CD25). Daclizumab (Zenapax®, F. Hoffmann-La Roche) is an FDA-approved humanized IgG1 mAb that binds to CD25. Traditionally used to inhibit T-cell proliferation in autoimmune disorders, it has recently been used to deplete Tregs in combination with a metastatic breast cancer vaccine. Daclizumab administration led to a marked and prolonged decrease in Tregs and boosted T-cell responses to all vaccine antigens in absence of autoimmunity [114]. Daclizumab is currently being evaluated in combination with a DC-based vaccine in ovarian cancer (NCT01132014). Another approach to targeting CD25 is through denileukin diftitox (Ontak®, Eisai), an FDA-approved engineered fusion protein of IL-2 and diphtheria toxin. In a recent phase II trial of 28 patients with epithelial ovarian cancer, denileukin diftitox administration was well tolerated and significantly depleted functional Tregs from blood and the TME, but showed no significant clinical efficacy [115]. Combination strategies with checkpoint blockade may improve clinical efficacy and have shown promise in preclinical studies [116].

Cyclophosphamide

Cyclophosphamide is a chemotherapeutic agent that has immunomodulatory activity when administered in repeated, low doses (metronomically). It depletes Tregs and restores T-cell function and has been used to augment antitumor immune responses of ACT and vaccination strategies [117]. In a phase I/II trial in 11 patients with recurrent ovarian cancer, a single low dose of cyclophosphamide was explored as an adjuvant to a vaccine regimen of peptide-pulsed DCs. While the 3-year OS was 90 %, the single dose of cyclophosphamide did not reduce the number of circulating Tregs, and no significant survival benefit over controls was observed [118]. In another phase II trial in patients with recurrent ovarian cancer, low-dose cyclophosphamide administered prior to each dose of the p53-SLP vaccine led to p53-specific IFN-γ-producing T cells in 90 % of evaluable patients after two immunizations [119].

Checkpoint Blockade

Immune checkpoints tightly regulate the intensity and duration of the T-cell response and are critical for avoiding autoimmunity. These include the T-cell surface molecules cytotoxic T-lymphocyte antigen 4 (CTLA-4), programmed death 1 (PD-1), T-cell immunoglobulin and mucin domain-containing protein 3 (TIM-3), and lymphocyte activation gene-3 (LAG-3). In addition, the metabolic enzyme indoleamine 2,3-dioxygenase (IDO), which catalyzes the rate-limiting step of the oxidative catabolism of the amino acid tryptophan, regulates T-cell activation. By depleting tryptophan and generating the toxic metabolite kynurenine, IDO can inhibit T-cell proliferation and trigger cell cycle arrest and apoptosis. Kynurenine can also induce naive CD4 T cells into Tregs [120–123].

Activation of immune checkpoint pathways in the TME, however, limits the antitumor immune response. TILs upregulating the expression of checkpoints are hyporesponsive or functionally exhausted [124]. In patients with ovarian cancer, a significant fraction of antigen-specific CD8 TILs co-express LAG-3 and PD-1 and demonstrate impaired effector function [125]. Additionally, Tregs naturally express checkpoints and employ them to suppress effector T cells [124]. Moreover, 56 % of ovarian tumors have demonstrated IDO expression, which correlated with a reduced number of CD8 TILs and with reduced survival in serous (but not other) ovarian cancer histologies [126, 127]. IDO expression was also found to inhibit NK cell intratumoral accumulation and to promote tumor angiogenesis [128]. Reversing TME-mediated immunosuppression via targeting checkpoints with mAbs or inhibitors, an approach coined "checkpoint blockade," was found to boost immune responses and is becoming increasingly valuable in the clinic.

Anti-CTLA-4 (Ipilimumab)

CTLA-4 (CD152) is an inhibitory co-receptor and member of the B7-CD28 immunoglobulin superfamily. It competes with the costimulatory receptor CD28 for the ligands (B7 molecules) on APCs, leading to downregulation of T-cell activation. Ipilimumab (Yervoy®, BMS) is an FDA-approved human IgG1 mAb that blocks the CTLA-4/B7 interaction to restore CD4 and CD8 effector T-cell activation and can also deplete tumor-infiltrating Tregs [129, 130]. Ipilimumab represents the first standard-of-care immune checkpoint inhibitor, and the majority of clinical experience is derived from studies in patients with melanoma. In a pilot study in two patients with advanced ovarian cancer previously vaccinated with GM-CSF-modified irradiated autologous tumor cells (GVAX), a single dose of ipilimumab triggered a decrease or stabilization of CA-125 levels for several months [131]. In a subsequent study in additional nine patients, three patients had SD, and the extent of therapy-induced tumor necrosis correlated with the intratumoral CD8 T-cell/Treg ratio [132]. An ongoing phase II trial is studying ipilimumab as monotherapy in patients with recurrent platinum-sensitive ovarian cancer (NCT01611558). The primary drawback of ipilimumab is the high frequency of immune-related adverse events (irAEs) like colitis or hypophysitis: approximately 25 % of patients experience an irAE, requiring aggressive management [133].

Anti-PD-1 (Nivolumab and Pembrolizumab) and Anti-PD-L1 (Several mAbs)

PD-1 is another co-inhibitory receptor member of the CD28/B7 immunoglobulin superfamily that binds to its ligands PD-L1 and PD-L2 (mainly expressed by epithelial cells, DCs, and macrophages) to down-modulate the immune response [124]. In addition to the high expression of PD-1 by TILs in ovarian tumors [10, 125], PD-L1 was also found to be highly expressed by ovarian tumor cells and is negatively correlated with CD8 TIL counts and with survival [11]. PD-L1 tumor expression has also been implicated in promoting peritoneal dissemination of ovarian cancer [12]. The blockade of the PD-1 inhibitory pathway is being clinically explored using mAbs targeting either the receptor or its ligands and has so far proven less immunotoxic than ipilimumab.

Nivolumab (Opdivo®, BMS) is an FDA-approved human IgG4 anti-PD-1 mAb that is being investigated in ovarian cancer. In a phase I trial in 15 patients with advanced platinum-resistant ovarian cancer (regardless of PD-L1 expression), nivolumab was well tolerated and led to 3 PR and 4 SD, with an ORR of 17 % [134]. In a recent update, 2 patients with CR survived without disease progression for 17 and 14 months each [135]. Another anti-PD-1 mAb is pembrolizumab (Keytruda®, Merck), an FDA-approved humanized IgG4 mAb. In a recent interim analysis of a phase Ib trial in 26 patients with heavily treated PD-L1$^+$ advanced ovarian cancer, pembrolizumab was well tolerated and achieved 1 CR, 2 PR, and 6 SD with a durable ORR of 11.5 % [136].

Several mAbs that block PD-L1 are being investigated in numerous clinical trials that include ovarian cancer patients. Examples include avelumab (MSB0010718C, human IgG1, Merck Serono), BMS-936559 (human IgG4, BMS-ONO), MPDL3280A (human IgG1, Roche/Genetech), and durvalumab (MEDI4736, human IgG1, MedImmune). In an ongoing phase Ib trial in 75 patients with platinum-resistant or chemotherapy-refractory ovarian cancer (regardless of PD-L1 expression), avelumab demonstrated an acceptable safety profile and had an ORR of 10.7 % in 67 evaluable patients [137]. In a phase I trial involving 17 patients with ovarian cancer, BMS-936559 demonstrated safety and led to 1 PR and 3 SD lasting at least 24 weeks [138].

IDO Inhibitors (Indoximod, GDC-0919, and Epacadostat)

Indoximod (D-1-methyl-tryptophan (D-1-MT), NewLink Genetics) is the first small-molecule IDO inhibitor to enter clinical trials. Preclinical studies in murine models of ovarian cancer have shown that IDO inhibition with the racemic compound 1-MT is synergistic with chemotherapy and that the D (but not the L) racemer is responsible for the majority of antitumor activity [139, 140]. Another IDO inhibitor is the second-generation GDC-0919 (formerly NLG919, NewLink Genetics/Genentech) which specifically inhibits IDO1. Both inhibitors are currently being examined in several clinical trials for solid tumors. A third is the IDO1 inhibitor epacadostat (INCB024360, Incyte Corporation) that is in several clinical trials for ovarian cancer either as monotherapy (NCT01685255 and NCT02042430) or in combination with peptide vaccines (NCT02166905 and NCT02575807) or checkpoint blockade (NCT02178722 and NCT02327078). In a phase I trial in patients with advanced malignancies including ovarian cancer, 90 % inhibition of IDO activity was achieved [141].

Combination Therapies

Combination immunotherapies can synergize to enhance clinical responses by enhancing different stages of the antitumor immune response (antigen uptake and presentation, T-cell activation, and T-cell response maintenance) and modifying various aspects in the TME (angiogenesis and immunosuppression). Combining checkpoint blockade with other immunotherapeutic strategies that have shown limited efficacy as monotherapies, such as vaccination, is an area of intensive research. For example, a phase I trial in six patients with recurrent ovarian cancer examined a DC-based autologous whole tumor lysate vaccine in combination with Treg-depleting metronomic cyclophosphamide, the antiangiogenic mAb bevacizumab, and ACT (vaccine-primed ex vivo CD3/CD28-costimulated peripheral blood autologous T cells). Antitumor immune responses (in the form of increased tumor-reactive T cells and reduced Tregs) and clinical benefit were observed in four patients, including 1 CR, 1 PR, and 2 SD [142]. Checkpoint inhibitors in combination are also being clinically tested. For example, an ongoing phase I trial in patients with advanced solid tumors (including ovarian cancer) is evaluating the combination of tremelimumab (a humanized IgG2 anti-CTLA-4 mAb) with durvalumab (anti-PD-L1) (NCT01975831) [143]. Identification of the optimal immunotherapy combination will require evaluation of not only synergistic mechanisms of action and ideal sequence of dosing but also overlapping toxicities in order to maximize clinical benefit.

Conclusions

Recent advances and rational immunotherapeutic combinations hold immense potential to improve outcomes for patients with ovarian cancer. Nonetheless, a number of challenges remain that are being critically addressed. Immunotherapies are typically administered in conjunction with or post chemotherapy. Several chemotherapeutic drugs utilized in ovarian cancer exert immunostimulatory effects. Examples include platinum compounds (which reduce PD-L2 expression on DCs), trabectedin (which inhibits monocyte differentiation into TAMs), and decitabine (which triggers a type I IFN response) [144–146]. Integrating immunotherapy with chemotherapy requires careful consideration of drugs, dosing, and schedule in order to neutralize the unwarranted immunosuppressive effects and maximize the immunostimulatory effects of chemotherapy [147]. A second challenge is to better characterize the TME not only to identify the rare somatic mutations that are immunogenic but also to understand host-tumor interactions. Like other cancers, ovarian cancer is heterogenic, and recent gene expression profiling studies have recognized several distinct molecular subtypes with markedly different prognoses [148]. Identifying dominant immunosuppressive pathways as well as collateral pathways can improve response rates in immunotherapy by improving the design of combination treatment regimens [149, 150]. Lastly, identification of biomarkers that predict response to immunotherapies will allow patients to be optimally matched with therapies that are expected to deliver the maximum benefit while minimizing unnecessary toxicity.

References

1. Zhang L, Conejo-Garcia JR, Katsaros D, Gimotty PA, Massobrio M, Regnani G, et al. Intratumoral T cells, recurrence, and survival in epithelial ovarian cancer. N Engl J Med. 2003;348(3):203–13. doi:348/3/203 [pii].
2. Sato E, Olson SH, Ahn J, Bundy B, Nishikawa H, Qian F, et al. Intraepithelial CD8+ tumor-infiltrating lymphocytes and a high CD8+/regulatory T cell ratio are associated with favorable prognosis in ovarian cancer. Proc Natl Acad Sci U S A. 2005;102(51):18538–43. doi:10.1073/pnas.0509182102.
3. Tomsová M, Melichar B, Sedláková I, Steiner I. Prognostic significance of CD3+ tumor-infiltrating lymphocytes in ovarian carcinoma. Gynecol Oncol. 2008;108(2):415–20. doi:10.1016/j.ygyno.2007.10.016.
4. Hwang WT, Adams SF, Tahirovic E, Hagemann IS, Coukos G. Prognostic significance of tumor-infiltrating T cells in ovarian cancer: a meta-analysis. Gynecol Oncol. 2012;124(2):192–8. doi:10.1016/j.ygyno.2011.09.039.
5. Curiel TJ, Coukos G, Zou L, Alvarez X, Cheng P, Mottram P, et al. Specific recruitment of regulatory T cells in ovarian carcinoma fosters immune privilege and predicts reduced survival. Nat Med. 2004;10(9):942–9. doi:10.1038/nm1093.
6. Chu CS, Kim SH, June CH, Coukos G. Immunotherapy opportunities in ovarian cancer. Expert Rev Anticancer Ther. 2008;8(2):243–57. doi:10.1586/14737140.8.2.243.
7. Walters CL, Arend RC, Armstrong DK, Naumann RW, Alvarez RD. Folate and folate receptor alpha antagonists mechanism of action in ovarian cancer. Gynecol Oncol. 2013;131(2):493–8. doi:10.1016/j.ygyno.2013.07.080.
8. Yakirevich E, Sabo E, Lavie O, Mazareb S, Spagnoli GC, Resnick MB. Expression of the MAGE-A4 and NY-ESO-1 cancer-testis antigens in serous ovarian neoplasms. Clini Cancer Res Off J Am Asso. 2003;9(17):6453–60.
9. Lin CK, Chao TK, Yu CP, Yu MH, Jin JS. The expression of six biomarkers in the four most common ovarian cancers: correlation with clinicopathological parameters. APMIS Acta Pathologica Micro Immunolo Scandinavica. 2009;117(3):162–75. doi:10.1111/j.1600-0463.2008.00003.x.
10. Webb JR, Milne K, Nelson BH. PD-1 and CD103 are widely coexpressed on prognostically favorable intraepithelial CD8 T cells in human ovarian cancer. Cancer Immunol Res. 2015;3(8):926–35. doi:10.1158/2326-6066.CIR-14-0239.
11. Hamanishi J, Mandai M, Iwasaki M, Okazaki T, Tanaka Y, Yamaguchi K, et al. Programmed cell death 1 ligand 1 and tumor-infiltrating CD8+ T lymphocytes are prognostic factors of human ovarian cancer. Proc Natl Acad Sci U S A. 2007;104(9):3360–5. doi:10.1073/pnas.0611533104.
12. Abiko K, Mandai M, Hamanishi J, Yoshioka Y, Matsumura N, Baba T, et al. PD-L1 on tumor cells is induced in ascites and promotes peritoneal dissemination of ovarian cancer through CTL dysfunction. Clini Cancer Res Off J Am Asso. 2013;19(6):1363–74. doi:10.1158/1078-0432.CCR-12-2199.
13. Makkouk A, Weiner GJ. Cancer immunotherapy and breaking immune tolerance: new approaches to an old challenge. Cancer Res. 2015;75(1):5–10. doi:10.1158/0008-5472.CAN-14-2538.
14. Martinez Forero I, Okada H, Topalian SL, Gajewski TF, Korman AJ, Melero I. Workshop on immunotherapy combinations. Society for Immunotherapy of Cancer annual meeting Bethesda, November 3, 2011. J Transl Med. 2012;10:108. doi:10.1186/1479-5876-10-108.

15. Geskin LJ. Monoclonal antibodies. Dermatol Clin. 2015;33(4):777–86. doi:10.1016/j.det.2015.05.015.
16. Vanneman M, Dranoff G. Combining immunotherapy and targeted therapies in cancer treatment. Nat Rev Cancer. 2012;12(4):237–51. doi:10.1038/nrc3237;10.1038/nrc3237.
17. Weiner GJ. Building better monoclonal antibody-based therapeutics. Nat Rev Cancer. 2015;15(6):361–70. doi:10.1038/nrc3930.
18. Siwak DR, Carey M, Hennessy BT, Nguyen CT, McGahren Murray MJ, Nolden L, et al. Targeting the epidermal growth factor receptor in epithelial ovarian cancer: current knowledge and future challenges. J Oncol. 2010;2010:568938. doi:10.1155/2010/568938.
19. Lu Y, Li X, Liang K, Luwor R, Siddik ZH, Mills GB, et al. Epidermal growth factor receptor (EGFR) ubiquitination as a mechanism of acquired resistance escaping treatment by the anti-EGFR monoclonal antibody cetuximab. Cancer Res. 2007;67(17):8240–7. doi:10.1158/0008-5472.CAN-07-0589.
20. Patel D, Lahiji A, Patel S, Franklin M, Jimenez X, Hicklin DJ, et al. Monoclonal antibody cetuximab binds to and down-regulates constitutively activated epidermal growth factor receptor vIII on the cell surface. Anticancer Res. 2007;27(5A):3355–66.
21. Schilder RJ, Pathak HB, Lokshin AE, Holloway RW, Alvarez RD, Aghajanian C, et al. Phase II trial of single agent cetuximab in patients with persistent or recurrent epithelial ovarian or primary peritoneal carcinoma with the potential for dose escalation to rash. Gynecol Oncol. 2009;113(1):21–7. doi:10.1016/j.ygyno.2008.12.003.
22. Secord AA, Blessing JA, Armstrong DK, Rodgers WH, Miner Z, Barnes MN, et al. Phase II trial of cetuximab and carboplatin in relapsed platinum-sensitive ovarian cancer and evaluation of epidermal growth factor receptor expression: a Gynecologic Oncology Group study. Gynecol Oncol. 2008;108(3):493–9. doi:10.1016/j.ygyno.2007.11.029.
23. Steffensen KD, Waldstrom M, Pallisgard N, Lund B, Bergfeldt K, Wihl J, et al. Panitumumab and pegylated liposomal doxorubicin in platinum-resistant epithelial ovarian cancer with KRAS wild-type: the PaLiDo study, a phase II nonrandomized multicenter study. Int J Gynecolo Cancer Off J. 2013;23(1):73–80. doi:10.1097/IGC.0b013e3182775fae.
24. Gordon AN, Fleagle JT, Guthrie D, Parkin DE, Gore ME, Lacave AJ. Recurrent epithelial ovarian carcinoma: a randomized phase III study of pegylated liposomal doxorubicin versus topotecan. J Clin Oncol. 2001;19(14):3312–22.
25. Tang Z, Qian M, Ho M. The role of mesothelin in tumor progression and targeted therapy. Anticancer Agents Med Chem. 2013;13(2):276–80.
26. Felder M, Kapur A, Gonzalez-Bosquet J, Horibata S, Heintz J, Albrecht R, et al. MUC16 (CA125): tumor biomarker to cancer therapy, a work in progress. Mol Cancer. 2014;13:129. doi:10.1186/1476-4598-13-129.
27. Hassan R, Cohen SJ, Phillips M, Pastan I, Sharon E, Kelly RJ, et al. Phase I clinical trial of the chimeric anti-mesothelin monoclonal antibody MORAb-009 in patients with mesothelin-expressing cancers. Clin Cancer Res. 2010;16(24):6132–8. doi:10.1158/1078-0432.CCR-10-2275.
28. Sabbatini P, Harter P, Scambia G, Sehouli J, Meier W, Wimberger P, et al. Abagovomab as maintenance therapy in patients with epithelial ovarian cancer: a phase III trial of the AGO OVAR, COGI, GINECO, and GEICO--the MIMOSA study. J Clin Oncol. 2013;31(12):1554–61. doi:10.1200/JCO.2012.46.4057.
29. Berek JS, Taylor PT, Gordon A, Cunningham MJ, Finkler N, Orr J, et al. Randomized, placebo-controlled study of oregovomab for consolidation of clinical remission in patients with advanced ovarian cancer. J Clin Oncol. 2004;22(17):3507–16. doi:10.1200/JCO.2004.09.016.
30. Berek J, Taylor P, McGuire W, Smith LM, Schultes B, Nicodemus CF. Oregovomab maintenance monoimmunotherapy does not improve outcomes in advanced ovarian cancer. J Clin Oncol. 2009;27(3):418–25. doi:10.1200/JCO.2008.17.8400.
31. Bagnoli M, Canevari S, Figini M, Mezzanzanica D, Raspagliesi F, Tomassetti A, et al. A step further in understanding the biology of the folate receptor in ovarian carcinoma. Gynecol Oncol. 2003;88(1 Pt 2):S140–4.

32. Lutz RJ. Targeting the folate receptor for the treatment of ovarian cancer. Transl Cancer Res. 2015;4(1):118–26. doi: 10.3978/j.issr2218-676X.2015.01.04.
33. Armstrong DK, White AJ, Weil SC, Phillips M, Coleman RL. Farletuzumab (a monoclonal antibody against folate receptor alpha) in relapsed platinum-sensitive ovarian cancer. Gynecol Oncol. 2013;129(3):452–8. doi:10.1016/j.ygyno.2013.03.002.
34. Drerup JM, Liu Y, Padron AS, Murthy K, Hurez V, Zhang B, et al. Immunotherapy for ovarian cancer. Curr Treat Options Oncol. 2015;16(1):317. doi:10.1007/s11864-014-0317-1.
35. Ferrara N, Gerber HP, LeCouter J. The biology of VEGF and its receptors. Nat Med. 2003;9(6):669–76. doi:nm0603-669 [pii].
36. Hata K, Watanabe Y, Nakai H, Hata T, Hoshiai H. Expression of the vascular endothelial growth factor (VEGF) gene in epithelial ovarian cancer: an approach to anti-VEGF therapy. Anticancer Res. 2011;31(2):731–7. doi:31/2/731 [pii].
37. Yang DH, Park JS, Jin CJ, Kang HK, Nam JH, Rhee JH, et al. The dysfunction and abnormal signaling pathway of dendritic cells loaded by tumor antigen can be overcome by neutralizing VEGF in multiple myeloma. Leuk Res. 2009;33(5):665–70. doi:10.1016/j.leukres.2008.09.006.
38. Shrimali RK, Yu Z, Theoret MR, Chinnasamy D, Restifo NP, Rosenberg SA. Antiangiogenic agents can increase lymphocyte infiltration into tumor and enhance the effectiveness of adoptive immunotherapy of cancer. Cancer Res. 2010;70(15):6171–80. doi:10.1158/0008-5472.CAN-10-0153.
39. Burger RA, Sill MW, Monk BJ, Greer BE, Sorosky JI. Phase II trial of bevacizumab in persistent or recurrent epithelial ovarian cancer or primary peritoneal cancer: a Gynecologic Oncology Group Study. J Clin Oncol. 2007;25(33):5165–71. doi:10.1200/JCO.2007.11.5345.
40. Cannistra SA, Matulonis UA, Penson RT, Hambleton J, Dupont J, Mackey H, et al. Phase II study of bevacizumab in patients with platinum-resistant ovarian cancer or peritoneal serous cancer. J Clin Oncol. 2007;25(33):5180–6. doi:10.1200/JCO.2007.12.0782.
41. McGonigle KF, Muntz HG, Vuky J, Paley PJ, Veljovich DS, Greer BE, et al. Combined weekly topotecan and biweekly bevacizumab in women with platinum-resistant ovarian, peritoneal, or fallopian tube cancer: results of a phase 2 study. Cancer. 2011;117(16):3731–40. doi:10.1002/cncr.25967.
42. Garcia AA, Hirte H, Fleming G, Yang D, Tsao-Wei DD, Roman L, et al. Phase II clinical trial of bevacizumab and low-dose metronomic oral cyclophosphamide in recurrent ovarian cancer: a trial of the California, Chicago, and Princess Margaret Hospital phase II consortia. J Clin Oncol. 2008;26(1):76–82. doi:10.1200/JCO.2007.12.1939.
43. Pujade-Lauraine E, Hilpert F, Weber B, Reuss A, Poveda A, Kristensen G, et al. Bevacizumab combined with chemotherapy for platinum-resistant recurrent ovarian cancer: the AURELIA open-label randomized phase III trial. J Clini Oncolo Offi J Am Soc. 2014;32(13):1302–8. doi:10.1200/JCO.2013.51.4489.
44. Sica A, Larghi P, Mancino A, Rubino L, Porta C, Totaro MG, et al. Macrophage polarization in tumour progression. Semin Cancer Biol. 2008;18(5):349–55. doi:10.1016/j.semcancer.2008.03.004.
45. Kawamura K, Komohara Y, Takaishi K, Katabuchi H, Takeya M. Detection of M2 macrophages and colony-stimulating factor 1 expression in serous and mucinous ovarian epithelial tumors. Pathol Int. 2009;59(5):300–5. doi:10.1111/j.1440-1827.2009.02369.x.
46. Takaishi K, Komohara Y, Tashiro H, Ohtake H, Nakagawa T, Katabuchi H, et al. Involvement of M2-polarized macrophages in the ascites from advanced epithelial ovarian carcinoma in tumor progression via Stat3 activation. Cancer Sci. 2010;101(10):2128–36. doi:10.1111/j.1349-7006.2010.01652.x.
47. Zhang M, He Y, Sun X, Li Q, Wang W, Zhao A, et al. A high M1/M2 ratio of tumor-associated macrophages is associated with extended survival in ovarian cancer patients. J Ovarian Res. 2014;7:19. doi:10.1186/1757-2215-7-19.
48. Hume DA, MacDonald KP. Therapeutic applications of macrophage colony-stimulating factor-1 (CSF-1) and antagonists of CSF-1 receptor (CSF-1R) signaling. Blood. 2012;119(8):1810–20. doi:10.1182/blood-2011-09-379214.

49. Ries CH, Cannarile MA, Hoves S, Benz J, Wartha K, Runza V, et al. Targeting tumor-associated macrophages with anti-CSF-1R antibody reveals a strategy for cancer therapy. Cancer Cell. 2014;25(6):846–59. doi:10.1016/j.ccr.2014.05.016.
50. Cassier PA, Gomez-Roca CA, Italiano A, Cannarile M, Ries C, Brillouet A, et al. Phase 1 study of RG7155, a novel anti-CSF1R antibody, in patients with locally advanced pigmented villonodular synovitis (PVNS). ASCO annual meeting abstract #10504. 2014. http://meetinglibrary.asco.org/content/131522-144.
51. Kryczek I, Wei S, Zou L, Zhu G, Mottram P, Xu H, et al. Cutting edge: induction of B7-H4 on APCs through IL-10: novel suppressive mode for regulatory T cells. J Immunol. 2006;177(1):40–4.
52. Kryczek I, Zou L, Rodriguez P, Zhu G, Wei S, Mottram P, et al. B7-H4 expression identifies a novel suppressive macrophage population in human ovarian carcinoma. J Exp Med. 2006;203(4):871–81. doi:10.1084/jem.20050930.
53. Kryczek I, Wei S, Zhu G, Myers L, Mottram P, Cheng P, et al. Relationship between B7-H4, regulatory T cells, and patient outcome in human ovarian carcinoma. Cancer Res. 2007;67(18):8900–5. doi:10.1158/0008-5472.CAN-07-1866.
54. Dangaj D, Lanitis E, Zhao A, Joshi S, Cheng Y, Sandaltzopoulos R, et al. Novel recombinant human b7-h4 antibodies overcome tumoral immune escape to potentiate T-cell antitumor responses. Cancer Res. 2013;73(15):4820–9. doi:10.1158/0008-5472.CAN-12-3457.
55. Litvinov SV, Bakker HA, Gourevitch MM, Velders MP, Warnaar SO. Evidence for a role of the epithelial glycoprotein 40 (Ep-CAM) in epithelial cell-cell adhesion. Cell Adhes Commun. 1994;2(5):417–28.
56. Bellone S, Siegel ER, Cocco E, Cargnelutti M, Silasi DA, Azodi M, et al. Overexpression of epithelial cell adhesion molecule in primary, metastatic, and recurrent/chemotherapy-resistant epithelial ovarian cancer: implications for epithelial cell adhesion molecule-specific immunotherapy. Int J Gynecolo Cancer Off J. 2009;19(5):860–6. doi:00009577-200907000-00011 [pii].
57. Köbel M, Kalloger SE, Boyd N, McKinney S, Mehl E, Palmer C, et al. Ovarian carcinoma subtypes are different diseases: implications for biomarker studies. PLoS Med. 2008;5(12):e232. doi:10.1371/journal.pmed.0050232.
58. Spizzo G, Went P, Dirnhofer S, Obrist P, Moch H, Baeuerle PA, et al. Overexpression of epithelial cell adhesion molecule (Ep-CAM) is an independent prognostic marker for reduced survival of patients with epithelial ovarian cancer. Gynecol Oncol. 2006;103(2):483–8. doi:10.1016/j.ygyno.2006.03.035.
59. Heiss MM, Murawa P, Koralewski P, Kutarska E, Kolesnik OO, Ivanchenko VV, et al. The trifunctional antibody catumaxomab for the treatment of malignant ascites due to epithelial cancer: results of a prospective randomized phase II/III trial. Int J Cancer. 2010;127(9):2209–21. doi:10.1002/ijc.25423.
60. Ruf P, Lindhofer H. Induction of a long-lasting antitumor immunity by a trifunctional bispecific antibody. Blood. 2001;98(8):2526–34.
61. Zeidler R, Mysliwietz J, Csánady M, Walz A, Ziegler I, Schmitt B, et al. The Fc-region of a new class of intact bispecific antibody mediates activation of accessory cells and NK cells and induces direct phagocytosis of tumour cells. Br J Cancer. 2000;83(2):261–6. doi:10.1054/bjoc.2000.1237.
62. Berek JS, Edwards RP, Parker LP, DeMars LR, Herzog TJ, Lentz SS, et al. Catumaxomab for the treatment of malignant ascites in patients with chemotherapy-refractory ovarian cancer: a phase II study. Int J Gynecol Cancer. 2014;24(9):1583–9. doi:10.1097/IGC.0000000000000286.
63. Erickson HK, Park PU, Widdison WC, Kovtun YV, Garrett LM, Hoffman K, et al. Antibody-maytansinoid conjugates are activated in targeted cancer cells by lysosomal degradation and linker-dependent intracellular processing. Cancer Res. 2006;66(8):4426–33. doi:10.1158/0008-5472.CAN-05-4489.
64. Golfier S, Kopitz C, Kahnert A, Heisler I, Schatz CA, Stelte-Ludwig B, et al. Anetumab ravtansine: a novel mesothelin-targeting antibody-drug conjugate cures tumors with

heterogeneous target expression favored by bystander effect. Mol Cancer Ther. 2014;13(6):1537–48. doi:10.1158/1535-7163.MCT-13-0926.
65. Liu J, Moore K, Birrer M, Berlin S, Matulonis U, Infante J, et al. Abstract LB-290: Targeting MUC16 with the antibody-drug conjugate (ADC) DMUC5754A in patients with platinum-resistant ovarian cancer: a phase I study of safety and pharmacokinetics. Cancer Res. 2013;73(8 Suppl):LB-290. doi:10.1158/1538-7445.AM2013-LB-290.
66. Ab O, Whiteman KR, Bartle LM, Sun X, Singh R, Tavares D, et al. IMGN853, a folate receptor-α (FRα)-targeting antibody-drug conjugate, exhibits potent targeted antitumor activity against FRα-expressing tumors. Mol Cancer Ther. 2015;14(7):1605–13. doi:10.1158/1535-7163.MCT-14-1095.
67. Moore KN, Martin LP, Seward SM, Bauer TM, O'Malley DM, Perez RP, et al. Preliminary single agent activity of IMGN853, a folate receptor alpha (FRα)-targeting antibody-drug conjugate (ADC), in platinum-resistant epithelial ovarian cancer (EOC) patients (pts): phase I trial. ASCO annual meeting abstract # 5518. 2015. http://meetinglibrary.asco.org/content/150377-156.
68. Martin LP, Moore KN, O'Malley DM, Seward SM, Bauer TM, Perez RP, et al. Association of folate receptor alpha (FRα) expression level and clinical activity of IMGN853 (mirvetuximab soravtansine), a FRα-targeting antibody-drug conjugate (ADC), in FRα -expressing platinum-resistant epithelial ovarian cancer (EOC) patients (pts). Proceedings of the 2015 AACR-NCI-EORTC international conference on molecular targets and cancer therapeutics, Nov 5–9. Boston: AACR; 2015.
69. Gattinoni L, Powell DJ, Rosenberg SA, Restifo NP. Adoptive immunotherapy for cancer: building on success. Nat Rev Immunol. 2006;6(5):383–93. doi:10.1038/nri1842.
70. Restifo NP, Dudley ME, Rosenberg SA. Adoptive immunotherapy for cancer: harnessing the T cell response. Nat Rev Immunol. 2012;12(4):269–81. doi:10.1038/nri3191.
71. Rosenberg SA, Yang JC, Restifo NP. Cancer immunotherapy: moving beyond current vaccines. Nat Med. 2004;10(9):909–15. doi:10.1038/nm1100.
72. Freedman RS, Edwards CL, Kavanagh JJ, Kudelka AP, Katz RL, Carrasco CH, et al. Intraperitoneal adoptive immunotherapy of ovarian carcinoma with tumor-infiltrating lymphocytes and low-dose recombinant interleukin-2: a pilot trial. J Immunother Emphasis Tumor Immunol. 1994;16(3):198–210.
73. Aoki Y, Takakuwa K, Kodama S, Tanaka K, Takahashi M, Tokunaga A, et al. Use of adoptive transfer of tumor-infiltrating lymphocytes alone or in combination with cisplatin-containing chemotherapy in patients with epithelial ovarian cancer. Cancer Res. 1991;51(7):1934–9.
74. Fujita K, Ikarashi H, Takakuwa K, Kodama S, Tokunaga A, Takahashi T, et al. Prolonged disease-free period in patients with advanced epithelial ovarian cancer after adoptive transfer of tumor-infiltrating lymphocytes. Clin Cancer Res. 1995;1(5):501–7.
75. Wefers C, Lambert LJ, Torensma R, Hato SV. Cellular immunotherapy in ovarian cancer: targeting the stem of recurrence. Gynecol Oncol. 2015;137(2):335–42. doi:10.1016/j.ygyno.2015.02.019.
76. Kershaw MH, Westwood JA, Parker LL, Wang G, Eshhar Z, Mavroukakis SA, et al. A phase I study on adoptive immunotherapy using gene-modified T cells for ovarian cancer. Clin Cancer Res. 2006;12(20 Pt 1):6106–15. doi:10.1158/1078-0432.CCR-06-1183.
77. Song DG, Ye Q, Carpenito C, Poussin M, Wang LP, Ji C, et al. In vivo persistence, tumor localization, and antitumor activity of CAR-engineered T cells is enhanced by costimulatory signaling through CD137 (4-1BB). Cancer Res. 2011;71(13):4617–27. doi:10.1158/0008-5472.CAN-11-0422.
78. Kandalaft LE, Powell DJ, Coukos G. A phase I clinical trial of adoptive transfer of folate receptor-alpha redirected autologous T cells for recurrent ovarian cancer. J Transl Med. 2012;10:157. doi:10.1186/1479-5876-10-157.
79. Tanyi JL, Haas AR, Beatty GL, Morgan MA, Stashwick, Caitlin J, O'Hara MH, et al. Safety and feasibility of chimeric antigen receptor modified T cells directed against mesothelin (CART-meso) in patients with mesothelin expressing cancers. Proceedings of the 106th

Annual Meeting of the American Association for Cancer Research; Apr 18–22; Philadelphia: AACR, 2015.
80. Hung CF, Wu TC, Monie A, Roden R. Antigen-specific immunotherapy of cervical and ovarian cancer. Immunol Rev. 2008;222:43–69. doi:10.1111/j.1600-065X.2008.00622.x.
81. Melief CJ, van Hall T, Arens R, Ossendorp F, van der Burg SH. Therapeutic cancer vaccines. J Clin Invest. 2015;125(9):3401–12. doi:10.1172/JCI80009.
82. Odunsi K, Jungbluth AA, Stockert E, Qian F, Gnjatic S, Tammela J, et al. NY-ESO-1 and LAGE-1 cancer-testis antigens are potential targets for immunotherapy in epithelial ovarian cancer. Cancer Res. 2003;63(18):6076–83.
83. Jäger E, Chen YT, Drijfhout JW, Karbach J, Ringhoffer M, Jäger D, et al. Simultaneous humoral and cellular immune response against cancer-testis antigen NY-ESO-1: definition of human histocompatibility leukocyte antigen (HLA)-A2-binding peptide epitopes. J Exp Med. 1998;187(2):265–70.
84. Odunsi K, Qian F, Matsuzaki J, Mhawech-Fauceglia P, Andrews C, Hoffman EW, et al. Vaccination with an NY-ESO-1 peptide of HLA class I/II specificities induces integrated humoral and T cell responses in ovarian cancer. Proc Natl Acad Sci U S A. 2007;104(31):12837–42. doi:10.1073/pnas.0703342104.
85. Diefenbach CS, Gnjatic S, Sabbatini P, Aghajanian C, Hensley ML, Spriggs DR, et al. Safety and immunogenicity study of NY-ESO-1b peptide and montanide ISA-51 vaccination of patients with epithelial ovarian cancer in high-risk first remission. Clin Cancer Res. 2008;14(9):2740–8. doi:10.1158/1078-0432.CCR-07-4619.
86. Sabbatini P, Tsuji T, Ferran L, Ritter E, Sedrak C, Tuballes K, et al. Phase I trial of overlapping long peptides from a tumor self-antigen and poly-ICLC shows rapid induction of integrated immune response in ovarian cancer patients. Clin Cancer Res. 2012;18(23):6497–508. doi:10.1158/1078-0432.CCR-12-2189.
87. Tsuji T, Sabbatini P, Jungbluth AA, Ritter E, Pan L, Ritter G, et al. Effect of Montanide and poly-ICLC adjuvant on human self/tumor antigen-specific CD4+ T cells in phase I overlapping long peptide vaccine trial. Cancer Immunol Res. 2013;1(5):340–50. doi:10.1158/2326-6066.CIR-13-0089.
88. Odunsi K, Matsuzaki J, James SR, Mhawech-Fauceglia P, Tsuji T, Miller A, et al. Epigenetic potentiation of NY-ESO-1 vaccine therapy in human ovarian cancer. Cancer Immunol Res. 2014;2(1):37–49. doi:10.1158/2326-6066.CIR-13-0126.
89. Vousden KH, Lu X. Live or let die: the cell's response to p53. Nat Rev Cancer. 2002;2(8):594–604. doi:10.1038/nrc864.
90. Nijman HW, Lambeck A, van der Burg SH, van der Zee AG, Daemen T. Immunologic aspect of ovarian cancer and p53 as tumor antigen. J Transl Med. 2005;3:34. doi:10.1186/1479-5876-3-34.
91. Goodell V, Salazar LG, Urban N, Drescher CW, Gray H, Swensen RE, et al. Antibody immunity to the p53 oncogenic protein is a prognostic indicator in ovarian cancer. J Clin Oncol. 2006;24(5):762–8. doi:10.1200/JCO.2005.03.2813.
92. Lambeck A, Leffers N, Hoogeboom BN, Sluiter W, Hamming I, Klip H, et al. P53-specific T cell responses in patients with malignant and benign ovarian tumors: implications for p53 based immunotherapy. Int J Cancer. 2007;121(3):606–14. doi:10.1002/ijc.22710.
93. Rahma OE, Ashtar E, Czystowska M, Szajnik ME, Wieckowski E, Bernstein S, et al. A gynecologic oncology group phase II trial of two p53 peptide vaccine approaches: subcutaneous injection and intravenous pulsed dendritic cells in high recurrence risk ovarian cancer patients. Cancer Immunol Immunother. 2012;61(3):373–84. doi:10.1007/s00262-011-1100-9.
94. Leffers N, Lambeck AJ, Gooden MJ, Hoogeboom BN, Wolf R, Hamming IE, et al. Immunization with a P53 synthetic long peptide vaccine induces P53-specific immune responses in ovarian cancer patients, a phase II trial. Int J Cancer. 2009;125(9):2104–13. doi:10.1002/ijc.24597.
95. Leffers N, Vermeij R, Hoogeboom BN, Schulze UR, Wolf R, Hamming IE, et al. Long-term clinical and immunological effects of p53-SLP® vaccine in patients with ovarian cancer. Int J Cancer. 2012;130(1):105–12. doi:10.1002/ijc.25980.

96. Disis ML, Gooley TA, Rinn K, Davis D, Piepkorn M, Cheever MA, et al. Generation of T-cell immunity to the HER-2/neu protein after active immunization with HER-2/neu peptide-based vaccines. J Clin Oncol. 2002;20(11):2624–32.
97. Disis ML, Goodell V, Schiffman K, Knutson KL. Humoral epitope-spreading following immunization with a HER-2/neu peptide based vaccine in cancer patients. J Clin Immunol. 2004;24(5):571–8. doi:10.1023/B:JOCI.0000040928.67495.52.
98. Kandalaft LE, Powell DJ, Singh N, Coukos G. Immunotherapy for ovarian cancer: what's next? J Clin Oncol. 2011;29(7):925–33. doi:10.1200/JCO.2009.27.2369.
99. Senzer N, Barve M, Kuhn J, Melnyk A, Beitsch P, Lazar M, et al. Phase I trial of "bi-shRNAi(furin)/GMCSF DNA/autologous tumor cell" vaccine (FANG) in advanced cancer. Mol Ther. 2012;20(3):679–86. doi:10.1038/mt.2011.269.
100. Oh J, Barve M, Grosen EA, Fine BA, Heffernan TP, Matthews CM, et al. Randomized phase II trial of maintenance autologous tumor cell vaccine (FANG™) following clinical complete response (cCR) in stage III/IV ovarian cancer: preliminary results. Gynecol Oncol. 2015;137(Supplement 1):2–3. doi:10.1016/j.ygyno.2015.01.003.
101. Palucka K, Banchereau J. Cancer immunotherapy via dendritic cells. Nat Rev Cancer. 2012;12(4):265–77. doi:10.1038/nrc3258.
102. Vlad AM, Diaconu I, Gantt KR. MUC1 in endometriosis and ovarian cancer. Immunol Res. 2006;36(1–3):229–36. doi:10.1385/IR:36:1:229.
103. Brossart P, Wirths S, Stuhler G, Reichardt VL, Kanz L, Brugger W. Induction of cytotoxic T-lymphocyte responses in vivo after vaccinations with peptide-pulsed dendritic cells. Blood. 2000;96(9):3102–8.
104. Gray HJ, Gargosky SE, Team C-S. Progression-free survival in ovarian cancer patients in second remission with mucin-1 autologous dendritic cell therapy. ASCO annual meeting abstract #5504. 2014. http://meetinglibrary.asco.org/content/134878-144.
105. Peethambaram PP, Melisko ME, Rinn KJ, Alberts SR, Provost NM, Jones LA, et al. A phase I trial of immunotherapy with lapuleucel-T (APC8024) in patients with refractory metastatic tumors that express HER-2/neu. Clin Cancer Res. 2009;15(18):5937–44. doi:10.1158/1078-0432.CCR-08-3282.
106. Hernando JJ, Park TW, Kübler K, Offergeld R, Schlebusch H, Bauknecht T. Vaccination with autologous tumour antigen-pulsed dendritic cells in advanced gynaecological malignancies: clinical and immunological evaluation of a phase I trial. Cancer Immunol Immunother. 2002;51(1):45–52. doi:10.1007/s00262-001-0255-1.
107. Baek S, Kim YM, Kim SB, Kim CS, Kwon SW, Kim Y, et al. Therapeutic DC vaccination with IL-2 as a consolidation therapy for ovarian cancer patients: a phase I/II trial. Cell Mol Immunol. 2015;12(1):87–95. doi:10.1038/cmi.2014.40.
108. Chiang CL, Kandalaft LE, Tanyi J, Hagemann AR, Motz GT, Svoronos N, et al. A dendritic cell vaccine pulsed with autologous hypochlorous acid-oxidized ovarian cancer lysate primes effective broad antitumor immunity: from bench to bedside. Clin Cancer Res. 2013;19(17):4801–15. doi:10.1158/1078-0432.CCR-13-1185.
109. Larocca C, Schlom J. Viral vector-based therapeutic cancer vaccines. Cancer J. 2011;17(5):359–71. doi:10.1097/PPO.0b013e3182325e63.
110. Gulley JL, Arlen PM, Tsang KY, Yokokawa J, Palena C, Poole DJ, et al. Pilot study of vaccination with recombinant CEA-MUC-1-TRICOM poxviral-based vaccines in patients with metastatic carcinoma. Clin Cancer Res. 2008;14(10):3060–9. doi:10.1158/1078-0432.CCR-08-0126.
111. Mohebtash M, Tsang KY, Madan RA, Huen NY, Poole DJ, Jochems C, et al. A pilot study of MUC-1/CEA/TRICOM poxviral-based vaccine in patients with metastatic breast and ovarian cancer. Clin Cancer Res. 2011;17(22):7164–73. doi:10.1158/1078-0432.CCR-11-0649.
112. Odunsi K, Matsuzaki J, Karbach J, Neumann A, Mhawech-Fauceglia P, Miller A, et al. Efficacy of vaccination with recombinant vaccinia and fowlpox vectors expressing NY-ESO-1 antigen in ovarian cancer and melanoma patients. Proc Natl Acad Sci U S A. 2012;109(15):5797–802. doi:10.1073/pnas.1117208109.

113. Zakharia Y, Rahma O, Khleif SN. Ovarian cancer from an immune perspective. Radiat Res. 2014;182(2):239–51. doi:10.1667/RR13741.1.
114. Rech AJ, Mick R, Martin S, Recio A, Aqui NA, Powell Jr DJ, et al. CD25 blockade depletes and selectively reprograms regulatory T cells in concert with immunotherapy in cancer patients. Sci Transl Med. 2012;4(134):134ra62. doi:10.1126/scitranslmed.3003330;10.1126/scitranslmed.3003330.
115. Curiel T, Thibodeaux S, Wall S, Pandeswara SL, Daniel B, Drerup J, et al. Denileukin diftitox depletes regulatory T cells without clinical benefit in advanced stage epithelial ovarian carcinoma (VAC3P.945). J Immunol. 2014;192(1 Suppl) 73.7.
116. Curiel T, Sareddy G, Hurez V, Qin K, Pandeswara SL, Vadlamudi R, et al. B7-H1 blockade improves efficacy of regulatory T cell depletion as cancer immunotherapy by reducing Treg regeneration, possibly through tumor B7-H1 effects (VAC3P.950). J Immunol. 2014;192(1 Suppl) 73.12.
117. Ghiringhelli F, Menard C, Puig PE, Ladoire S, Roux S, Martin F, et al. Metronomic cyclophosphamide regimen selectively depletes CD4+CD25+ regulatory T cells and restores T and NK effector functions in end stage cancer patients. Cancer Immunol Immunother. 2007;56(5):641–8. doi:10.1007/s00262-006-0225-8.
118. Chu CS, Boyer J, Schullery DS, Gimotty PA, Gamerman V, Bender J, et al. Phase I/II randomized trial of dendritic cell vaccination with or without cyclophosphamide for consolidation therapy of advanced ovarian cancer in first or second remission. Cancer Immunol Immunother. 2012;61(5):629–41. doi:10.1007/s00262-011-1081-8.
119. Vermeij R, Leffers N, Hoogeboom BN, Hamming IL, Wolf R, Reyners AK, et al. Potentiation of a p53-SLP vaccine by cyclophosphamide in ovarian cancer: a single-arm phase II study. Int J Cancer. 2012;131(5):E670–80. doi:10.1002/ijc.27388.
120. Takikawa O. Biochemical and medical aspects of the indoleamine 2,3-dioxygenase-initiated l-tryptophan metabolism. Biochem Biophys Res Commun. 2005;338(1):12–9. doi:10.1016/j.bbrc.2005.09.032.
121. Frumento G, Rotondo R, Tonetti M, Damonte G, Benatti U, Ferrara GB. Tryptophan-derived catabolites are responsible for inhibition of T and natural killer cell proliferation induced by indoleamine 2,3-dioxygenase. J Exp Med. 2002;196(4):459–68.
122. Munn DH, Shafizadeh E, Attwood JT, Bondarev I, Pashine A, Mellor AL. Inhibition of T cell proliferation by macrophage tryptophan catabolism. J Exp Med. 1999;189(9):1363–72.
123. Chen W, Liang X, Peterson AJ, Munn DH, Blazar BR. The indoleamine 2,3-dioxygenase pathway is essential for human plasmacytoid dendritic cell-induced adaptive T regulatory cell generation. J Immunol Baltimore Md 1950. 2008;181(8):5396–404. doi:181/8/5396 [pii].
124. Topalian SL, Drake CG, Pardoll DM. Immune checkpoint blockade: a common denominator approach to cancer therapy. Cancer Cell. 2015;27(4):450–61. doi:10.1016/j.ccell.2015.03.001.
125. Matsuzaki J, Gnjatic S, Mhawech-Fauceglia P, Beck A, Miller A, Tsuji T, et al. Tumor-infiltrating NY-ESO-1-specific CD8+ T cells are negatively regulated by LAG-3 and PD-1 in human ovarian cancer. Proc Natl Acad Sci U S A. 2010;107(17):7875–80. doi:10.1073/pnas.1003345107.
126. Inaba T, Ino K, Kajiyama H, Yamamoto E, Shibata K, Nawa A, et al. Role of the immunosuppressive enzyme indoleamine 2,3-dioxygenase in the progression of ovarian carcinoma. Gynecol Oncol. 2009;115(2):185–92. doi:10.1016/j.ygyno.2009.07.015.
127. Takao M, Okamoto A, Nikaido T, Urashima M, Takakura S, Saito M, et al. Increased synthesis of indoleamine-2,3-dioxygenase protein is positively associated with impaired survival in patients with serous-type, but not with other types of, ovarian cancer. Oncol Rep. 2007;17(6):1333–9.
128. Nonaka H, Saga Y, Fujiwara H, Akimoto H, Yamada A, Kagawa S, et al. Indoleamine 2,3-dioxygenase promotes peritoneal dissemination of ovarian cancer through inhibition of natural killer cell function and angiogenesis promotion. Int J Oncol. 2011;38(1):113–20.
129. Hoos A, Ibrahim R, Korman A, Abdallah K, Berman D, Shahabi V, et al. Development of ipilimumab: contribution to a new paradigm for cancer immunotherapy. Semin Oncol. 2010;37(5):533–46. doi:10.1053/j.seminoncol.2010.09.015.

130. Simpson TR, Li F, Montalvo-Ortiz W, Sepulveda MA, Bergerhoff K, Arce F, et al. Fc-dependent depletion of tumor-infiltrating regulatory T cells co-defines the efficacy of anti-CTLA-4 therapy against melanoma. J Exp Med. 2013;210(9):1695–710. doi:10.1084/jem.20130579.
131. Hodi FS, Mihm MC, Soiffer RJ, Haluska FG, Butler M, Seiden MV, et al. Biologic activity of cytotoxic T lymphocyte-associated antigen 4 antibody blockade in previously vaccinated metastatic melanoma and ovarian carcinoma patients. Proc Natl Acad Sci U S A. 2003;100(8):4712–7. doi:10.1073/pnas.0830997100.
132. Hodi FS, Butler M, Oble DA, Seiden MV, Haluska FG, Kruse A, et al. Immunologic and clinical effects of antibody blockade of cytotoxic T lymphocyte-associated antigen 4 in previously vaccinated cancer patients. Proc Natl Acad Sci U S A. 2008;105(8):3005–10. doi:10.1073/pnas.0712237105.
133. Postow MA, Callahan MK, Wolchok JD. Immune checkpoint blockade in cancer therapy. J Clin Oncol. 2015;33(17):1974–82. doi:10.1200/JCO.2014.59.4358.
134. Hamanishi J, Mandai M, Ikeda T, Minami M, Kawaguchi A, Matsumura N, et al. Efficacy and safety of anti-PD-1 antibody (Nivolumab: BMS-936558, ONO-4538) in patients with platinum-resistant ovarian cancer. ASCO annual meeting abstract #5570. 2014.
135. Hamanishi J, Mandai M, Ikeda TI, Minami M, Kawaguchi A, Matsumura N, et al. Durable tumor remission in patients with platinum-resistant ovarian cancer receiving nivolumab. ASCO annual meeting abstract# 5511. 2015.
136. Varga A, Piha-Paul SA, Ott PA, Mehnert JM, Berton-Rigaud D, Johnson EA, et al. Antitumor activity and safety of pembrolizumab in patients (pts) with PD-L1 positive advanced ovarian cancer: interim results from a phase Ib study. ASCO annual meeting abstract #268. 2015.
137. Disis ML, Patel MR, Pant S, Infante JR, Lockhart C, Kelly K, et al. Avelumab (MSB0010718C), an anti-PD-L1 antibody, in patients with previously treated, recurrent or refractory ovarian cancer: a phase Ib, open-label expansion trial. ASCO annual meeting abstract #5509. 2015.
138. Brahmer JR, Tykodi SS, Chow LQ, Hwu WJ, Topalian SL, Hwu P, et al. Safety and activity of anti-PD-L1 antibody in patients with advanced cancer. N Engl J Med. 2012;366(26):2455–65. doi:10.1056/NEJMoa1200694.
139. Muller AJ, DuHadaway JB, Donover PS, Sutanto-Ward E, Prendergast GC. Inhibition of indoleamine 2,3-dioxygenase, an immunoregulatory target of the cancer suppression gene Bin1, potentiates cancer chemotherapy. Nat Med. 2005;11(3):312–9. doi:10.1038/nm1196.
140. Hou DY, Muller AJ, Sharma MD, DuHadaway J, Banerjee T, Johnson M, et al. Inhibition of indoleamine 2,3-dioxygenase in dendritic cells by stereoisomers of 1-methyl-tryptophan correlates with antitumor responses. Cancer Res. 2007;67(2):792–801. doi:10.1158/0008-5472.CAN-06-2925.
141. Newton RC, Scherle PA, Bowman K, Liu X, Beatty GL, O'Dwyer PJ, et al. Pharmacodynamic assessment of INCB024360, an inhibitor of indoleamine 2,3-dioxygenase 1 (IDO1), in advanced cancer patients. ASCO annual meeting abstract #2500. 2012.
142. Kandalaft LE, Powell DJ, Chiang CL, Tanyi J, Kim S, Bosch M, et al. Autologous lysate-pulsed dendritic cell vaccination followed by adoptive transfer of vaccine-primed ex vivo co-stimulated T cells in recurrent ovarian cancer. Oncoimmunol. 2013;2(1):e22664. doi:10.4161/onci.22664.
143. Ott PA, Callahan MK, Odunsi K, Park AJ, Pan LS, Venhaus RR, et al. A phase I study to evaluate the safety and tolerability of MEDI4736, an anti-programmed cell death-ligand-1 (PD-L1) antibody, in combination with tremelimumab in patients with advanced solid tumors. ASCO annual meeting abstract #TPS3099. 2015. http://meetinglibrary.asco.org/content/149819-156.
144. Lesterhuis WJ, Punt CJ, Hato SV, Eleveld-Trancikova D, Jansen BJ, Nierkens S, et al. Platinum-based drugs disrupt STAT6-mediated suppression of immune responses against cancer in humans and mice. J Clin Invest. 2011;121(8):3100–8. doi:10.1172/JCI43656.
145. Allavena P, Signorelli M, Chieppa M, Erba E, Bianchi G, Marchesi F, et al. Anti-inflammatory properties of the novel antitumor agent yondelis (trabectedin): inhibition of macrophage

differentiation and cytokine production. Cancer Res. 2005;65(7):2964–71. doi:10.1158/0008-5472.CAN-04-4037.
146. Chiappinelli KB, Strissel PL, Desrichard A, Li H, Henke C, Akman B, et al. Inhibiting DNA methylation causes an interferon response in cancer via dsRNA including endogenous retroviruses. Cell. 2015;162(5):974–86. doi:10.1016/j.cell.2015.07.011.
147. Galluzzi L, Buqué A, Kepp O, Zitvogel L, Kroemer G. Immunological effects of conventional chemotherapy and targeted anticancer agents. Cancer Cell. 2015;28(6):690–714. doi:10.1016/j.ccell.2015.10.012.
148. Tothill RW, Tinker AV, George J, Brown R, Fox SB, Lade S, et al. Novel molecular subtypes of serous and endometrioid ovarian cancer linked to clinical outcome. Clin Cancer Res. 2008;14(16):5198–208. doi:10.1158/1078-0432.CCR-08-0196.
149. Topalian SL, Wolchok JD, Chan TA, Mellman I, Palucka K, Banchereau J, et al. Immunotherapy: the path to win the war on cancer? Cell. 2015;161(2):185–6.
150. Chester C, Dorigo O, Berek JS, Kohrt H. Immunotherapeutic approaches to ovarian cancer treatment. J Immunother Cancer. 2015;3:7. doi:10.1186/s40425-015-0051-7.

Part II

Particular Types of Ovarian Cancers

For each: histology and molecular specificities, specificity for surgery and management in first line and relapse

12 High-Grade Carcinomas, BRCA Mutations and the Role of PARP Inhibitors

Jonathan A. Ledermann

Abstract

Mutations in the BRCA gene are associated with a defect in the repair of DNA damage. These cells have a deficiency in the homologous recombination repair pathway. In ovarian cancer patients with a BRCA-mutated tumour, PARP (poly(ADP-ribose) polymerase) inhibitors prevent alternative pathway repair of DNA damage leading to synthetic lethality of tumour cells. Significant antitumour activity occurs in BRCA-mutated ovarian cancer treated with a PARP inhibitor; the greatest benefit seen thus far has been with maintenance therapy with olaparib following platinum-based chemotherapy for relapsed ovarian cancer. This leads to a significant delay in tumour progression with some patients remaining on treatment for several years with few side effects from treatment. Whilst the greatest benefit is in patients with a BRCA mutation, PARP inhibitors have also been shown to be active in 'platinum-sensitive' tumours without a BRCA mutation. Ongoing clinical trials with different PARP inhibitors are exploring the effect of maintenance therapy in patients with or without a BRCA mutation. In the EU, olaparib has now been licensed as maintenance therapy for 'platinum-sensitive' BRCA-mutated high-grade serous cancer after platinum-based therapy. In the USA the licence is based on the activity of olaparib in patients with a BRCA mutation who have received 3 or more prior lines of chemotherapy. Ongoing trials are now exploring the combination of different PARP inhibitors with chemotherapy or other molecularly targeted therapies to build on the benefit seen with olaparib. A BRCA mutation is the first predictive marker in ovarian cancer, identifying patients who are likely to derive a significant benefit from PARP inhibitor therapy.

J.A. Ledermann
UCL Cancer Institute, Cancer Research UK and UCL Cancer Trials Centre,
University College London, 90 Tottenham Court Road, London W1T 4TJ, UK
e-mail: j.ledermann@ucl.ac.uk

E. Pujade-Lauraine et al. (eds.), *Ovarian Cancers*,
DOI 10.1007/978-3-319-32110-3_12

Introduction

One key characteristic of ovarian cancer is its responsiveness to chemotherapy. A large proportion of women with advanced disease will enter a remission following surgery and chemotherapy, but most will relapse. Platinum-based therapy is central to the initial management and also to treatment of recurrence, as the majority of patients will relapse more than 6 months after completing first-line therapy and will usually respond to further treatments. Intervals between treatments of subsequent relapses become shorter as drug resistance increases, eventually leading to the failure of not only platinum-based therapies but also non-platinum drugs. Historically, all types of ovarian cancer have been treated in a similar fashion, yet we know that among the most commonly described histiotypes, there are significant differences in survival and a variability in the sensitivity to chemotherapy drugs. Recent data have shown that ovarian cancers have different pathways of development, and it is important that such biological differences are taken into account as new therapies are developed. In particular, the most common subtype, high-grade serous cancer, has a distinct evolution, and it is this subtype that is most commonly, but not exclusively, associated with BRCA mutations.

BRCA Mutations

The *BRCA1* gene was identified in 1990 and was cloned 4 years later [1], around the same time that the *BRCA2* gene was discovered [2]. *BRCA1* mutations are more common, occurring approximately twice as frequently as *BRCA2*. Women who inherit a deleterious *BRCA1* or *BRCA2* mutation have up to a 40 % and 20 % lifetime risk, respectively, of developing ovarian cancer and higher risks of developing breast cancer [3]. It is estimated that *BRCA* mutations are found in about 10–15 % of patients with ovarian cancer [4], but this may be an underestimate as testing for mutations has historically been based on identifying a family history of breast or ovarian cancer. Among the Western population, it is estimated that about 1 in 400 persons carries a germ-line mutation, but in some ethnic groups, such as the Ashkenazi Jewish population, the prevalence is ten times higher. Furthermore, the distribution of BRCA-related ovarian cancer differs among the commonly reported histiotypes. It is more commonly found in patients with high-grade serous ovarian cancer (HGSOC) [5–7]. In one series where 17 % of patients with HGSOC were found to carry a *BRCA* mutation, almost half (44 %) of these women had no family history of cancer [5]. BRCA mutations have also been described in association with clear-cell tumours, but the association with this subtype is less common [8].

Until recently knowledge of these mutations has not led to a change in the management of women with ovarian cancer. Observational clinical studies in women with ovarian cancer have shown that BRCA-mutated cancers have a better outcome following surgery and platinum-based chemotherapy than patients without a BRCA mutation [9, 10]. These tumours have impaired DNA repair due to a defect in the homologous recombination pathway, and this may explain an increase in sensitivity to DNA cross-linking drugs such as the platinum analogues [11]. How can such knowledge of biological differences in BRCA-mutated tumours be exploited to improve treatment?

DNA Repair as a Target for BRCA-Mutated Ovarian Cancer

The accurate and efficient repair of DNA damage is essential for cell survival. Complex processes have evolved to ensure that cells, which constantly sustain DNA damage, are repaired effectively to ensure genomic stability and cell survival. Poly(ADP-ribose) polymerase (PARP) is an enzyme that has an important role in the repair of single-strand DNA breaks. Double-strand DNA breaks (DSB) require a more complex repair mechanism to ensure high-fidelity repair, and without such a process, lethal genomic damage can arise. The two primary DSB repair pathways in humans are nonhomologous end joining (NHEJ) and homologous recombination repair (HRR). HRR is the preferred pathway as it is an error-free mechanism. HRR requires the presence of a variety of proteins including functioning BRCA1 and BRCA2 [12]. Thus, deficiencies in BRCA1 or BRCA2 result in defective HRR and subsequent loss of efficient and effective DNA DSB repair. The PARP pathway of repair remains intact for BRCA-mutated cells, but further disruption of DNA repair by PARP inhibitors leads to genomic instability and cell death through a process called synthetic lethality [13]. Preclinical models have clearly shown this; inhibition of PARP-1 activity in homozygous BRCA-deficient cells that have HRR deficiency leads to significant cell death [14, 15]. Thus, the hypothesis was developed that PARP inhibitors may have therapeutic activity in BRCA-mutated ovarian cancer.

Clinical Development of PARP Inhibitors in Ovarian Cancer

Early-Phase Trials with Olaparib

Initially, the development strategy for PARP inhibitors was to use the drugs to potentiate treatment with chemotherapy or radiotherapy [16]. However, given the results of preclinical models in BRCA-mutated tumours, development has revolved around exploring PARP inhibitors as single-agent therapy. Some of the earliest information is derived from the phase I studies with AZD2281 (olaparib). Significant activity with low levels of toxicity was seen in women with heavily pretreated BRCA-mutated ovarian cancer [17]. In an expanded phase I trial in BRCA-mutated ovarian cancer, there was a 40 % RECIST and/or CA125 response rate; some other patients had disease stabilisation leading to a 46 % overall clinical benefit rate [18]. Clinical activity was confirmed in a phase II study of two dose cohorts; a response rate of 33 % was seen in multiply pretreated women with BRCA1 or BRCA2 mutations at the higher dose of olaparib, 400 mg bd [19]. The main side effects observed were fatigue, nausea and anaemia.

Randomised Clinical Trials of Olaparib and Integration into Clinical Care

Following the promising results of early-phase studies, randomised trials were developed to undertake further study of olaparib in ovarian cancer. In the first trial, 'study 12', patients with BRCA-mutated recurrent ovarian cancer were randomised to treatment with either olaparib (200 or 400 mg bd) or pegylated liposomal doxorubicin (PLD) 50 mg/m^2. Patients in this trial had either 'platinum-resistant' or 'partially platinum-sensitive' recurrent ovarian cancer. The median progression-free survival (PFS) was 8.8 months with olaparib 400 mg bd, 6.5 months with olaparib 200 mg bd and 7.1 months with PLD [20]. Olaparib was clearly active but the median PFS with PLD was better than expected, illustrating that the biology of tumours in patients with a BRCA mutation is different and the response to cytotoxic drugs other than platinum analogues may be better than in the general population. The evidence emerging from single-agent studies suggested that tumour response rates appeared greater in patients with 'platinum-sensitive' disease [21], so further randomised trials focussed on this population. One hypothesis was that olaparib might augment the activity of carboplatin. This was tested in a randomised trial, 'study 41', in which patients with 'platinum-sensitive' ovarian cancer were randomised to carboplatin and paclitaxel with or without olaparib. Olaparib was continued as maintenance therapy [22]. A BRCA mutation was not required for entry into this trial. The dose of carboplatin was reduced to an AUC 4 and the schedule and dose of olaparib were altered (200 mg bd days 1–10) during each cycle of chemotherapy to manage the increased myelosuppression seen when olaparib was combined with these drugs. During the maintenance phase olaparib was given in full dose, 400 mg bd. Patients on olaparib had a median PFS of 12.2 months, significantly longer than the 9.6 months in the chemotherapy alone group (HR 0.51 [95 % CI 0.34–0.77]; $p=0.0012$). However, no difference in PFS was seen during the chemotherapy phase. The second trial was a randomised maintenance study of olaparib in patients with 'platinum-sensitive' high-grade serous cancer who had responded to platinum-based therapy. The trial, 'study 19' (ClinicalTrials.gov NCT00753546), was designed to include patients with or without a BRCA mutation to test the hypothesis that HRR deficiency, or 'BRCAness', may be present in a broader group of women with HGSOC and that these women in addition to those with a germ-line BRCA mutation may benefit from olaparib [11]. This was subsequently supported by evidence from the Cancer Genome Atlas study [6] and the demonstration that olaparib was active as a single agent in patients without a BRCA mutation [21]. 'Study 19' randomised 265 patients with HGSOC to olaparib or placebo maintenance within 8 weeks of completing a second or greater line of platinum-based therapy for relapsed ovarian cancer. The primary endpoint was PFS measured by response evaluation criteria in solid tumours (RECIST). BRCA status was known in 36.6 % of patients, and a BRCA1 or BRCA2 mutation was known to be present in 22.2 % of the study population. There was a statistically significant improvement in PFS in patients receiving olaparib compared with placebo, leading to a 3.6-month increase in the median PFS from the start of trial drug. The median PFS on maintenance therapy was 4.8 months on placebo and 8.4 months for patients treated with olaparib (hazard ratio [HR] 0.35; 95 % confidence interval [CI] 0.25–0.49; $p<0.0001$) [23].

However, no difference in overall survival (OS) was seen in an interim analysis with only 38 % of death events. Although these data were immature, the results in December 2011 led to a temporary cessation in the development of olaparib in ovarian cancer. A planned subgroup analysis suggested there was a greater effect of olaparib in patients with a BRCA mutation, and as a result, BRCA mutational analysis was performed on blood samples and archival tumour to determine BRCA status (germ-line or somatic mutations) in 63.4 % of patients who entered the trial with an unknown BRCA status. Consent had previously been obtained and information on BRCA mutation status became available in 95.8 % of patients. A reanalysis of PFS and updated OS was performed for the overall population and by BRCA mutation status [24]. The clinical benefit of olaparib was greatest in the BRCA mutation group. In this subset of 136 patients, the median PFS post chemotherapy was 11.2 months in patients receiving olaparib compared with 4.3 months for those treated with placebo (HR 0.18; 95 % CI 0.10–0.31; $p<0.0001$). A significant but smaller benefit in PFS was seen in BRCA wild-type patients taking olaparib. The median PFS increased from 5.5 months on placebo to 7.4 months on olaparib (HR 0.54; 95 % CI 0.34–0.85; $p=0.0075$). All sensitivity analyses and centralised computed tomography (CT) scan assessments confirmed the observed increase in PFS in patients with a BRCA mutation receiving olaparib compared with placebo (blinded independent central review: PFS HR 0.22; 95 % CI 0.12–0.40; $p<0.0001$). In 18 patients there was a somatic mutation of BRCA, and within this small group (8 of whom received olaparib) the effect on PFS appeared similar to those with a germ-line mutation of the BRCA gene.

Survival data are still immature (58 % of patients have died), but there is a trend towards an improved OS for patients with a BRCA mutation taking olaparib (HR 0.73; 95 % CI 0.45–1.17; $p=0.19$). No difference was seen in the BRCA wild-type patients. However, the OS results may have been confounded by crossover in patients with BRCA mutation randomised to placebo. Subsequent PARP inhibitor use occurred in 23 % of these patients compared with no patients receiving olaparib. In an attempt to control for this effect, a post hoc exploratory OS analysis was performed excluding patients from all study sites where at least one patient received post-progression treatment with a PARP inhibitor. This resulted in a numerical improvement in the OS HR in all groups (olaparib versus placebo; overall population, median OS 29.8 versus 26.6 months, respectively, HR 0.80; 95 % CI 0.55–1.16; $p=0.243$; BRCA mutation population, median OS 34.9 versus 26.6 months, respectively, HR 0.52; 95 % CI 0.28–0.97; $p=0.039$) [25]. Whilst awaiting the final OS analysis (85 % maturity), two exploratory clinical secondary endpoint analyses were performed to investigate the outcome of patients post progression. These were time to first subsequent therapy or death (TFST; a clinically relevant interpretation of PFS, representing the clinical decision made by investigators to initiate a further course of chemotherapy) and the time to second subsequent therapy or death (TSST), an approximation to the PFS2 (time to progression after subsequent treatment). The median TFST was 15.6 months in those who had received olaparib and 6.2 months in those who had received placebo (HR 0.33; $p < 0.00001$). The value of this exploratory endpoint is that it provides greater clinical meaning to the interpretation of progression. Patients in a trial with RECIST progression often have no symptoms of progression, and the time at which a decision is made to restart a patient on treatment could be considered more clinically meaningful. Trial drug allocation was not 'unblinded' on progression and this helped to avoid bias in these decisions. The median TSST takes account of post-progression therapy to examine whether the effect of olaparib is maintained beyond progression. It was 23.8 months compared with 15.2 months for patients receiving olaparib and placebo, respectively (HR 0.44; $p = 0.00013$). Thus, the benefit seen following subsequent therapy demonstrates that a positive effect of olaparib continues beyond progression and persists at least until the second subsequent treatment. In summary, olaparib treatment does not compromise subsequent therapy, and the 9.4-month median difference in delay in restarting chemotherapy (TFST) in patients with a BRCA mutation treated with olaparib is clinically meaningful and raises the possibility that the pattern of clinical relapse is different in the two groups of patients [24].

Toxicity and Tolerability of Olaparib Therapy

The trials described above demonstrate that for many patients, olaparib can be given as a long-term therapy. Maintenance therapy is given following a partial or complete response to chemotherapy, and it is important that long-term use of drugs does not produce significant adverse effects on symptoms. The toxicity analysis in study 19 showed that in general olaparib was well tolerated. The main adverse events were fatigue, nausea and anaemia. Fatigue and nausea usually appeared soon after the start of treatment [26]. Clinical experience suggests that nausea was often self-limiting, although the intermittent collection of data on each clinical visit can make this sort of information difficult to capture. Patients received 400 mg bd. Currently this is the capsule preparation which involves taking 16 capsules per day. Treatment breaks were sometimes used to manage adverse events; 36 % had dose interruptions and 42 % had a dose reduction (16 % and 22 %, respectively, in the placebo group. Nine patients in the olaparib group and two on placebo discontinued treatment due to an adverse event [24]. It should be noted that adverse events were not infrequent in patients taking placebo, highlighting that these patients with recurrent ovarian cancer may have disease-related symptoms following a partial response to chemotherapy. Corroborative data for tolerability was obtained through measurement of quality of life. These were only measured until progression, but there were no statistically significant or clinically relevant differences in health-related quality of life endpoints between treatment groups in the overall or BRCA-mutated populations demonstrating that olaparib has no detrimental effect on patients' quality of life [27]. In summary, it appears that olaparib is a well-tolerated drug that can be used long term. This is important as 25 % of patients on study 19 took the drug for more than 2 years, and 17 % of patients remained on olaparib for more than 3 years.

Clinical Studies with Other PARP Inhibitors

There are now at least four other PARP inhibitors undergoing clinical trials in ovarian cancer (see Table 12.1). Niraparib (MK 4827) and rucaparib have both been shown to have activity as a single agent in patients with a BRCAm [28, 29]. Randomised maintenance trials are now in progress with both drugs. The NOVA study (NCT01847274) of niraparib and the ARIEL3 study of rucaparib include cohorts of patients with a BRCA mutation as maintenance therapy following platinum-based treatment for 'platinum-sensitive' ovarian cancer. A companion diagnostic is being developed to identify patients without a germ-line BRCA mutation who are likely to benefit from a PARP inhibitor. Veliparib (ABT888) is being developed in combination with carboplatin and paclitaxel [30] and will be taken forward in a randomised trial in first-line therapy. Talazoparib (BMN-673) is a potent PARP inhibitor that has been tested more extensively in breast cancer but has demonstrable activity in ovarian cancer [31]. Table 12.1 summarises the ongoing clinical trials and includes the SOLO programme, two studies with olaparib, using the tablet preparation, rather than capsules (300 mg), in patients with a BRCA mutation. The trials include high-grade endometrioid as well as serous cancers and are evaluating maintenance olaparib in the first-line (SOLO-1) or 'platinum-sensitive' recurrent disease setting (SOLO-2).

Table 12.1 PARP inhibitors under investigation in ovarian cancer

PARP inhibitor	Company	PARP inhibition	Details
Olaparib (AZD2281)	AstraZeneca	PARP 1/2/3	Licensed in EU for maintenance BRCAm; ≥3rd line (FDA) in BRCAm. Phase III trials with tablet formulation – first line (*SOLO-1*) and maintenance in 'platinum-sensitive' recurrence (*SOLO-2*)
Rucaparib (AG-014699; CO-338)	Clovis oncology	PARP 1/2	Ongoing phase II and III studies in BRCAm, BRCAwt (*ARIEL2; ARIEL3*)
Veliparib (ABT-888)	AbbVie	PARP 1/2	First line phase III planned with chemotherapy
Niraparib (MK4827)	Tesaro	PARP 1/2	Ongoing phase III (*NOVA*) maintenance in BRCAm and BRCAwt; plans for first line
Talazoparib (BMN-673)	BioMarin Pharmaceutical	PARP 1/2	Ovarian cancer strategy unclear

BRCAm BRCA mutation, *BRCAwt* BRCA wild type

Challenges for Integrating PARP Inhibitors into Clinical Care

In the EU, olaparib is now licensed for maintenance therapy in BRCA-mutated HGSOC that has responded to platinum-based therapy. The licence is based on the analysis of the BRCA-mutated population in study 19 and includes those patients with a somatic mutation. This indication has not been accepted by the FDA in the USA, where the licence for olaparib is for single-agent therapy in patients with a BRCA mutation and active disease in need of treatment. The indication is based on an 'unmet need' in this group of women who have received 3 or more lines of chemotherapy and is derived from composite data from 223 patients with a germ-line BRCA mutation, 137 of whom had measurable disease (FDA olaparib data). The details of some of these patients are described in the 193 patients in the ovarian cohort in 'study 42'. The response rate was 34 % and the median progression-free survival was 7.9 months [32]. These two differing indications can be a source of confusion for some patients and indeed physicians outside the EU and USA. However, there is for the first time a molecularly targeted therapy for ovarian cancer based on genomics – the presence of a BRCA mutation. Although the cost of treatment is high, it is only applicable to a relatively small population of women with ovarian cancer. It is also clear that BRCA mutations have historically been under-diagnosed, and strategies need to be developed to ensure that patients with high-grade tumours are tested for a BRCA mutation. This is not as simple as it sounds. Historically, the responsibility for testing for germ-line mutations has been with cancer genetics departments; the indications are based largely on family history and the aim is to identify unaffected relatives. As we now know that the absence of family history is a poor negative predictor for a positive test, there needs to be a more widespread programme to test all patients. For some funders, this represents a significant resource issue. Although the cost of testing for a BRCA mutation is falling, many genetics departments do not have the resources to see and test all patients. For this reason in many areas, locally arranged consent and testing are performed within the context of gynaecology/oncology clinics, and only patients who are tested positive are referred to genetics departments for counselling so that a decision can be made about family testing. Opinion varies about the best time to test for a BRCA mutation, but it should be done either at diagnosis or after the completion of first-line therapy so that information is available at the time of first recurrence. There is also no consensus on the age limit of gene testing. The probability of detecting a germ-line BRCA-positive tumour falls off beyond the age of 60 years; there will be an even lower probability of finding a germ-line BRCA gene mutation in women over 70 years. However, testing only for germ-line mutations will miss somatic mutations estimated to be present in 6–8 % of tumours. For this reason, some advocate tumour testing of all patients with germ-line testing of those women who have a BRC mutation in the tumour. This presents additional resource and logistic issues that will need to be addressed.

Future Directions for PARP Inhibitor Therapy

Within a few years the results of three additional maintenance therapy trials in patients with 'platinum-sensitive tumours' (SOLO-2, NOVA, ARIEL3) will be available. In addition, the trials with niraparib and rucaparib will report on the use of maintenance therapy in patients without a BRCA mutation who are 'BRCA-like' by virtue of impaired HRR. Ongoing studies with rucaparib in BRCA-mutated tumours will provide a greater body of evidence of single-agent activity of this drug [29]. The results of the SOLO-1 trial, a randomised placebo-controlled trial of 2 years of maintenance olaparib following first-line therapy in patients with a BRCA mutation, will also be available. If this trial is positive, there will be three situations where olaparib can be used, creating a challenge for clinicians to select the appropriate time to use this drug. The results so far have shown that resistance to PARP inhibitors occurs in most patients with recurrent ovarian cancer. In a few situations, it has been shown that a revertant (functional) mutation occurs [33], but its importance as a factor underlying resistance to PARP inhibitors is unknown. Patients will respond to further chemotherapy after becoming resistant to a PARP inhibitor [34]. Following patients to the time of a second subsequent treatment after the treatment following failure of olaparib has shown that a benefit from the drug is maintained during subsequent treatment [24]. More information will emerge as the ongoing maintenance trials will measure the 'PFS2', the second progression-free survival after the subsequent treatment following progression on the trial drug. It is unknown whether patients will respond again to a (different) PARP inhibitor at a later point in their treatment, and it is important that strategies such as this are explored. Not all PARP inhibitors have an identical mode of action or potency. For example, in vitro data have shown that talazoparib (BMN-673) has greater potency than several other PARP inhibitors [35].

It is also becoming clear that there may be opportunities to combine PARP inhibitors with other molecularly targeted therapies. Synergy has been demonstrated between anti-angiogenic agents and PARP inhibitors [36]. The first indications of an additive or synergistic effect have come from a randomised trial comparing olaparib with a combination of cediranib, a VEGF receptor tyrosine kinase inhibitor [37] and olaparib in women with 'platinum-sensitive' relapsed ovarian cancer. The PFS was significantly improved in women receiving the combination and the magnitude of the effect was similar to that seen with conventional cytotoxic drugs. Trials are being planned to explore this combination further. One conducted through the NCI-CTEP will compare the combination with platinum-based chemotherapy, and the other, a UK-led study (ICON 9), will investigate the combination in a maintenance setting after chemotherapy. There are data to show that olaparib can be given safely with bevacizumab [38], and there will soon be a first-line trial (PAOLA-1) to evaluate the effect of adding olaparib to bevacizumab during the maintenance phase of treatment. Studies combining bevacizumab with niraparib in the second-line setting are also being planned. Other molecularly targeted agents, particularly those interfering with cell cycle replication, present additional opportunities for combination studies, and these are under discussion.

In summary, it is now clear that a BRCA mutation is the first predictive marker for molecularly targeted therapy of ovarian cancer and that PARP inhibitors represent a highly active new class of drug for this disease. The indication for their use will most likely expand, particularly if reliable predictive markers for defective HRR are found. The results so far have clearly demonstrated that treatment of ovarian cancer needs to be tailored to its biology.

References

1. Miki Y, Swensen J, Shattuck-Eidens D, Futreal PA, Harshman K, Tavtigian S, et al. A strong candidate for the breast and ovarian cancer susceptibility gene BRCA1. Science. 1994; 266(5182):66–71.
2. Wooster R, Neuhausen SL, Mangion J, Quirk Y, Ford D, Collins N, et al. Localization of a breast cancer susceptibility gene, BRCA2, to chromosome 13q12-13. Science. 1994; 265(5181):2088–90.
3. Chen S, Parmigiani G. Meta-analysis of BRCA1 and BRCA2 penetrance. J Clin Oncol. 2007;25(11):1329–33.
4. Risch HA, McLaughlin JR, Cole DE, Rosen B, Bradley L, Kwan E, et al. Prevalence and penetrance of germline BRCA1 and BRCA2 mutations in a population series of 649 women with ovarian cancer. Am J Hum Genet. 2001;68(3):700–10.
5. Alsop K, Fereday S, Meldrum C, deFazio A, Emmanuel C, George J, et al. BRCA mutation frequency and patterns of treatment response in BRCA mutation-positive women with ovarian cancer: a report from the Australian ovarian cancer study group. J Clin Oncol. 2012; 30(21):2654–63.
6. Bell D, Berchuck A, Birrer M, Chien J, Cramer DW, Dao F, et al. Integrated genomic analyses of ovarian carcinoma. Nature. 2011;474(7353):609–15.
7. Risch HA, McLaughlin JR, Cole DE, Rosen B, Bradley L, Fan I, et al. Population BRCA1 and BRCA2 mutation frequencies and cancer penetrances: a kin-cohort study in Ontario, Canada. J Natl Cancer Inst. 2006;98(23):1694–706.
8. Goodheart MJ, Rose SL, Hattermann-Zogg M, Smith BJ, De Young BR, Buller RE. BRCA2 alteration is important in clear cell carcinoma of the ovary. Clin Genet. 2009;76(2):161–7.
9. Bolton KL, Chenevix-Trench G, Goh C, Sadetzki S, Ramus SJ, Karlan BY, et al. Association between BRCA1 and BRCA2 mutations and survival in women with invasive epithelial ovarian cancer. JAMA. 2012;307(4):382–90.
10. Zhong Q, Peng H-L, Zhao X, Zhang L, Hwang W-T. Effects of BRCA1- and BRCA2-related mutations on ovarian and breast cancer survival: a meta-analysis. Clin Cancer Res. 2015;21(1):211–20.
11. Tan DSP, Rothermundt C, Thomas K, Bancroft E, Eeles R, Shanley S, et al. 'BRCAness' syndrome in ovarian cancer: a case-control study describing the clinical features and outcome of patients with epithelial ovarian cancer associated with BRCA1 and BRCA2 mutations. J Clin Oncol. 2008;26(34):5530–6.
12. Gudmundsdottir K, Ashworth A. The roles of BRCA1 and BRCA2 and associated proteins in the maintenance of genomic stability. Oncogene. 2006;25(43):5864–74.
13. Helleday T, Petermann E, Lundin C, Hodgson B, Sharma RA. DNA repair pathways as targets for cancer therapy. Nat Rev Cancer. 2008;8(3):193–204.
14. Bryant HE, Schultz N, Thomas HD, Parker KM, Flower D, Lopez E, et al. Specific killing of BRCA2-deficient tumours with inhibitors of poly(ADP-ribose) polymerase. Nature. 2005;434(7035):913–7.
15. Farmer H, McCabe N, Lord CJ, Tutt AN, Johnson DA, Richardson TB, et al. Targeting the DNA repair defect in BRCA mutant cells as a therapeutic strategy. Nature. 2005;434(7035): 917–21.

16. Ferraris DV. Evolution of poly(ADP-ribose) polymerase-1 (PARP-1) inhibitors. From concept to clinic. J Med Chem. 2010;53(12):4561–84.
17. Fong PC, Boss DS, Yap TA, Tutt A, Wu P, Mergui-Roelvink M, et al. Inhibition of poly(ADP-ribose) polymerase in tumors from BRCA mutation carriers. N Engl J Med. 2009; 361(2):123–34.
18. Fong PC, Yap TA, Boss DS, Carden CP, Mergui-Roelvink M, Gourley C, et al. Poly(ADP)-ribose polymerase inhibition: frequent durable responses in BRCA carrier ovarian cancer correlating with platinum-free interval. J Clin Oncol. 2010;28(15):2512–9.
19. Audeh MW, Carmichael J, Penson RT, Friedlander M, Powell B, Bell-McGuinn KM, et al. Oral poly(ADP-ribose) polymerase inhibitor olaparib in patients with BRCA1 or BRCA2 mutations and recurrent ovarian cancer: a proof-of-concept trial. Lancet. 2010;376(9737): 245–51.
20. Kaye SB, Lubinski J, Matulonis U, Ang JE, Gourley C, Karlan BY, et al. Phase II, open-label, randomized, multicenter study comparing the efficacy and safety of olaparib, a poly (ADP-ribose) polymerase inhibitor, and pegylated liposomal doxorubicin in patients with BRCA1 or BRCA2 mutations and recurrent ovarian cancer. J Clin Oncol. 2012;30(4):372–9.
21. Gelmon KA, Tischkowitz M, Mackay H, Swenerton K, Robidoux A, Tonkin K, et al. Olaparib in patients with recurrent high-grade serous or poorly differentiated ovarian carcinoma or triple-negative breast cancer: a phase 2, multicentre, open-label, non-randomised study. Lancet Oncol. 2011;12(9):852–61.
22. Oza AM, Cibula D, Benzaquen AO, Poole C, Mathijssen RH, Sonke GS, et al. Olaparib combined with chemotherapy for recurrent platinum-sensitive ovarian cancer: a randomised phase 2 trial. Lancet Oncol. 2015;16:87–97.
23. Ledermann J, Harter P, Gourley C, Friedlander M, Vergote I, Rustin G, et al. Olaparib maintenance therapy in platinum-sensitive relapsed ovarian cancer. N Engl J Med. 2012; 366(15):1382–92.
24. Ledermann J, Harter P, Gourley C, Friedlander M, Vergote I, Rustin G, et al. Olaparib maintenance therapy in patients with platinum-sensitive relapsed serous ovarian cancer: a preplanned retrospective analysis of outcomes by BRCA status in a randomised phase 2 trial. Lancet Oncol. 2014;15(8):852–61.
25. Matulonis U, Harter P, Gourley C, Friedlander M, Vergote IB, Rustin GJS, et al. Analysis of intermediate clinical endpoints from a phase II trial of olaparib maintenance therapy in patients with platinum-sensitive relapsed serous ovarian cancer (PSR SOC). Gynecol Oncol. 2015;137(Suppl1):5–6.
26. Matulonis U, Friedlander M, du Bois A, Gourley C, Vergote IB, Rustin G, et al. Frequency, severity and timing of common adverse events (AEs) with maintenance olaparib in patients (pts) with platinum-sensitive relapsed serous ovarian cancer (PSR SOC). J Clin Oncol. 2015;33(Suppl; abstr 5550).
27. Ledermann JA, Harter P, Gourley C, Friedlander M, Vergote IB, Rustin GJS, et al. 885PD. Health-related Quality of Life (HRQOL) during olaparib maintenance therapy in patients with platinum-sensitive relapsed serous ovarian cancer (PSR SOC) and a BRCA mutation (BRCAm). Ann Oncol. 2014;25(Suppl 4):iv308–iv9.
28. Sandhu SK, Schelman WR, Wilding G, Moreno V, Baird RD, Miranda S, et al. The poly(ADP-ribose) polymerase inhibitor niraparib (MK4827) in BRCA mutation carriers and patients with sporadic cancer: a phase 1 dose-escalation trial. Lancet Oncol. 2013;14(9):882–92.
29. Shapira-Frommer R, Oza A, Domchek S, Balmaña J, Patel MR, Chen L, et al. A phase II open-label, multicenter study of single-agent rucaparib in the treatment of patients with relapsed ovarian cancer and a deleterious BRCA mutation. J Clin Oncol. 2015;22(Supple; abstr 5513).
30. Bell-McGuinn K, Brady W, Schilder R, Fracasso P, Moore K, Walker J, et al. A phase I study of continuous veliparib in combination with IV carboplatin/paclitaxel or IV/IP paclitaxel/cisplatin and bevacizumab in newly diagnosed patients with previously untreated epithelial ovarian, fallopian tube, or primary peritoneal cancer: an NRG Oncology/Gynecologic Oncology Group study. J Clin Oncol. 2015;33(Suppl; abstr 5507).

31. Ramanathan R, Wainberg Z, Mina L, Byers L, Chugh R, Zhang C, et al. PARP inhibition with BMN 673 in ovarian and breast cancer patients with deleterious mutations of BRCA1 and BRCA2. Eur J Cancer. 2013;49(Suppl 3; abstr # 29).
32. Kaufman B, Shapira-Frommer R, Schmutzler RK, Audeh MW, Friedlander M, Balmana J, et al. Olaparib monotherapy in patients with advanced cancer and a germline BRCA1/2 mutation. J Clin Oncol. 2015;33(3):244–50.
33. Edwards SL, Brough R, Lord CJ, Natrajan R, Vatcheva R, Levine DA, et al. Resistance to therapy caused by intragenic deletion in BRCA2. Nature. 2008;451(7182):1111–5.
34. Ang JE, Gourley C, Powell CB, High H, Shapira-Frommer R, Castonguay V, et al. Efficacy of chemotherapy in BRCA1/2 mutation carrier ovarian cancer in the setting of PARP inhibitor resistance: a multi-institutional study. Clin Cancer Res. 2013;19(19):5485–93.
35. Shen Y, Rehman FL, Feng Y, Boshuizen J, Bajrami I, Elliott R, et al. BMN 673, a novel and highly potent PARP1/2 inhibitor for the treatment of human cancers with DNA repair deficiency. Clin Cancer Res. 2013;19(18):5003–15.
36. Chan N, Pires IM, Bencokova Z, Coackley C, Luoto KR, Bhogal N, et al. Contextual synthetic lethality of cancer cell kill based on the tumor microenvironment. Cancer Res. 2010; 70(20):8045–54.
37. Liu JF, Barry WT, Birrer M, Lee J-M, Buckanovich RJ, Fleming GF, et al. Combination cediranib and olaparib versus olaparib alone for women with recurrent platinum-sensitive ovarian cancer: a randomised phase 2 study. Lancet Oncol. 2014;15:1207–14.
38. Dean E, Middleton MR, Pwint T, Swaisland H, Carmichael J, Goodege-Kunwar P, et al. Phase I study to assess the safety and tolerability of olaparib in combination with bevacizumab in patients with advanced solid tumours. Br J Cancer. 2012;106(3):468–74.

Serous Tumors of Low Malignant Potential and Low-Grade Serous Carcinomas of the Ovary or Peritoneum

13

David M. Gershenson

Abstract
Serous tumors of low malignant potential (LMP) and invasive low-grade serous carcinoma exist on a continuum. Pathological criteria for diagnosis for both entities are well described. For both, the mitogen-activated protein kinase pathway appears to play a prominent role in their pathogenesis. Surgery is the cornerstone of treatment. Fertility-sparing surgery is commonly performed for serous LMP tumors. While stage I serous LMP tumors have an excellent prognosis, at least 20 % of serous LMP tumors associated with peritoneal implants relapse, most as low-grade serous carcinoma. Low-grade serous carcinoma is characterized by young age at diagnosis, relative chemoresistance, and prolonged survival compared with high-grade serous carcinoma. Standard postoperative treatment for low-grade serous carcinoma consists of platinum/taxane chemotherapy. Treatment of recurrence includes options for chemotherapy, hormonal therapy, and targeted agents such as bevacizumab. MEK inhibitor therapy has had promising activity in a phase II trial, and multiple phase III trials of MEK inhibitor therapy for recurrent low-grade serous carcinoma are ongoing.

Introduction

Evidence to date, including histopathologic, clinical, and molecular/genetic information, strongly suggests that low-grade serous and high-grade serous carcinomas develop along two different pathways and that serous tumors of low malignant potential (serous

D.M. Gershenson, MD
Department of Gynecologic Oncology and Reproductive Medicine,
Unit 1362, The University of Texas MD Anderson Cancer Center,
1515 Holcombe Boulevard, Houston, TX 77030, USA
e-mail: dgershen@mdanderson.org

E. Pujade-Lauraine et al. (eds.), *Ovarian Cancers*,
DOI 10.1007/978-3-319-32110-3_13

borderline tumors) and low-grade serous carcinomas lie along the same developmental continuum [1–12]. This chapter will focus only on these latter two low-grade serous tumor entities, with emphasis on our current understanding based on the past 25 years of investigations, their clinical behavior, and current management.

Serous Tumors of Low Malignant Potential

Background

Taylor first described serous tumors of low malignant potential in 1929, classifying them as a "semi-malignant" or "hyperplastic type" of cystadenoma [13]. However, it was not until 1973 that this group of tumors was incorporated into the classification system of the International Federation of Gynecology and Obstetrics as "carcinoma of low malignant potential" and into that of the World Health Organization as "borderline ovarian tumor" [14, 15]. Only since the 1990s have we begun to understand the clinical behavior and molecular underpinnings of these fascinating neoplasms.

Epidemiology

Tumors of low malignant potential account for approximately 10–20 % of all epithelial ovarian neoplasms [16]. The most common histologic subtype is serous [17, 18]. Women with tumors of low malignant potential (LMP) are, on average, significantly younger than those with invasive epithelial ovarian cancer, and approximately one-third are less than 40 years of age [17, 19]. In addition, there is evidence that obesity or unopposed estrogen replacement may increase a woman's risk of serous tumors of LMP [20].

Diagnosis

Serous tumors of LMP are generally diagnosed on pelvic examination or by pelvic ultrasound. Approximately 60 % of women with stage I serous LMP tumor and 85 % of women with stage II–IV serous LMP tumor have abnormal serum CA 125 levels [21]. A definitive diagnosis is made on histopathologic review of tumor removed at surgery.

Pathology

There are two distinct histologic patterns in serous LMP tumors: (1) typical and (2) micropapillary/cribriform. The typical pattern consists of (1) stratification of the epithelial lining of the papillae; (2) formation of microscopic papillary projections or tufts, often detached, arising from the epithelial lining of the papillae; (3) varying degrees of nuclear atypia; and (4) absence of frank stromal invasion [3]. The micropapillary/cribriform pattern consists of (1) elongate filiform micropapillae that arise in a nonhierarchical manner from cyst walls or from large fibrous or edematous papillae, have cores containing little or no connective tissue, and are most frequently lined by cuboidal cells with scant cytoplasm, (2) a high nuclear-to-cytoplasmic ratio, and (3) mildly to moderately atypical round nuclei [22–25]. In some cases, the two patterns may be admixed. In addition, within the primary ovarian serous LMP tumor, microinvasion may be present. Microinvasion is defined as a focus or foci, each less than 3 mm in greatest dimension, of tumor cells that infiltrate the stroma as single cells, nests of cells, or papillae [26, 27].

Peritoneal implants are classified as either noninvasive or invasive [27, 28]. Noninvasive implants have features similar to the primary serous LMP tumor and are subclassified into epithelial or desmoplastic types. Invasive implants are defined by the presence of irregular infiltration into adjacent tissue and are composed of glands with extensive bridging or small solid epithelial nests.

Molecular Biology

The molecular biology of serous LMP tumors has been extensively studied. Serous LMP tumors have a high frequency of estrogen receptor (ER) and progesterone receptor (PR) positivity. Arias-Pulido et al. reported that in 22 serous LMP tumors, 63.6 % were positive for ER and 81.8 % were positive for PR [29]. Unlike high-grade serous carcinomas but similar to low-grade serous carcinomas, serous LMP tumors have a low frequency of p53 mutations. Singer et al. reported that only 8 % of 25 serous LMP tumors contained a p53 mutation [30].

The mitogen-activated protein kinase (MAPK) pathway appears to play a prominent role in the pathogenesis of serous LMP tumors. Singer et al. reported *KRAS* mutations in 33 % of 51 serous LMP tumors and *BRAF* mutations in 28 % [11]. In a subsequent study of 45 cases of advanced-stage serous LMP tumors from Denmark, Ardighieri and colleagues demonstrated *KRAS* mutations in 34 (61.8 %) and *BRAF* mutations in eight (14.5 %) of 55 serous LMP tumors [31]. Mutational analysis was also performed in 56 peritoneal implants and revealed *KRAS* mutations in 60.7 % and *BRAF* mutations in 12.5 % of these implants. These findings supported the theory that peritoneal implants are largely derived from the primary serous LMP tumor. In a recent report of gene expression profiling of serous LMP tumors, Curry et al. identified 50 genes that appear to separate these tumors into benign and malignant subtypes [32].

Clinical Behavior and Treatment

The presentation for women with a serous LMP tumor is generally a pelvic mass palpated on examination or found on ultrasound. Considerations regarding surgical approach include stage distribution and frequency of bilaterality. Stage I accounts for at least 60 % of cases in most series, and the incidence of ovarian bilaterality is approximately 50 %. Two large European studies indicated that stage I serous LMP tumors account for approximately 76–85 % of all serous LMP tumors [18, 33]. In the Danish cohort, 34.7 % of 1042 cases were bilateral [33].

Surgery is the primary treatment. One of the initial considerations in contemplating surgery for a pelvic mass is the surgical approach—minimally invasive or open technique. Factors to be considered in the selection of minimally invasive surgical approaches (laparoscopic or robotic) include size of the ovarian mass(es), extent of tumor metastasis, number and type or previous operations, and body habitus. Several reports have documented the feasibility and safety of the minimally invasive approach when appropriately used [34–37].

Since a large proportion of patients with serous LMP tumors are young and have not completed childbearing, fertility-sparing surgery is widely practiced. For women with unilateral ovarian involvement, either ovarian cystectomy or unilateral salpingo-oophorectomy is appropriate. For those with bilateral ovarian involvement, the most common intraoperative procedures are unilateral salpingo-oophorectomy and ovarian cystectomy or bilateral ovarian cystectomy, depending on the findings. Following ovarian cystectomy, recurrence of a serous LMP tumor in the ipsilateral or contralateral ovary occurs in approximately 12–36 % [38–40]. Several further reports have indicated that after fertility-sparing surgery, the most common site of recurrence is in the residual ovary(ies) [41–44]. In most cases, a repeat surgical procedure is the treatment of choice, and adjuvant therapy is unnecessary. Following removal of the ovary(ies) or portions thereof, frozen section examination for confirmation is recommended. However, accuracy is somewhat limited, and the surgeon should factor into his/her intraoperative decision-making the possibility of a final diagnosis of invasive cancer [45].

A major question in the treatment of serous LMP tumors involves the role of comprehensive surgical staging. Since the presence of peritoneal implants has prognostic significance, and the most common sites of implants include the omentum and peritoneal surfaces, surgical staging consisting of omentectomy and peritoneal biopsies is generally recommended [3, 46]. However, comprehensive surgical staging remains somewhat controversial for serous LMP tumors. For instance, because the incidence of lymph node involvement is quite low, routine pelvic and para-aortic lymphadenectomy is not recommended by most [47]. However, if lymphadenopathy is noted, resection is appropriate. Even more controversial is the role of surgical restaging for a patient who undergoes surgery with final diagnosis of serous LMP tumor but without surgical staging. Although restaging surgery is associated with a significant rate of detection of extraovarian peritoneal implants, it may provide only prognostic information and no therapeutic value [48, 49]. If surgical restaging is performed following adequate counseling, a minimally invasive surgical approach is preferred.

Outcome is influenced by several factors, including pathological and clinical factors. Pathological factors that may be associated with an increased risk of relapse include the presence of the micropapillary/cribriform pattern or microinvasion in the primary ovarian serous LMP tumor or the presence of peritoneal implants [3–6, 23, 24, 27, 28, 50–54]. For instance, the presence of noninvasive peritoneal implants is associated with a 20 % or greater lifetime risk of relapse [3, 6], whereas the presence of invasive peritoneal implants is associated with a 50 % or greater lifetime risk of relapse

[4]. Although still somewhat controversial, the consensus is that lymph node involvement with serous LMP tumors does not significantly influence outcome [55–57]. Clinical factors that also influence prognosis include FIGO stage, which is obviously associated with the presence or absence of peritoneal implants, and preoperative serum CA 125 level [53, 54, 58–61]. Women with stage I serous LMP tumors have an excellent prognosis, with a relapse rate of 1 % or less [19, 53, 61].

For women who undergo fertility-sparing surgery, successful pregnancies have been reported in several series [62, 63]. In addition, in selected patients prior to or following surgery for serous LMP tumor or prior to adjuvant chemotherapy for invasive peritoneal implants or recurrent disease, in vitro fertilization techniques may be discussed and recommended. There is no standard approach in these situations, and options and recommendation must be individualized.

Despite the fact that several clinicopathologic factors for relapse are known, postoperative chemotherapy is recommended very seldom. Historically, platinum-based chemotherapy for women with peritoneal implants—both noninvasive and invasive—was recommended. However, no reports have indicated either a decreased risk of relapse or survival advantage associated with this approach [3, 4, 64]. On the other hand, because of the high risk of relapse for women who have serous LMP tumors and invasive peritoneal implants, platinum/taxane chemotherapy continues to be recommended in several centers.

Treatment of Recurrent Disease

Clinicopathologic risk factors are discussed above. As noted, the most powerful factor associated with recurrence following a diagnosis of serous LMP tumor is stage or the presence of peritoneal implants. As discussed above, following conservative or fertility-sparing surgery, women may develop a "recurrence" or second primary lesion in the residual ovarian tissue. The histology of this type of lesion is almost always another serous LMP tumor and can be managed with surgery alone. However, most relapses involve extraovarian sites, and the majority of these recurrences are not serous LMP tumor, but rather invasive low-grade serous carcinoma [3–7, 27]. In a report of 49 women with recurrent serous LMP tumors with known histology, 27 % had serous LMP tumors and 73 % had invasive low-grade serous carcinoma [5]. Initial treatment of low-grade serous carcinoma is generally combination platinum/taxane chemotherapy, as discussed below. In rare cases, serous LMP tumors may recur as high-grade serous carcinoma [65, 66].

Low-Grade Serous Carcinoma

Background

The convergence of two major factors over the past 10–15 years combined to propel the study of low-grade serous carcinoma of the ovary or peritoneum: (1) the development and reporting of the binary grading system for serous carcinoma to replace the grading system of the International Federation of Gynecology and Obstetrics (FIGO) [67–74] and (2) the accelerated understanding of its associated molecular biology and genetics [1, 8–12, 30, 67–88]. Concomitantly, studies of the clinical behavior of low-grade serous carcinoma have underscored its distinct character compared to high-grade serous carcinoma [89–102].

One of the leaders in this transformation has been the Rare Tumor Committee of the Gynecologic Oncology Group (GOG), which was established in 2005. In 2014, the GOG merged with other cooperative groups to form the new NRG Oncology cooperative group. Since 2005, several clinical trials for rare ovarian/peritoneal cancer subtypes—clear-cell carcinomas, mucinous carcinomas, and low-grade serous carcinomas and non-epithelial tumors—have been activated.

The overarching principles by which the GOG (NRG) Rare Tumor Committee has operated have included the following: (1) separate clinical trials for distinct histologic subtypes; (2) investigation of novel targeted agents based on promising preclinical studies, whenever possible; and (3) inclusion of robust tissue acquisition and translational research components within each trial.

Nevertheless, the study of rare ovarian cancers remains logistically challenging for a variety of reasons. Small patient numbers within each of the subtypes represent a threat to meeting accrual targets. This realization has led to strategies to overcome this limitation, including intergroup trials and international consortia or other collaborations. Additional issues include the implementation of novel trial designs with which to efficiently study these rare tumors and accurate pathological diagnostic criteria for eligibility. For example, prospective digital pathology review rather than the usual post hoc central pathology review is necessary for trial screening in most of such investigations. Furthermore, the financial, regulatory, and nursing and data management efforts associated with opening any clinical trials are particularly burdensome when one considers that any single institution may accrue a relatively small number of patients to a multi-institutional or cooperative group trial of a rare tumor.

Epidemiology

Approximately 10 % of patients with invasive serous carcinoma of the ovary/peritoneum have low-grade serous carcinoma [89, 101]. The stage distribution is very similar to that of high-grade serous carcinoma, with over 70 % of cases in the stage III or IV category [89, 101]. On the other hand, the median age of women with low-grade serous carcinoma is significantly younger than those with high-grade serous carcinoma [89, 101]. In addition, the median overall survival for women with low-grade serous carcinoma is significantly longer than the median overall survival times reported for women with high-grade serous carcinoma [89].

Although there appears to be indirect evidence that estrogen or hormonal stimulation may somehow play a role in the pathogenesis of low-grade serous carcinoma, we are far from understanding this relationship. In a report of a large, international collaborative study consisting of 7911 women with invasive ovarian cancer and

13,226 controls, self-reported endometriosis was associated with a significantly increased risk of a number of subtypes of ovarian cancer, including low-grade serous carcinoma [103].

Diagnosis

Low-grade serous carcinoma is thought to present either after an original diagnosis of advanced-stage serous tumor of low malignant potential (see above) or de novo. The clinical presentation for low-grade serous carcinoma does not differ from that of other ovarian cancer subtypes and may include any or all of the following symptoms: abdominal or pelvic pain, bloating, or bowel or bladder dysfunction. Initial diagnostic studies may include serum CA 125, sonography, or computed tomography of the abdomen/pelvis. Serum CA 125 at the time of diagnosis appears to be elevated in approximately 85 % of women with stage II–IV low-grade serous carcinoma [89, 98].

A definitive diagnosis is usually made at the time of primary surgery. However, if a patient has extensive metastatic tumor, neoadjuvant chemotherapy may be recommended prior to interval cytoreductive surgery. In the latter case, a tissue biopsy, which can be obtained via a CT-guided fine needle aspiration/core biopsy or laparoscopic procedure, is always recommended.

Pathology

The binary grading system for serous carcinoma is based primarily on the assessment of nuclear atypia with the mitotic count used as a secondary criterion [2]. In comparison with the FIGO grading system, all but one of the 36 FIGO grade 1 cases were classified as low grade, and all of the 11 FIGO grade 3 cases were classified as high grade. However, of the 53 FIGO grade 2 cases, 15 were classified as low grade and 38 as high grade. The results of this study simply underscore the confusion surrounding the FIGO grade 2 category and why migrating to a two-tier grading system makes so much sense. A further important finding of this study was the coexistence of serous tumor of low malignant potential and low-grade serous carcinoma in 60 % of cases. Subsequent reports only further strengthened the observation that the FIGO grading system is flawed and the wisdom surrounding dichotomization of the grading system for serous carcinoma [68, 69, 71, 72]. For instance, in the study of Bodurka et al., there was no difference in clinical outcome in patients with grade 2 or 3 tumors in multivariate analysis [72].

Molecular Biology

Molecular and genetic investigations over the past decade have brought the biology of low-grade serous carcinoma into much sharper focus. Based on available evidence, we currently believe that low-grade serous carcinoma may arise following an

Table 13.1 Frequency of mutations in serous tumors of low malignant potential and low-grade serous carcinomas

Gene mutation	Serous tumor of LMP	Low-grade serous carcinoma	References
TP53	0–8 %	0–8.3 %	[30, 82]
KRAS	33–61.8 %	19–41 %	[11, 31, 82, 108]
BRAF	14.5–28 %	2–33 %	[11, 31, 82, 108]

initial diagnosis of serous tumor of low malignant potential or de novo [3–7, 89]. The weight of evidence further suggests that the mitogen-activated protein kinase (MAPK) pathway plays a prominent role in the pathogenesis of both entities. Genomic profiling studies have demonstrated that low-grade serous carcinomas segregate from high-grade serous carcinomas but are similar to serous tumors of low malignant potential [8, 9]. Compared with high-grade serous carcinomas, low-grade serous carcinomas have a much lower frequency of p53 mutations or p53 expression [30, 77], greater expression of ER and PR [79], greater expression of PAX2 [81], overexpression of anterior gradient homolog 3 (AGR3) [104], and overexpression of IGF-1 [105]. And, although germ-line BRCA mutations occur in a relatively high proportion of women with high-grade serous carcinoma, low-grade serous carcinoma does not appear to be part of the hereditary breast-ovarian cancer syndrome [106, 107].

In 2003, Singer et al. reported their study of 182 ovarian tumors, including 51 serous tumors of low malignant potential and 21 low-grade serous carcinomas [11]. *KRAS* mutations were reported in 33 % of serous tumors of low malignant potential and in 35 % of low-grade serous carcinomas, and *BRAF* mutations were found in 28 % and 33 %, respectively. Subsequent reports of low-grade serous carcinoma, however, seemed to confirm a 20–40 % frequency of *KRAS* mutations but a much lower frequency of *BRAF* mutations—2–6 % [82, 108]. Based on their findings, Wong et al. concluded that the low frequency of *BRAF* mutations in advanced-stage low-grade serous carcinomas compared with serous tumors of low malignant potential suggested that the former are more likely derived from serous tumors of low malignant potential without *BRAF* mutations [82]. A more recent study appeared to confirm these observations [85]. In other words, the presence of a *BRAF* mutation in an advanced-stage serous tumor of low malignant potential may somehow protect against the development of a subsequent low-grade serous carcinoma. Table 13.1 summarizes the frequency of known mutations in serous tumors of low malignant potential and low-grade serous carcinomas. In a study of 23 patients with an original diagnosis of serous tumor of low malignant potential who subsequently recurred with low-grade serous carcinoma, patients with *KRAS G12V* mutations had shorter survival times than those with either *KRAS G12D*, wild-type, or rare *KRAS* variants ($HR = 4.77$; $p = 0.023$) [86] And, although it appears that aberrations of the PI3K/AKT/mTOR pathway are relatively rare in low-grade serous carcinoma [84], there is some evidence that dual blockade of the MAP kinase and PI3K/AKT/mTOR pathways may be associated with enhanced activity compared with MAP kinase pathway blockade alone (see below).

Clinical Behavior and Treatment

Surgery is a major modality of treatment in low-grade serous carcinoma, as it is in all histologic subtypes. For most patients, primary surgery, including comprehensive surgical staging for patients with apparent early-stage disease and cytoreductive surgery for those with metastatic disease, is the initial treatment. Fertility-sparing surgery is an option for selected young patients. For selected women with extensive metastatic tumor or significant comorbidities, neoadjuvant chemotherapy with interval cytoreductive surgery may be recommended. In such cases, either fine needle aspiration/core biopsy or a minimally invasive surgical procedure to establish an accurate diagnosis is performed prior to starting chemotherapy.

Several predominant themes have emerged from studies of the clinical course of low-grade serous carcinoma of the ovary or peritoneum. In an ancillary study of Gynecologic Oncology Group (GOG) protocol 182, Fader et al. reported the details regarding 189 patients with FIGO grade 1 serous carcinoma (a surrogate for low-grade serous carcinoma) [96]. On multivariate analysis, only residual disease status following primary surgery was significantly associated with overall survival. Patients with microscopic residual had a significantly longer median progression-free (33.2 months) and overall survival (96.9 months) compared with those with residual 0.1–1.0 cm (14.7 months and 44.5 months, respectively) and more than 1.0 cm of residual disease (14.1 months and 42.0 months, respectively). The overall pattern of these results closely resembles that of epithelial ovarian cancer in general. In a second study from the same dataset, serum CA 125 values were analyzed [98]. Although pretreatment CA 125 was not prognostic of outcome, patients with CA 125 levels that normalized after one to three cycles of chemotherapy were 60–64 % less likely to experience disease progression as compared to those who never normalized or normalized after 4 cycles ($p \leq 0.024$). Normalization of CA 125 levels before the second cycle was negatively associated with death, with an HR of 0.45 ($p = 0.025$).

Previs et al. reported the Duke experience with 81 women with low-grade serous carcinoma of the ovary [100]. On multivariate analysis, obesity (HR = 2.8) and optimal tumor debulking (HR = 0.05) were significant predictors of overall survival. Additionally obesity was not associated with worse disease-specific survival, suggesting that mortality of obese patients may have been attributable to other comorbidities.

In the initial systematic study of metastatic low-grade serous carcinoma of the ovary, major features included relatively young age at diagnosis (median age = 43 years), prolonged overall survival (median OS = 82 months), and relative chemoresistance as reflected by the surrogate marker of persistent tumor at completion of primary treatment (48 % of patients) [89]. After adjusting for other variables, persistent disease after primary chemotherapy was associated with a shorter PFS time (HR = 2.64; $P = 0.03$). The theme of relative chemoresistance, thought to be related to the indolent nature of low-grade serous carcinoma, was subsequently also observed in reports of patients treated with neoadjuvant chemotherapy [90], patients with primary peritoneal low-grade serous carcinoma [92], and patients with

Table 13.2 Molecular biomarkers and potential targets in low-grade serous carcinoma of the ovary or peritoneum

Gene or pathway	Frequency	Potential active agents	References
KRAS	20–40 %	MEKi	[11, 82, 84–86, 108]
BRAF	2–6 %	BRAFi	[11, 82, 84–86, 108]
IGF-1R	Overexpressed compared to STLMP and HGSC	IGF-1Ri	[105]
Angiogenesis (e.g., VEGF)	–	Antiangiogenesis agents (e.g., bevacizumab)	[99, 116]
PI3K/AKT/mTOR	Rare	PI3Ki AKTi mTORi	[84]

Abbreviations: *STLMP* serous tumors of low malignant potential, *HGSC* high-grade serous carcinoma

recurrent disease [91]. Nevertheless, chemotherapy generally remains the standard therapy for women with stage II–IV low-grade serous carcinoma until such time that it is replaced by evidence-based alternative treatment. In addition, in the report of chemotherapy for recurrent low-grade serous carcinoma, 60 % of women had stable disease for a period of time. Whether the frequency of stable disease is more related to tumor biology or a therapeutic effect remains unresolved (Table 13.2).

For some women, hormonal therapy may offer a greater benefit than chemotherapy with less associated toxicity [95]. In a report of 64 women with recurrent low-grade serous carcinoma who received 89 separate hormonal therapy regimens, 9 % of patient regimens resulted in an objective response, and 62 % of patient regimens resulted in stable disease [95]. In addition, ER/PR expression data were available in 50 patients in this study. Patients with ER+/PR- tumors had a shorter time to progression (HR = 1.8) than patients with ER+/PR+ tumors; however, this observation approached but did not reach statistical significance ($p = 0.056$). Thus, hormonal therapy remains a reasonable and potentially active treatment for women with metastatic low-grade serous carcinoma.

Given the realization that cytotoxic chemotherapy has limited activity in low-grade serous carcinoma, a search for more effective systemic therapies is warranted. As with most cancer types, investigators have principally focused on the study of targeted therapies over the past few years. Coupled with these efforts is the continued study of the molecular biology of low-grade serous carcinoma through additional basic science and translational research studies.

Targeted Therapeutics

Based on preclinical research findings, potential genes or pathways for targeting low-grade serous carcinoma include the MAPK pathway, IGF-1R, the angiogenesis pathway, and possibly the PI3K/AKT/mTOR pathway. The MAPK signaling pathway is one of the most activated and best characterized in cancer [109]. The MAPK cascade is triggered by the binding of a ligand that ultimately leads to phosphorylation of *ERK* [110, 111]. Thus, *MEK* is a good candidate for targeted therapy, and a number of MEKi have been developed in the past few years [112, 113]. Preclinical studies of ovarian cancer demonstrated significant growth inhibition in cell lines with *KRAS* or *BRAF* mutations compared with cell lines with wild-type cells [114, 115]. In view of the cumulative data indicating mutations within the MAPK pathway, as discussed above, exploration of MEKi in patients with low-grade serous carcinoma was a natural progression.

In a landmark GOG phase II trial (GOG 0239), Farley et al. demonstrated promising results with an MEKi, selumetinib [108]. Fifty-two women with recurrent low-grade serous carcinoma were enrolled in this trial and treated with the MEKi, selumetinib 50 mg twice daily. The overall response rate was 15 %, with one complete response and seven partial responses. Another 65 % of patients in the trial had stable disease. The median PFS was 11.0 months. The most common toxicities were gastrointestinal (13), dermatologic (nine), and metabolic (seven). Three patients experienced grade 4 toxicities—one each cardiac, pain, and pulmonary. Mutational analysis was conducted on formalin-fixed, paraffin-embedded tumor samples from 34 patients in this trial. The primary tumor accounted for 82 % of the cases. In these 34 cases, there were two (6 %) *BRAF* mutations and 14 (41 %) *KRAS* mutations. In this study, there was no correlation between mutations of *BRAF* or *KRAS* and objective response. Subsequently, the promising results of this trial in the context of the relatively low response rates of low-grade serous carcinoma to either chemotherapeutic or hormonal agents prompted further investigations.

Three ongoing phase II or III clinical trials have emerged from this experience. Each of these trials includes a different MEKi. The MILO trial (NCT01849874) is an open-label phase III protocol that randomizes patients with recurrent low-grade serous carcinoma to either chemotherapy (physician's choice of pegylated liposomal doxorubicin, paclitaxel, or topotecan) or MEK162. A second trial (NCT01936363) has a randomized phase II design and includes the MEKi, pimasertib, with either placebo or SAR245409 (a PI3K/mTOR inhibitor). And GOG 0281 is a randomized phase II/III trial (NCT02101788) that has been activated through NRG Oncology. This trial includes a randomization between standard of care (physician's choice of letrozole, tamoxifen, pegylated liposomal doxorubicin, weekly paclitaxel, or topotecan) and MEKi monotherapy, trametinib. This trial also includes a robust translational research component, with fresh and archival FFPE tissue for next-generation sequencing and proteomics as well as cell-free DNA and pharmacokinetic studies.

As noted above, the angiogenesis pathway may also be a target in patients with low-grade serous carcinoma. Bidus et al. reported three patients with apparent recurrent low-grade serous carcinomas (one with primary peritoneal low-grade serous carcinoma, one with ovarian low-grade serous carcinoma, and another with a mixed low-grade serous-endometrioid carcinoma) treated with bevacizumab [116]. All three patients experienced a sustained response—two partial responses and one complete response. Subsequently, Grisham et al. reported on 17 patients with low-grade serous carcinoma of the ovary or peritoneum who received bevacizumab [99]. Two patients were treated with single-agent bevacizumab and the others with a combination of bevacizumab and chemotherapy. Fifteen patients were evaluable for response, and six (40 %) had a partial response. An additional five (33.3 %) had stable disease lasting 3 months or longer.

To date, there have been no clinical trials exploring the role of IGF-1R targeted therapy in women with low-grade serous carcinoma. Likewise, although an agent targeting the PI3K/AKT/mTOR pathway in combination with an MEKi was administered to a proportion of women on one of the three trials above (NCT01936363), the results of this trial are pending, and no AKTi, PI3Ki, or mTORi monotherapy trials specifically for patients with low-grade serous carcinoma have been developed.

References

1. Shih I-M, Kurman RJ. Ovarian tumorigenesis. Am J Pathol. 2010;164(5):1511–8. American Society for Investigative Pathology.
2. Malpica A, Deavers MT, Lu K, Bodurka DC, Atkinson EN, Gershenson DM, et al. Grading ovarian serous carcinoma using a two-tier system. Am J Surg Pathol. 2004;28(4):496–504.
3. Gershenson DM, Silva EG, Tortolero-Luna G, Levenback C, Morris M, Tornos C. Serous borderline tumors of the ovary with noninvasive peritoneal implants. Cancer. 1998;83(10): 2157–63.
4. Gershenson DM, Silva EG, Levy L, Burke TW, Wolf JK, Tornos C. Ovarian serous borderline tumors with invasive peritoneal implants. Cancer. 1998;82(6):1096–103.
5. Crispens MA, Bodurka D, Deavers M, Lu K, Silva EG, Gershenson DM. Response and survival in patients with progressive or recurrent serous ovarian tumors of low malignant potential. Obstet Gynecol. 2002;99(1):3–10.
6. Silva EG, Gershenson DM, Malpica A, Deavers M. The recurrence and the overall survival rates of ovarian serous borderline neoplasms with noninvasive implants is time dependent. Am J Surg Pathol. 2006;30(11):1367–71.
7. Shvartsman HS, Sun CC, Bodurka DC, Mahajan V, Crispens M, Lu KH, et al. Comparison of the clinical behavior of newly diagnosed stages II-IV low-grade serous carcinoma of the ovary with that of serous ovarian tumors of low malignant potential that recur as low-grade serous carcinoma. Gynecol Oncol. 2007;105(3):625–9.
8. Bonome T, Lee J-Y, Park D-C, Radonovich M, Pise-Masison C, Brady J, et al. Expression profiling of serous low malignant potential, low-grade, and high-grade tumors of the ovary. Cancer Res. 2005;65(22):10602–12. American Association for Cancer Research.
9. Meinhold-Heerlein I, Bauerschlag D, Hilpert F, Dimitrov P, Sapinoso LM, Orlowska-Volk M, et al. Molecular and prognostic distinction between serous ovarian carcinomas of varying grade and malignant potential. Oncogene. 2004;24(6):1053–65.
10. Singer G, Kurman RJ, Chang H-W, Cho SKR, Shih I-M. Diverse tumorigenic pathways in ovarian serous carcinoma. Am J Pathol. 2002;160(4):1223–8.
11. Singer G, Oldt R, Cohen Y, Wang BG, Sidransky D, Kurman RJ, et al. Mutations in BRAF and KRAS characterize the development of low-grade ovarian serous carcinoma. J Natl Cancer Inst. 2003;95(6):484–6.
12. Singer G, Shih I-M, Truskinovsky A, Umudum H, Kurman RJ. Mutational analysis of K-ras segregates ovarian serous carcinomas into two types: invasive MPSC (low-grade tumor) and conventional serous carcinoma (high-grade tumor). Int J Gynecol Pathol. 2003;22(1):37–41.
13. Taylor HC. Malignant and semimalignant tumors of the ovary. Surg Gynecol Obstet. 1929;48:206–30.

14. Kottmeier HL, Kolstad P, mcGarrity KA. Annual report on results of treatment in gynecologic cancer, vol. 17. Statements of results obtained in 1969-1972, inclusive. FIGO. Stockholm: Editorial office, Radiumhemmet; 1973.
15. Serov SF, Scully RE, Sobin LH. Histological typing of ovarian tumours, International histological classification of tumors, vol. 9. Geneva: World Health Organization; 1973.
16. Skírnisdóttir I, Garmo H, Wilander E, Holmberg L. Borderline ovarian tumors in Sweden 1960-2005: trends in incidence and age at diagnosis compared to ovarian cancer. Int J Cancer. 2008;123(8):1897–901. Wiley Subscription Services, Inc., A Wiley Company.
17. Åkeson M, Zetterqvist BM, Dahllöf K, Jakobsen AM, Brännström M, Horvath G. Population-based cohort follow-up study of all patients operated for borderline ovarian tumor in western Sweden during an 11-year period. Int J Gynecol Cancer. 2008;18(3):453–9.
18. duBois A, Ewald-Riegler N, de Gregorio N, Reuss A, Mahner S, Fotopoulou C, et al. Borderline tumours of the ovary: a cohort study of the Arbeitsgmeinschaft Gynäkologische Onkologie (AGO) study group. Eur J Cancer. 2013;49(8):1905–14.
19. Tropé CG, Kaern J, Davidson B. Borderline ovarian tumours. Best Pract Res Clin Obstet Gynaecol. 2012;26(3):325–36.
20. Riman T, Dickman PW, Nilsson S, Correia N, Nordlinder H, Magnusson CM, et al. Risk factors for epithelial borderline ovarian tumors: results of a Swedish case–control study. Gynecol Oncol. 2001;83(3):575–85.
21. Kolwijck E, Thomas CMG, Bulten J, Massuger LFAG. Preoperative CA-125 levels in 123 patients with borderline ovarian tumors. Int J Gynecol Cancer. 2009;19(8):1335–8.
22. Seidman JD, Kurman RJ. Subclassification of serous borderline tumors of the ovary into benign and malignant types. A clinicopathologic study of 65 advanced stage cases. Am J Surg Pathol. 1996;20(11):1331–45.
23. Eichhorn JH, Bell DA, Young RH, Scully RE. Ovarian serous borderline tumors with micropapillary and cribriform patterns: a study of 40 cases and comparison with 44 cases without these patterns. Am J Surg Pathol. 1999;23(4):397–409.
24. Deavers MT, Gershenson DM, Tortolero-Luna G, Malpica A, Lu KH, Silva EG. Micropapillary and cribriform patterns in ovarian serous tumors of low malignant potential: a study of 99 advanced stage cases. Am J Surg Pathol. 2002;26(9):1129–41.
25. Bell DA, Longacre TA, Prat J, Kohn EC, Soslow RA, Ellenson LH, et al. Serous borderline (low malignant potential, atypical proliferative) ovarian tumors: Workshop perspectives. Hum Pathol. 2004;35(8):934–48.
26. Bell DA, Scully RE. Ovarian serous borderline tumors with stromal microinvasion: a report of 21 cases. Hum Pathol. 1990;21(4):397–403.
27. Longacre TA, McKenney JK, Tazelaar HD, Kempson RL, Hendrickson MR. Ovarian serous tumors of low malignant potential (borderline tumors): outcome-based study of 276 patients with long-term (> or =5-year) follow-up. Am J Surg Pathol. 2005;29(6): 707–23.
28. Bell DA, Weinstock MA, Scully RE. Peritoneal implants of ovarian serous borderline tumors. Histologic features and prognosis. Cancer. 1988;62(10):2212–22.
29. Arias-Pulido H, Smith HO, Joste NE, et al. Estrogen and progesterone receptor status and outcome in epithelial ovarian cancers and low malignant potential tumors. Gynecol Oncol. 2009;114(3):480–5.
30. Singer G, Stöhr R, Cope L, Dehari R, Hartmann A, Cao D-F, et al. Patterns of p53 mutations separate ovarian serous borderline tumors and low- and high-grade carcinomas and provide support for a new model of ovarian carcinogenesis: a mutational analysis with immunohistochemical correlation. Am J Surg Pathol. 2005;29(2):218–24.
31. Ardighieri L, Zeppernick F, Hannibal CG, et al. Mutational analysis of BRAF and KRAS in ovarian serous borderline (atypical proliferative) tumours and associated peritoneal implants. J Pathol. 2013;232(1):16–22.
32. Curry EW, Stronach EA, Rama NR, Wang YY, Gabra H, El-Bahrawy MA. Molecular subtypes of serous borderline ovarian tumor show distinct expression patterns of benign tumor and malignant tumor-associated signatures. Mod Pathol. 2013;27:433–42.

33. Hannibal CG, Vang R, Junge J, et al. A nationwide study of serous "borderline" ovarian tumors in Denmark 1978–2002: Centralized pathology review and overall survival compared with the general population. Gynecol Oncol. 2014;134(2):267–73.
34. Maneo A, Vignali M, Chiari S, Colombo A, Mangioni C, Landoni F. Are borderline tumors of the ovary safely treated by laparoscopy? Gynecol Oncol. 2004;94(2):387–92.
35. Deffieux X, Morice P, Camatte S, Fourchotte V, Duvillard P, Castaigne D. Results after laparoscopic management of serous borderline tumor of the ovary with peritoneal implants. Gynecol Oncol. 2005;97(1):84–9.
36. Desfeux P, Camatte S, Chatellier G, Blanc B, Querleu D, Lécuru F. Impact of surgical approach on the management of macroscopic early ovarian borderline tumors. Gynecol Oncol. 2005;98(3):390–5.
37. Romagnolo C, Gadducci A, Sartori E, Zola P, Maggino T. Management of borderline ovarian tumors: results of an Italian multicenter study. Gynecol Oncol. 2006;101(2):255–60.
38. Tazelaar HD, Bostwick DG, Ballon SC, et al. Conservative treatment of borderline ovarian tumors. Obstet Gynecol. 1985;66:417–22.
39. Lim-Tan SK, Cajigas HE, Scully RE. Ovarian cystectomy for serous borderline tumors: a follow-up study of 35 cases. Obstet Gynecol. 1988;72:775–81.
40. Morice P, Camatte S, El Hassan J, Pautier P, Duvillard P, Castaigne D. Clinical outcomes and fertility after conservative treatment of ovarian borderline tumors. Fertil Steril. 2001;75(1): 92–6.
41. Park J-Y, Kim D-Y, Kim J-H, Kim Y-M, Kim Y-T, Nam J-H. Surgical management of borderline ovarian tumors: the role of fertility-sparing surgery. Gynecol Oncol. 2009;113(1): 75–82.
42. Rao GG, Skinner EN, Gehrig PA, Duska LR, Miller DS, Schorge JO. Fertility-sparing surgery for ovarian low malignant potential tumors. Gynecol Oncol. 2005;98(2):263–6.
43. Song T, Choi CH, Park HS, et al. Fertility-sparing surgery for borderline ovarian tumors. Int J Gynecol Cancer. 2011;21(4):640–6.
44. Uzan C, Kane A, REY A, Gouy S, Duvillard P, Morice P. Outcomes after conservative treatment of advanced-stage serous borderline tumors of the ovary. Ann Oncol. 2009;21(1): 55–60.
45. Song T, Choi CH, Kim H-J, et al. Accuracy of frozen section diagnosis of borderline ovarian tumors. Gynecol Oncol. 2011;122(1):127–31.
46. Fotopoulou C, Schumacher G, Schefold JC, Denkert C, Lichtenegger W, Sehouli J. Systematic evaluation of the intraoperative tumor pattern in patients with borderline tumor of the ovary. Int J Gynecol Cancer. 2009;19(9):1550–5.
47. Rao GG, Skinner E, Gehrig PA, Duska LR, Coleman RL, Schorge JO. Surgical staging of ovarian Low malignant potential tumors. Obstet Gynecol. 2004;104(2):261–6.
48. Lin PS, Gershenson DM, Bevers MW, Lucas KR, Burke TW, Silva EG. The current status of surgical staging of ovarian serous borderline tumors. Cancer. 1999;85(4):905–11.
49. Fauvet R, Boccara J, Dufournet C, David-Montefiore E, Poncelet C, Daraï E. Restaging surgery for women with borderline ovarian tumors. Cancer. 2004;100(6):1145–51.
50. Buttin BM, Herzog TJ, Powell MA, Rader JS, Mutch DG. Epithelial ovarian tumors of low malignant potential: the role of microinvasion. Obstet Gynecol. 2002;99(1):11–7.
51. McKenney JK, Balzer BL, Longacre TA. Patterns of stromal invasion in ovarian serous tumors of low malignant potential (borderline tumors): a reevaluation of the concept of stromal microinvasion. Am J Surg Pathol. 2006;30(10):1209–21.
52. Ren J, Peng Z, Yang K. A clinicopathologic multivariate analysis affecting recurrence of borderline ovarian tumors. Gynecol Oncol. 2008;110(2):162–7.
53. Shih KK, Zhou Q, Huh J, et al. Risk factors for recurrence of ovarian borderline tumors. Gynecol Oncol. 2011;120(3):480–4.
54. Song T, Lee Y-Y, Choi CH, et al. Risk factors for progression to invasive carcinoma in patients with borderline ovarian tumors. Int J Gynecol Cancer. 2014;24(7):1206–14.
55. Lesieur B, Kane A, Duvillard P, et al. Prognostic value of lymph node involvement in ovarian serous borderline tumors. Am J Obstet Gynecol. 2011;204(5):438.e1–7.

56. McKenney JK, Balzer BL, Longacre TA. Lymph node involvement in ovarian serous tumors of low malignant potential (borderline tumors): pathology, prognosis, and proposed classification. Am J Surg Pathol. 2006;30(5):614–24.
57. Djordjevic B, Malpica A. Lymph node involvement in ovarian serous tumors of low malignant potential: a clinicopathologic study of thirty-six cases. Am J Surg Pathol. 2010; 34(1):1–9.
58. Ayhan A, Guvendag Guven ES, Guven S, Kucukali T. Recurrence and prognostic factors in borderline ovarian tumors. Gynecol Oncol. 2005;98(3):439–45.
59. Tang A, Chennakesavan SK, Ngan H, et al. Prognostic value of elevated preoperative serum CA125 in ovarian tumors of low malignant potential: a multinational collaborative study (ANZGOG0801). Gynecol Oncol. 2012;126(1):36–40.
60. Obermair A, Tang A, Kondalsamy-Chennakesavan S, et al. Nomogram to predict the probability of relapse in patients diagnosed with borderline ovarian tumors. Int J Gynecol Cancer. 2013;23(2):264–7.
61. Wu T-I, Lee C-L, Wu M-Y, et al. Prognostic factors predicting recurrence in borderline ovarian tumors. Gynecol Oncol. 2009;114(2):237–41.
62. Morris RT, Gershenson DM, Silva EG, Follen M, Morris M, Wharton JT. Outcome and reproductive function after conservative surgery for borderline ovarian tumors. Obstet Gynecol. 2000;95(4):541–7.
63. Boran N, Cil AP, Tulunay G, et al. Fertility and recurrence results of conservative surgery for borderline ovarian tumors. Gynecol Oncol. 2005;97(3):845–51.
64. Shih KK, Zhou QC, Aghajanian C, et al. Patterns of recurrence and role of adjuvant chemotherapy in stage II–IV serous ovarian borderline tumors. Gynecol Oncol. 2010;119(2): 270–3.
65. Dehari R, Kurman RJ, Logani S, Shih I-M. The development of high-grade serous carcinoma from atypical proliferative (borderline) serous tumors and low-grade micropapillary serous carcinoma: a morphologic and molecular genetic analysis. Am J Surg Pathol. 2007; 31(7):1007–12.
66. Boyd C, McCluggage WG. Low-grade ovarian serous neoplasms (low-grade serous carcinoma and serous borderline tumor) associated with high-grade serous carcinoma or undifferentiated carcinoma: report of a series of cases of an unusual phenomenon. Am J Surg Pathol. 2012;36(3):368–75.
67. Silva EG, Gershenson DM. Standardized histologic grading of epithelial ovarian cancer: elusive after all these years. Gynecol Oncol. 1998;70(1):1.
68. Seidman JD, Horkayne-Szakaly I, Cosin JA, Ryu HS, Haiba M, Boice CR, et al. Testing of two binary grading systems for FIGO stage III serous carcinoma of the ovary and peritoneum. Gynecol Oncol. 2006;103(2):703–8.
69. Malpica A, Deavers MT, Tornos C, et al. Interobserver and intraobserver variability of a two-tier system for grading ovarian serous carcinoma. Am J Surg Pathol. 2007;31(8):1168–74.
70. Roth LM. Two-tier grading system for ovarian epithelial cancer: has its time arrived? Am J Surg Pathol. 2007;31(8):1285–7.
71. Vang R, Shih I-M, Salani R, Sugar E, Ayhan A, Kurman RJ. Subdividing ovarian and peritoneal serous carcinoma into moderately differentiated and poorly differentiated does not have biologic validity based on molecular genetic and in vitro drug resistance data. Am J Surg Pathol. 2008;32(11):1667–74.
72. Bodurka DC, Deavers MT, Tian C, Sun CC, Malpica A, Coleman RL, et al. Reclassification of serous ovarian carcinoma by a 2-tier system: a Gynecologic Oncology Group Study. Cancer. 2012;118(12):3087–94.
73. Bell DA. Low-grade serous tumors of ovary. Int J Gynecol Pathol. 2014;33(4):348–56.
74. Kurman RJ, Carcangiu ML, Herrington CS, Young RH. WHO classification of tumours of female reproductive organs. Lyon: International Agency for Research on Cancer (IARC); 2013.
75. Gilks CB. Subclassification of ovarian surface epithelial tumors based on correlation of histologic and molecular pathologic data. Int J Gynecol Pathol. 2004;23(3):200–5.

76. Sieben NL, Macropoulos P, Roemen GM, Kolkman-Uljee SM, Jan Fleuren G, Houmadi R, et al. In ovarian neoplasms, BRAF, but not KRAS, mutations are restricted to low-grade serous tumours. J Pathol. 2004;202(3):336–40.
77. O'Neill CJ, Deavers MT, Malpica A, Foster H, McCluggage WG. An immunohistochemical comparison between low-grade and high-grade ovarian serous carcinomas: significantly higher expression of p53, MIB1, BCL2, HER-2/neu, and C-KIT in high-grade neoplasms. Am J Surg Pathol. 2005;29(8):1034–41.
78. Szymanska-Pasternak J, Szymanska A, Medrek K, Imyanitov EN, Cybulski C, Gorski B, et al. CHEK2 variants predispose to benign, borderline and low-grade invasive ovarian tumors. Gynecol Oncol. 2006;102(3):429–31.
79. Wong K-K, Lu KH, Malpica A, Bodurka DC, Shvartsman HS, Schmandt RE, et al. Significantly greater expression of ER, PR, and ECAD in advanced-stage low-grade ovarian serous carcinoma as revealed by immunohistochemical analysis. Int J Gynecol Pathol. 2007;26(4):404–9.
80. Kuo KT, Guan B, Feng Y, Mao TL, Chen X, Jinawath N, et al. Analysis of DNA copy number alterations in ovarian serous tumors identifies new molecular genetic changes in low-grade and high-grade carcinomas. Cancer Res. 2009;69(9):4036–42.
81. Tung CS, Mok SC, Tsang YTM, Zu Z, Song H, Liu J, et al. PAX2 expression in low malignant potential ovarian tumors and low-grade ovarian serous carcinomas. Mod Pathol. 2009;22(9):1243–50. Nature Publishing Group.
82. Wong K-K, Tsang YTM, Deavers MT, Mok SC, Zu Z, Sun C, et al. BRAF mutation is rare in advanced-stage low-grade ovarian serous carcinomas. Am J Pathol. 2010;177(4):1611–7.
83. May T, Virtanen C, Sharma M, Milea A, Begley H, Rosen B, et al. Low malignant potential tumors with micropapillary features are molecularly similar to low-grade serous carcinoma of the ovary. Gynecol Oncol. 2010;117(1):9–17.
84. Jones S, Wang T-L, Kurman RJ, Nakayama K, Velculescu VE, Vogelstein B, et al. Low-grade serous carcinomas of the ovary contain very few point mutations. J Pathol. 2011;226(3):413–20.
85. Grisham RN, Iyer G, Garg K, DeLair D, Hyman DM, Zhou Q, et al. BRAF Mutation is associated with early stage disease and improved outcome in patients with low-grade serous ovarian cancer. Cancer. 2012;119(3):548–54.
86. Tsang YT, Deavers MT, Sun CC, Kwan S-Y, Kuo E, Malpica A, et al. KRAS(but not BRAF) mutations in ovarian serous borderline tumour are associated with recurrent low-grade serous carcinoma. J Pathol. 2013;231(4):449–56.
87. Escobar J, Klimowicz AC, Dean M, Chu P, Nation JG, Nelson GS, et al. Quantification of ER/PR expression in ovarian low-grade serous carcinoma. Gynecol Oncol. 2013;128(2):371–6. Elsevier Inc.
88. Burotto M, Chiou VL, Lee J-M, Kohn EC. The MAPK pathway across different malignancies: a new perspective. Cancer. 2014;120(22):3446–56.
89. Gershenson DM, Sun CC, Lu KH, Coleman RL, Sood AK, Malpica A, et al. Clinical behavior of stage II-IV low-grade serous carcinoma of the ovary. Obstet Gynecol. 2006;108(2):361–8.
90. Schmeler KM, Sun CC, Bodurka DC, Deavers MT, Malpica A, Coleman RL, et al. Neoadjuvant chemotherapy for low-grade serous carcinoma of the ovary or peritoneum. Gynecol Oncol. 2008;108(3):510–4.
91. Gershenson DM, Sun CC, Bodurka D, Coleman RL, Lu KH, Sood AK, et al. Recurrent low-grade serous ovarian carcinoma is relatively chemoresistant. Gynecol Oncol. 2009;114(1):48–52. Elsevier Inc.
92. Schmeler KM, Sun CC, Malpica A, Deavers MT, Bodurka DC, Gershenson DM. Low-grade serous primary peritoneal carcinoma. Gynecol Oncol. 2011;121(3):482–6. Elsevier Inc.
93. Schlumbrecht MP, Sun CC, Wong KN, Broaddus RR, Gershenson DM, Bodurka DC. Clinicodemographic factors influencing outcomes in patients with low-grade serous ovarian carcinoma. Cancer. 2011;117(16):3741–9.
94. Diaz-Padilla I, Malpica AL, Minig L, Chiva LM, Gershenson DM, Gonzalez-Martin A. Ovarian low-grade serous carcinoma: a comprehensive update. Gynecol Oncol. 2012;126(2):279–85. Elsevier Inc.

95. Gershenson DM, Sun CC, Iyer RB, Malpica AL, Kavanagh JJ, Bodurka DC, et al. Hormonal therapy for recurrent low-grade serous carcinoma of the ovary or peritoneum. Gynecol Oncol. 2012;125(3):661–6. Elsevier Inc.
96. Nickles Fader A, Java J, Ueda S, Bristow RE, Armstrong DK, Bookman MA, et al. Survival in women with grade 1 serous ovarian carcinoma. Obstet Gynecol. 2013;122(2, PART 1):225–32.
97. Romero I, Sun CC, Wong KK, Bast RC, Gershenson DM. Low-grade serous carcinoma: new concepts and emerging therapies. Gynecol Oncol. 2013;130(3):660–6.
98. Fader AN, Java J, Krivak TC, Bristow RE, Tergas AI, Bookman MA, et al. The prognostic significance of pre- and post-treatment CA-125 in grade 1 serous ovarian carcinoma: a gynecologic Oncology Group study. Gynecol Oncol. 2014;132(3):560–5.
99. Grisham RN, Iyer G, Sala E, Zhou Q, Iasonos A, DeLair D, et al. Bevacizumab shows activity in patients with low-grade serous ovarian and primary peritoneal cancer. Int J Gynecol Cancer. 2014;24(6):1010–4.
100. Previs RA, Kilgore J, Craven R, Broadwater G, Bean S, Wobker S, et al. Obesity is associated with worse overall survival in women with low-grade papillary serous epithelial ovarian cancer. Int J Gynecol Cancer. 2014;24(4):670–5.
101. Plaxe SC. Epidemiology of low-grade serous ovarian cancer. Am J Obstet Gynecol. 2008;198(4):459.e1–8; discussion 459.e8–9.
102. Crane EK, Sun CC, Ramirez PT, Schmeler KM, Malpica A, Gershenson DM. The role of secondary cytoreduction in low-grade serous ovarian cancer or peritoneal cancer. Gynecol Oncol. 2015;136(1):25–9.
103. Pearce CL, Templeman C, Rossing MA, Lee A. Association between endometriosis and risk of histological subtypes of ovarian cancer: a pooled analysis of case–control studies. Lancet Oncol. 2012;13:385–94.
104. King ER, Tung CS, Tsang YTM, Zu Z, Lok GTM, Deavers MT, et al. The anterior gradient homolog 3 (AGR3) gene is associated with differentiation and survival in ovarian cancer. Am J Surg Pathol. 2011;35(6):904–12.
105. King ER, Zu Z, Tsang YTM, Deavers MT, Malpica A, Mok SC, et al. The insulin-like growth factor 1 pathway is a potential therapeutic target for low-grade serous ovarian carcinoma. Gynecol Oncol. 2011;123(1):13–8.
106. Press JZ, De Luca A, Boyd N, Young S, Troussard A, Ridge Y, et al. Ovarian carcinomas with genetic and epigenetic BRCA1 loss have distinct molecular abnormalities. BMC Cancer. 2008;8(1):17. BioMed Central Ltd.
107. Vineyard MA, Daniels MS, Urbauer DL, Deavers MT, Sun CC, Boerwinkle E, et al. Is low-grade serous ovarian cancer part of the tumor spectrum of Hereditary Breast and Ovarian Cancer? Gynecol Oncol. 2011;120(2):229–32. Elsevier Inc.
108. Farley JH, Brady WE, Vathipadiekal V, et al. Selumetinib in women with recurrent low-grade serous carcinoma of the ovary or peritoneum: an open-label, single-arm, phase 2 study. Lancet Oncol. 2013;14(2):134–40. Elsevier Ltd.
109. McCubrey JA, Steelman LS, Chappell WH, Abrams SL, Wong EWT, Chang F, et al. Roles of the Raf/MEK/ERK pathway in cell growth, malignant transformation and drug resistance. Biochim Biophys Acta. 2007;1773(8):1263–84.
110. Friday BB, Adjei AA. Advances in targeting the Ras/Raf/MEK/Erk mitogen-activated protein kinase cascade with MEK inhibitors for cancer therapy. Clin Cancer Res. 2008;14(2):342–6. American Association for Cancer Research.
111. Jing J, Greshock J, Holbrook JD, Gilmartin A, Zhang X, McNeil E, et al. Comprehensive predictive biomarker analysis for MEK inhibitor GSK1120212. Mol Cancer Ther. 2012;11(3):720–9.
112. Neuzillet C, Tijeras-Raballand A, de Mestier L, Cros J, Faivre S, Raymond E. MEK in cancer and cancer therapy. Pharmacol Ther. 2014;141(2):160–71. Elsevier Inc.
113. Miller CR, Oliver KE, Farley JH. MEK1/2 inhibitors in the treatment of gynecologic malignancies. Gynecol Oncol. 2014;133(1):128–37.
114. Pohl G, Ho C-L, Kurman RJ, Bristow R, Wang T-L, Shih I-M. Inactivation of the mitogen-activated protein kinase pathway as a potential target-based therapy in ovarian serous tumors

with KRAS or BRAF mutations. Cancer Res. 2005;65(5):1994–2000. American Association for Cancer Research.
115. Nakayama N, Nakayama K, Yeasmin S, Ishibashi M, Katagiri A, Iida K, et al. KRAS or BRAF mutation status is a useful predictor of sensitivity to MEK inhibition in ovarian cancer. Br J Cancer. 2008;99(12):2020–8.
116. Bidus MA, Webb JC, Seidman JD, Rose GS, Boice CR, Elkas JC. Sustained response to bevacizumab in refractory well-differentiated ovarian neoplasms. Gynecol Oncol. 2006; 102(1):5–7.

Clear Cell Carcinoma 14

Masashi Takano, Satoshi Takakura, and Keiichi Fujiwara

Abstract

Clear cell carcinoma (CCC) is a unique entity of adenocarcinoma of the ovary. In this chapter, we discuss the clinicopathological and molecular biological characteristics of CCC. The results of clinical trials conducted in the past strongly imply the chemoresistance of CCC, and clinical trials using targeted agents are ongoing.

Introduction

Clear cell carcinoma of the ovary (CCC) was first described as "mesonephroma ovarii" by Schiller in 1939. The tumor cell of CCC resembled renal cell carcinoma, and it was believed to be originated from mesonephric structure. In 1973, CCC was

M. Takano, MD, PhD (✉)
Department of Clinical Oncology, National Defense Medical College Hospital, 3-2 Namiki, Tokorozawa, Saitama 359-8513, Japan
e-mail: mastkn@ndmc.ac.jp

S. Takakura, MD, PhD
Department of Obstetrics and Gynecology, Dokkyo Medical University Koshigaya Hospital, 2-1-5-Minamikoshigaya, Koshigaya, Saitama 343-8555, Japan
e-mail: stakakur@dokkyomed.ac.jp

K. Fujiwara, MD, PhD
Department of Gynecologic Oncology, Saitama Medical University International Medical Center, 1397-1 Yamane, Hidaka-city, Saitama 350-1298, Japan
e-mail: fujiwara@saitama-med.ac.jp

E. Pujade-Lauraine et al. (eds.), *Ovarian Cancers*,
DOI 10.1007/978-3-319-32110-3_14

strictly classified as a histological subtype in ovarian cancers by the World Health Organization classification. Pathological features of CCC are characterized by clear cells growing in solid/tubular or glandular patterns as well as hobnail cells. There have been many publications that suggested distinctive clinical behavior of CCC, such as platinum-resistant phenotype, and worse prognosis in comparison with other histological subtypes [1–3]. However, until now, the treatment modality for CCC has been the same as other subtypes of ovarian cancers. The characteristics of CCC are described in this chapter, including clinical and molecular characteristics of the tumor.

Clinical Characteristics of CCC

Association with Endometriosis and Prognostic Factor in Early-Staged Disease

Recently, a marked ethnic difference of has been recognized in the incidence of CCC, although the reason for this difference is not clear [2]. The incidence of CCC is less than 10 % in Europe and North America [4]. However, in Japan, the prevalence of CCC is increasing, and now approximately 25 % of epithelial ovarian cancer is CCC according to the Japan Society of Obstetrics and Gynecology tumor registry in 2014.

Association with endometriosis and neoplastic tumor is often reported in CCC and endometrioid adenocarcinoma of the ovary. Recently, both atypical endometriosis and atypical adenofibroma of the ovary have been considered as precancerous lesions [5, 6]. The ovarian cancer risk was significantly elevated in the patients with endometrioma of the ovary (relative risk = 12.4) [5]. The risk increased significantly when the patients were diagnosed at elder age, especially over the age of fifties, suggesting that malignant change of endometriosis occurs near menopause stage. K-ras mutation was recognized as one of the triggers of malignant change of endometriosis [7]. Additionally, PTEN mutations are also frequently observed (27.3 %) in CCC, suggesting them to be carcinogenesis-related genetic changes [8]. On the other hand, unlike high-grade serous (HGS) tumors, CCC are generally p53 wild type and have a lower frequency of BRCA 1 and BRCA 2 mutations [9].

Most of CCC tumors are unilateral, and the mean size of CCC is approximately 15 cm. Additionally, CCC is frequently diagnosed at early-staged disease, and the proportion of stage I/II tumors was reported to be about 60 % of all staged CCC [9, 10]. In stage I ovarian cancer of all histological subtypes, the incidence of lymph node metastasis was reported to range from 5.1 to 20 % [11–13]. On the other hand, serous ovarian cancers had a higher incidence of lymph node metastasis than non-serous tumors [14]. A study of a large number of clear cell carcinomas revealed lymph node metastasis was observed in 9.1 % in stage Ia tumors, 7.1 % in stage Ic tumors, and 10.8 % in pT2 tumors [9]. Approximately, 10 % of clinical stage I/II tumors would be upstaged as stage IIICA 1 [9] based on lymph node status.

The incidence of thromboembolic complications in CCC, such as deep venous thrombosis and pulmonary embolism, is reported to be higher than other epithelial ovarian cancers (16.9–27.3 % vs. 0–6.8 %) and is considered as an independent prognostic factor [5, 6].

Impact of retroperitoneal lymph node status on prognosis in early-staged ovarian cancer patients is still controversial. Some retrospective reports showed positive relationship: survival rates with node-positive disease were significantly lower in clinical stage I and II disease [11]. In contrast, another report showed that the prognoses for clinical stage I/II patients with or without lymph node metastasis were similar [15]. However, in patients with clinical stage I CCC, lymph node involvement was identified as a stronger prognostic factor [9]. It is suggested that it is important to evaluate the lymph node status through complete surgical staging procedures in CCC patients. Also, complete resection with no macroscopic residual tumors could be often achievable in CCC. On the other hand, serous cystadenocarcinoma patients often present at advanced-stage tumors and harbor measurable disease after initial cytoreductive surgery [2].

Fertility-sparing surgery (FSS) is generally accepted in ovarian cancer patients with stage IA and grade 1/2 histology. CCC is regarded as grade 3 tumors, and FSS is not recommended even when the patient had Stage IA CCC disease. A multi-institutional retrospective study revealed that recurrence was documented in no case in 15 cases with stage IA CCC tumors and 4 cases (27 %) in stage IC CCC disease, suggesting that FSS could be an optional surgical technique in stage IA CCC cases [16]. Another observational study reported that recurrence was observed in a case (4 %) in 23 stage IA CCC and 6 cases (26 %) in stage IC CCC, respectively, and concluded that stage IA CCC patients might be treated with FSS [17]. Although further analyses are needed, FSS can be an optional treatment at least in stage IA CCC cases.

The impact of peritoneal cytology in stage I ovarian cancers still remain undetermined. A recent report showed no statistical significant difference between stages Ic preoperative versus intraoperative rupture by analyzing prognosis of 94 carcinoma cases including 25 CCC cases (26.6 %) [18]. But another report including higher ratio of CCC patients showed that stage Ic intraoperative rupture patients showed significantly poorer survival than stage Ia patients [19]. The impact of peritoneal cytology was confirmed in a study analyzing CCC cases only; tumor progression was observed in 11 % of stage Ic intraoperative rupture tumors and 3 % of stage Ia tumors [9]. These results implied the importance to remove ovarian tumor mass without intraoperative rupture and implantation of tumor cells, especially in clear cell carcinoma patients. Progression-free survival of the patients with stage Ic (ascites/malignant washing) and Ic (ovarian surface) was significantly worse than that of stage Ic (capsule ruptured) ($p = 0.04$) [9]. These results suggested that positive peritoneal cytology could be related with microscopic implantation of CCC cells which potentially harbored resistant clones for anticancer agent drugs, and these diagnoses would lead to early relapse of the disease despite postoperative chemotherapy.

Response to Platinum-Based Therapy and Prognosis of CCC and Prognostic Factor for Advanced-Stage CCC

Several publications with relatively small sample number have identified that CCC often showed resistance to platinum-based chemotherapy, and the response rate of primary therapy was extremely lower in CCC compared with serous adenocarcinomas [1, 2]. The response rate by combination therapy with paclitaxel and carboplatin was also lower, ranging from 18 to 56 %, reported by Enomoto at ASCO 2003. Although there is no larger phase II study confirming these results, clear cell carcinoma clearly showed resistance to paclitaxel and platinum as well as conventional platinum-based chemotherapy.

From a large retrospective cooperative study, 5-year progression-free survival and overall survival was 84 % and 88 % in stage I, 57 % and 70 % in stage II, 25 % and 33 % in stage III, and 0 % and 0 % in stage IV, respectively [9]. In advanced ovarian tumors, it is well known that optimal surgery achieving residual tumor diameter less than 1 cm improved survival of the patients. Since 1986, the Gynecologic Oncology Group (GOG) has used the definition, "less than 1 cm," in GOG studies [1]. In the analysis of CCC-specific cases, median progression-free survival duration was 39 months in the patients with no residual tumor, 7 months in those with the tumor diameter <1 cm, and 5 months in those with residual tumor diameter >1 cm, respectively [9]. Only the patients with complete resection could achieve a longer survival in advanced-stage cases. From these results, it is suggested that cytoreductive surgery achieving no residual tumor could only improve the prognosis of advanced CCC. "Optimal" cytoreduction in CCC had better be defined as "no residual tumor."

Adjuvant Radiotherapy for CCC

Postoperative whole abdominal radiotherapy (WAR) had been generally used for ovarian cancer patients for many years since 1970s [20]. However, many gynecologists changed postoperative radiotherapy to platinum-based chemotherapy, although there was no randomized clinical trial to compare WAR with chemotherapy. So far, there are a few centers around the world that performed postoperative WAR for ovarian cancers. A historical-control study revealed that overall survival and disease-free survival of CCC patients that received postoperative WAR were significantly better compared with those that treated with platinum-based chemotherapy [21]. Additionally, a report including a large number of CCC cases that received radiotherapy revealed that radiation therapy achieved almost similar disease-free survival compared with Japanese cohorts that mainly treated with chemotherapy [22]. Additionally, it was suggested that radiotherapy was more effective than chemotherapy in a subset of patients with stage IC 2/3 and stage II disease. As a relative lack of efficacy of chemotherapy has been well-known in CCC, potential benefit of radiotherapy would be further evaluated in clinical trials.

Molecular Pathology of CCC

There are many publications describing molecular markers highly expressed in CCC compared with other histology. Mutation in p53 is much less frequent in clear cell carcinoma than in other histological types of epithelial ovarian cancers, suggesting that there is another carcinogenesis mechanism in the development of clear cell carcinoma [23]. Wilms' tumor suppressor 1 gene (WT1) and WT1-antisense promoter were significantly methylated in CCC (88.2 %) compared with serous adenocarcinoma (24 %) [24]. Multidrug resistance protein 3 (MRP3), a well-known resistance marker to anticancer drug, is also highly expressed in CCC [25]. Also, hepatocyte nuclear factor 1beta (HNF-1beta) is highly expressed and has anti-apoptotic effects in clear cell carcinoma [26]. Gain of 17q21-q24 and consequent overexpression of two potential targets, PPM1D and APPBP2, are associated with malignant phenotypes of CCC, and these markers were reported as a predictor for prognosis [27]. More recently, frequent alteration of ARID1A [28] and PIK3CA [29] has been reported. Mutation of ARID1A was observed in approximately half of all cases with CCC, and PIK3Ca mutation was detected in about 40 % of CCC cases, respectively. Gene expression analysis revealed that CCC showed a specific expression pattern compared with other subtypes of ovarian cancers [30]. These genetic background combined with cell growth activity could be correlated with the distinct behavior of clear cell carcinoma. Suppression of the genes as shown above or acceleration of cell cycle might be a useful strategy for the future treatment of clear cell carcinoma of the ovary.

Results of Challenges to Improve the Prognosis of CCC in the Past

Several prospective studies or meta-analysis suggested that CCC is resistant to TC chemotherapy. In the JGOG trial, weekly administration of paclitaxel in a dose-dense manner with three-week administration of carboplatin significantly improved OS and PFS; however, it was not the case for CCC [31]. Intraperitoneal (IP) chemotherapy using cisplatin and paclitaxel improved the OS in optimally debulked stage III ovarian cancer, but survival benefit of IP chemotherapy was not observed in CCC and mucinous adenocarcinoma [32]. In 2014, JGOG presented the results of a randomized clinical trial that evaluated the efficacy and safety of combination chemotherapy using cisplatin and CPT-11 (CPT-P) versus TC. Unfortunately, the CPT-P regimen did not show PFS or OS benefit in stages I–IV CCC compared to TC.

These results strongly suggest that changing the conventional cytotoxic chemotherapy regimen does not improve the survival of CCC and the necessity of new innovative approach to establish an effective strategy for CCC.

Ongoing Clinical Trials and Future Directions

Based on the molecular profile pattern of CCC, the therapeutic target that is of the most interest is AKT-mTOR pathway. The first clinical trial using mTOR inhibitor is the GOG268 study (a phase II evaluation of temsirolimus (CCI-779) (NCI supplied agent: NSC# 683864, IND# 61010) in combination with carboplatin and paclitaxel followed by temsirolimus (CCI-779) consolidation as first–line therapy in the treatment of stage III-IV clear cell carcinoma of the ovary). In this study, one of the mTOR inhibitors, temsirolimus is being evaluated. The primary objective of this study is to assess the benefit of temsirolimus as measured by the proportion of patients who are alive and progression-free for at least 12 months after study entry in patients with newly diagnosed stage III or IV CCC. The most interesting proportion of this study is to compare PFS in CCC patients in Japan versus patients in the USA and worldwide (outside of Japan). Secondary objectives include to characterize the duration of OS and PFS in each population, to examine the frequency and serenity of adverse events, and to estimate the rate of objective tumor response in patients with measurable disease. Exploratory objectives of this study are to explore whether immunohistochemical expression of components of the mTOR signaling pathway (PTEN, total and phosphorylated AKT, and ABCC3 (MRP3), ABCF2, cyclin E, and VEGF) is associated with outcome, nationality, or clinical characteristics and to explore whether there are any differences in differential gene expression profiles between Japan versus the USA and worldwide (outside of Japan). The result of this study will be matured late 2015.

Anti-angiogenetic agents are also under investigation as a therapeutic target for CCC. GOG254 study (a phase II evaluation of SU11248 (sunitinib malate) (IND# 74019, NSC# 736511) in the treatment of persistent or recurrent clear cell ovarian carcinoma) evaluates the efficacy and safety of sunitinib. Sunitinib is a highly potent selective multiple tyrosine kinase inhibitor. The primary endpoints of this phase II study are to evaluate the antitumor activity and to examine the nature and degree of toxicity. Secondary endpoints are to characterize the distribution of progression-free survival and overall survival. This study also has translational research objectives. First translational objective is to determine the pre-cycle 1, pre-cycle 4, and off-treatment levels of pro-angiogenic proteins (e.g., angiogenin, soluble VCAM-I, bFGF, PDGF, PlGF, VEGF, and HIF1-alpha). The second objective is to identify changes in serum and plasma angiogenesis markers at baseline (pre-cycle 1), during treatment (cycle 4), and at progression in association with primary and secondary clinical endpoints associated with clinical response or progression-free survival. The result of this study was presented at the Society of Gynecologic Oncology Meeting in 2015 showing that sunitinib was minimally active in the second- and third-line treatments of persistent or recurrent CCC.

Another anti-angiogenetic agent that will be tested for CCC is nintedanib. A Scottish group is testing this agent as randomized phase II study comparing PLD, weekly paclitaxel, or weekly topotecan in 90 patients with platinum-resistant recurrent CCC. The primary endpoint is PFS, and secondary endpoints include OS, toxicity, response rate, and QOL.

References

1. Omura GA, Brady MF, Homesley HD, Yordan E, Major FJ, Buchsbaum HJ, Park RC. Long-term follow-up and prognostic factor analysis in advanced ovarian carcinoma: the Gynecologic Oncology Group experience. J Clin Oncol. 1991;9:1138–50.
2. Sugiyama T, Kamura T, Kigawa J, Terakawa N, Kikuchi Y, Kita T, Suzuki M, Sato I, Taguchi K. Clinical characteristics of clear cell carcinoma of the ovary: a distinct histologic type with poor prognosis and resistance to platinum-based chemotherapy. Cancer. 2000;88: 2584–9.
3. Pectasides D, Fountzilas G, Aravantinos G, Kalofonos C, Efstathiou H, Farmakis D, Skarlos D, Pavlidis N, Economopoulos T, Dimopoulos MA. Advanced stage clear-cell epithelial ovarian cancer: the Hellenic Cooperative Oncology Group experience. Gynecol Oncol. 2006; 102:285–91.
4. del Carmen MG, Birrer M, Schorge JO. Clear cell carcinoma of the ovary: a review of the literature. Gynecol Oncol. 2012;126:481–90.
5. Kobayashi H, Sumimoto K, Moniwa N, Imai M, Takakura K, Kuromaki T, Morioka E, Arisawa K, Terao T. Risk of developing ovarian cancer among women with ovarian endometrioma: a cohort study in Shizuoka, Japan. Int J Gynecol Cancer. 2007;17:37–43.
6. Yamamoto S, Tsuda H, Takano M, Hase K, Tamai S, Matsubara O. Clear-cell adenofibroma can be a clonal precursor for clear-cell adenocarcinoma of the ovary: a possible alternative ovarian clear-cell carcinogenic pathway. J Pathol. 2008;216:103–10.
7. Sekizawa A, Amemiya S, Otsuka J, Saito H, Farina A, Okai T, Tachikawa T. Malignant transformation of endometriosis: application of laser microdissection for analysis of genetic alterations according to pathological changes. Med Electron Microsc. 2004;37:97–100.
8. Sato N, Tsunoda H, Nishida M, Morishita Y, Takimoto Y, Kubo T, Noguchi M. Loss of heterozygosity on 10q23.3 and mutation of the tumor suppressor gene PTEN in benign endometrial cyst of the ovary: possible sequence progression from benign endometrial cyst to endometrioid carcinoma and clear cell carcinoma of the ovary. Cancer Res. 2000;60:7052–6.
9. Takano M, Kikuchi Y, Yaegashi N, Kuzuya K, Ueki M, Tsuda H, Suzuki M, Kigawa J, Takeuchi S, Tsuda H, Moriya T, Sugiyama T. Clear cell carcinoma of the ovary: a retrospective multicentre experience of 254 patients with complete surgical staging. Br J Cancer. 2006;94:1369–74.
10. Heintz AP, Odicino F, Maisonneuve P, Quinn MA, Benedet JL, Creasman WT, Ngan HY, Pecorelli S, Beller U. Carcinoma of the ovary. FIGO 26th Annual Report on the Results of Treatment in Gynecological Cancer. Int J Gynaecol Obstet. 2006;95 Suppl 1:S161–92.
11. Sakuragi N, Yamada H, Oikawa M, Okuyama K, Fujino T, Sagawa T, Fujimoto S. Prognostic significance of lymph node metastasis and clear cell histology in ovarian carcinoma limited to the pelvis (pT1M0 and pT2M0). Gynecol Oncol. 2000;79:251–5.
12. Cass I, Li AJ, Runowicz CD, Fields AL, Goldberg GL, Leuchter RS, Lagasse LD, Karlan BY. Pattern of lymph node metastases in clinically unilateral stage I invasive epithelial ovarian carcinomas. Gynecol Oncol. 2001;80:56–61.
13. Morice P, Joulie F, Camatte S, Atallah D, Rouzier R, Pautier P, Pomel C, Lhomme C, Duvillard P, Castaigne D. Lymph node involvement in epithelial ovarian cancer: analysis of 276 pelvic and paraaortic lymphadenectomies and surgical implications. J Am Coll Surg. 2003;197:198–205.
14. Takeshima N, Hirai Y, Umayahara K, Fujiwara K, Takizawa K, Hasumi K. Lymph node metastasis in ovarian cancer: difference between serous and non-serous primary tumors. Gynecol Oncol. 2005;99:427–31.
15. Onda T, Yoshikawa H, Yasugi T, Mishima M, Nakagawa S, Yamada M, Matsumoto K, Taketani Y. Patients with ovarian carcinoma upstaged to stage III after systematic lymphadenctomy have similar survival to Stage I/II patients and superior survival to other Stage III patients. Cancer. 1998;83:1555–60.

16. Satoh T, Hatae M, Watanabe Y, Yaegashi N, Ishiko O, Kodama S, Yamaguchi S, Ochiai K, Takano M, Yokota H, Kawakami Y, Nishimura S, Ogishima D, Nakagawa S, Kobayashi H, Shiozawa T, Nakanishi T, Kamura T, Konishi I, Yoshikawa H. Outcomes of fertility-sparing surgery for stage I epithelial ovarian cancer: a proposal for patient selection. J Clin Oncol. 2010;28:1727–32.
17. Kajiyama H, Shibata K, Mizuno M, Hosono S, Kawai M, Nagasaka T, Kikkawa F. Fertility-sparing surgery in patients with clear-cell carcinoma of the ovary: is it possible? Hum Reprod. 2011;26:3297–302.
18. Leitao Jr MM, Boyd J, Hummer A, Olvera N, Arroyo CD, Venkatraman E, Baergen RN, Dizon DS, Barakat RR, Soslow RA. Clinicopathologic analysis of early-stage sporadic ovarian carcinoma. Am J Surg Pathol. 2004;28:147–59.
19. Mizuno M, Kikkawa F, Shibata K, Kajiyama H, Ino K, Kawai M, Nagasaka T, Nomura S. Long-term follow-up and prognostic factor analysis in clear cell adenocarcinoma of the ovary. J Surg Oncol. 2006;94:138–43.
20. Dembo AJ, Bush RS, Beale FA, Bean HA, Pringle JF, Sturgeon J, Reid JG. Ovarian carcinoma: improved survival following abdominopelvic irradiation in patients with a completed pelvic operation. Am J Obstet Gynecol. 1979;134:793–800.
21. Nagai Y, Inamine M, Hirakawa M, Kamiyama K, Ogawa K, Toita T, Murayama S, Aoki Y. Postoperative whole abdominal radiotherapy in clear cell adenocarcinoma of the ovary. Gynecol Oncol. 2007;107:469–73.
22. Hoskins PJ, Le N, Gilks B, Tinker A, Santos J, Wong F, Swenerton KD. Low-stage ovarian clear cell carcinoma: population-based outcomes in British Columbia, Canada, with evidence for a survival benefit as a result of irradiation. J Clin Oncol. 2012;30:1656–62.
23. Ho ES, Lai CR, Hsieh YT, Chen JT, Lin AJ, Hung MH, Liu FS. p53 mutation is infrequent in clear cell carcinoma of the ovary. Gynecol Oncol. 2001;80:189–93.
24. Kaneuchi M, Sasaki M, Tanaka Y, Shiina H, Yamada H, Yamamoto R, Sakuragi N, Enokida H, Verma M, Dahiya R. WT1 and WT1-AS genes are inactivated by promoter methylation in ovarian clear cell adenocarcinoma. Cancer. 2005;104:1924–30.
25. Ohishi Y, Oda Y, Uchiumi T, Kobayashi H, Hirakawa T, Miyamoto S, Kinukawa N, Nakano H, Kuwano M, Tsuneyoshi M. ATP-binding cassette superfamily transporter gene expression in human primary ovarian carcinoma. Clin Cancer Res. 2002;8:3767–75.
26. Tsuchiya A, Sakamoto M, Yasuda J, Chuma M, Ohta T, Ohki M, Yasugi T, Taketani Y, Hirohashi S. Expression profiling in ovarian clear cell carcinoma: identification of hepatocyte nuclear factor-1 beta as a molecular marker and a possible molecular target for therapy of ovarian clear cell carcinoma. Am J Pathol. 2003;163:2503–12.
27. Hirasawa A, Saito-Ohara F, Inoue J, Aoki D, Susumu N, Yokoyama T, Nozawa S, Inazawa J, Imoto I. Association of 17q21-q24 gain in ovarian clear cell adenocarcinomas with poor prognosis and identification of PPM1D and APPBP2 as likely amplification targets. Clin Cancer Res. 2003;9:1995–2004.
28. Wiegand KC, Shah SP, Al-Agha OM, Zhao Y, Tse K, Zeng T, Senz J, McConechy MK, Anglesio MS, Kalloger SE, Yang W, Heravi-Moussavi A, Giuliany R, Chow C, Fee J, Zayed A, Prentice L, Melnyk N, Turashvili G, Delaney AD, Madore J, Yip S, McPherson AW, Ha G, Bell L, Fereday S, Tam A, Galletta L, Tonin PN, Provencher D, Miller D, Jones SJ, Moore RA, Morin GB, Oloumi A, Boyd N, Aparicio SA, Shih Ie M, Mes-Masson AM, Bowtell DD, Hirst M, Gilks B, Marra MA, Huntsman DG. ARID1A mutations in endometriosis-associated ovarian carcinomas. N Engl J Med. 2010;363:1532–43.
29. Kuo KT, Mao TL, Jones S, Veras E, Ayhan A, Wang TL, Glas R, Slamon D, Velculescu VE, Kuman RJ, Shih IM. Frequent activating mutations of PIK3CA in ovarian clear cell carcinoma. Am J Pathol. 2009;174:1597–601.
30. Yamaguchi K, Mandai M, Oura T, Matsumura N, Hamanishi J, Baba T, Matsui S, Murphy SK, Konishi I. Identification of an ovarian clear cell carcinoma gene signature that reflects inherent disease biology and the carcinogenic processes. Oncogene. 2010;29:1741–52.

31. Katsumata N, Yasuda M, Isonishi S, Takahashi F, Michimae H, Kimura E, Aoki D, Jobo T, Kodama S, Terauchi F, Sugiyama T, Ochiai K, Japanese Gynecologic Oncology G. Long-term results of dose-dense paclitaxel and carboplatin versus conventional paclitaxel and carboplatin for treatment of advanced epithelial ovarian, fallopian tube, or primary peritoneal cancer (JGOG 3016): a randomised, controlled, open-label trial. Lancet Oncol. 2013;14:1020–6.
32. Tewari D, Java JJ, Salani R, Armstrong DK, Markman M, Herzog T, Monk BJ, Chan JK. Long-term survival advantage and prognostic factors associated with intraperitoneal chemotherapy treatment in advanced ovarian cancer: a gynecologic oncology group study. J Clin Oncol. 2015;33:1460–6.

Endometrioid Carcinoma of the Ovary 15

Laure de Cock, Gerlinde Averous, Philippe Barthélémy, and Jean-Emmanuel Kurtz

Abstract

Ovarian epithelial tumor is a complex disease involving several subgroups. Ovarian endometrioid carcinoma (OEC) ranks second in terms of incidence, occurs in perimenopausal women and is generally diagnosed at early stage. Low grade carcinoma arises from endometriotic cysts, with an early loss of ARID1A. PTEN and KRAS mutations are also frequent in low grade ECO, although there is no data supporting the involvement of NRAS. Conversely, high grade OEC is associated with atypical endometriosis and is characterized by genetic instability and TP53 and CCNE mutations.

OEC shares morphological features of endometrioid tissues as immunochemistry shows strong and diffuse expression of estrogen and progesteron receptors, vimentine, and wild type p53. Grading is similar to that of endometrioid adenocarcinoma of the uterus. Differential diagnosis of low grade OEC include sex cords stromal tumors, clear cell carcinomas and carcinosarcoma. Grade 3 EOC can be confused with serous carcinoma and metastasis of colorectal adenocarcinoma.

EOC seems to have a better prognosis than high grade serous tumors even in advanced stages. Platinum-based combination chemotherapy with paclitaxel and bevacizumab is the standard frontline treatment in the setting of advanced disease although data in the OEC subgroup remains scarce.

G. Averous
Département de Pathologie, Hôpitaux Universitaires de Strasbourg,
1, Avenue Molière, Strasbourg 67200, France

J.-E. Kurtz (✉) • P. Barthélémy • L. de Cock
Service d'Oncologie, Hôpitaux Universitaires de Strasbourg,
1, Avenue Molière, Strasbourg 67200, France
e-mail: j-emmanuel.kurtz@chru-strasbourg.fr; jemkurtz@yahoo.fr

E. Pujade-Lauraine et al. (eds.), *Ovarian Cancers*,
DOI 10.1007/978-3-319-32110-3_15

Introduction

Epithelial ovarian carcinoma is a complex disease that involves different entities, including serous, mucinous, clear-cell, and endometrioid subtypes, alongside ovarian carcinosarcoma with different prognoses and outcomes. Although these tumors originate from the surface of the ovary, they have distinct molecular carcinogenesis pathways. As current advances in cancer care rely on the deciphering of molecular pathways, one can anticipate that new classifications of ovarian tumors will distinguish subtypes in which specific targeted therapies may be active. Although high-grade serous ovarian cancer is the most prominent subtype, endometrioid cancer is not uncommon and deserves in-depth investigations to enhance the patients' outcomes.

Epidemiology of Ovarian Endometrioid Carcinoma

Ovarian epithelial tumors represent a melting pot where several tumors coexist, having different origins and outcomes (for a review of histologic subtypes, see [1]). Endometrioid carcinoma of the ovary ranks second in terms of incidence of epithelial tumors, after the serous subtype, accounting for 10–20 % of ovarian cancers [2–4]. According to the SEER database, the incidence of ECO was 2.11 cases/100.000 women over the 1992–1999 period [5]. ECO preferentially occurs in perimenopausal women and is generally diagnosed at early stages, especially in low-grade tumors that grow slowly and may remain confined to the ovary for a long time [6, 7]. Of note, ECO also (in part) belong to the spectrum of malignancies encountered in the Lynch syndrome (or hereditary nonpolyposis colon cancer syndrome), associated to DNA mismatch repair abnormalities [8]. Finally, ECO may be bilateral in 28 % of cases and coexist with nonmalignant lesions such as endometriosis or even endometrioid carcinoma of the endometrium [9]. Indeed, coexistence of endometrioid endometrial and ovarian cancer routinely raises the question of simultaneous primaries versus metastatic disease that may be resolved by gene expression analysis as discussed below. Endometrioid and clear-cell carcinoma of the ovary share a number of molecular alterations, but also express molecular differences. Moreover, from the clinical point of view, several risk factors have been identified for these two entities, such as obesity with a twofold increased risk for clear-cell versus endometrioid carcinoma, whereas the risk decreased in smokers and educated patients [10].

Carcinogenesis of Ovarian Endometrioid Carcinoma

Over the last years, an outstanding effort has been made to reclassify epithelial ovarian cancer owing to both molecular events and pathologic precursor lesions. Two classes of epithelial tumors have been identified, consisting in the following: for class I tumors, low-grade serous, low-grade endometrioid, clear-cell carcinoma, and mucinous tumors and, for class II tumors, high-grade serous, high-grade endometrioid tumors, as well as carcinosarcoma [7, 11]. It is important to acknowledge that endometrioid carcinoma of the ovary may fall in both classes, making of outmost importance an adequate grading by the pathologist.

Carcinogenesis of Low-Grade Endometrioid Ovarian Carcinoma (ECO)

Most ECO are low-grade tumors, originating from endometriotic cysts (endometriomas), whereas high-grade ECO are morphologically close to the high-grade serous subtype, with a consistent gene expression profile [3, 12]. The transition from endometriotic cyst to clear-cell or endometrioid carcinoma requires the early loss of ARID1A, a gene involved in chromatin remodeling [13, 14]. Indeed, ARID1A mutations appear in 46 and 30 % of clear-cell and endometrioid carcinomas, contrasting with 0 % in high-grade serous carcinomas [15]. Other mutations, such as the phosphatase and tensin homolog PTEN can be found in endometriotic cysts at significant (57 %) rates [16] reinforcing the link between both endometrioid and clear-cell carcinomas and endometriotic cysts. However, these two conditions, although strongly associated with endometriosis, are distinct diseases, given the poor prognosis of the latter, certainly owing to different molecular characteristics, including the gene methylation profile [17, 18]. Low-grade tumors are characterized by the presence of KRAS mutations [19, 20].

Conversely to colorectal cancer, there is at the moment no data in the literature supporting the involvement of NRAS in this subtype. Okuda et al. analyzed the frequency of KRAS mutations in a series of 64 clear-cell and endometrioid ovarian cancers and found that these mutations occurred in 3.7 and 16.2 % of endometrioid and clear-cell carcinomas, respectively [21]. These relatively low numbers are however intriguing, but no data regarding to the tumor grade appeared in the report. Moreover, clear-cell tumors are more frequent in Eastern countries, and these data may not apply to Western countries' population. Other mutations in type I (low-grade) ECO carcinogenesis involve the Wnt pathway with CNNTB1 (beta-catenin) and the PI3K/Akt pathway with PI3KCA (phosphoinositide 3 kinase) and PTEN (phosphatase and tensin homolog).

Carcinogenesis of High-Grade Endometrioid Ovarian Carcinoma (ECO)

Conversely to the common precursor found in low-grade endometrioid carcinomas of the ovary, high-grade endometrioid and clear-cell tumors share a different common precursor lesion, i.e., atypical endometriosis [22]. Atypical endometriosis differs from typical endometriosis by dysplastic characteristics and is present in 8 % of endometriotic patients [23, 24].

High-grade endometrioid carcinomas are characterized (as other class II tumors) by genetic instability, as well as the presence of TP53 and CCNE (cyclin E1) mutations [7, 20]. Okuda et al. found that the occurrence of p53 mutations was a predictor of poorer survival in endometrioid carcinomas [21]. This might however simply reflect a subgroup of high-grade patients in their patient's population, since high levels of p53 mutations were found (63 %) that is contradictory to the molecular characteristics of type I tumors. Hence, given to such a separate carcinogenesis pathway, it is likely that there is no transition from low-grade to high-grade endometrioid carcinoma.

Morphology and Immunophenotype of Endometrioid Ovarian Carcinoma

Ovarian endometrioid carcinomas (OEC) have a mean size of 15 cm with mostly a smooth outer surface. On the cut surface, the tumor tissue is friable, soft, possibly hemorrhagic, or necrotic, sometimes forming polypus masses protruding into cystic spaces.

Microscopically OEC shares the morphological features of its endometrial counterpart: most low-grade tumors show a back-to-back arrangement of glands with high-columnar pseudostratified epithelium with grade 1 or 2 nuclei and confluent, cribriform to solid, or villoglandular architecture.

Immunohistochemical features of EOC are strong and diffuse expression of estrogen (ER) and progesterone receptors (PR), coexpression of low-molecular-weight cytokeratins and vimentine, absent or weak focal expression of CEA, heterogeneous and patchy p16 staining, as well as "wild-type" p53 expression, but aberrant p53 expression has been reported in up to 11 % of the tumors. According to the genetic mutations underlying carcinogenesis, EOC shows loss of PTEN expression and/or nuclear β-catenin expression and in Lynch syndrome loss of DNA MMR protein expression of MSH2, MSH6, MLH-1, and PMS2.

Grading of EOC is the same as for endometrioid adenocarcinoma of the uterus.

Tumors with less than 5 % solid architecture are considered grade 1 (Fig. 15.1), those with 6–50 % solid growth grade 2, and those with over 50 % solid growth grade 3 (Fig. 15.2). Nuclear grading is important as the presence of grade 3 nuclei involving greater than 50 % of the tumor indicates increased aggressiveness and upgrades the carcinoma by one grade.

Adequate sampling of the tumors should enable to establish whether EOC arises in endometriosis, adenofibromatous endometrioid precursors, or de novo. It should allow correct grading and evaluation of tumor extension for staging and give information about presence or absence of lymphovascular invasion.

Differential Diagnosis

Low-grade tumors (grades 1 and 2) display a variety of histological patterns such as squamous differentiation with morules (30–50 %); clear-cell changes; mucinous glands; sex cord-like, mucin rich, ciliated cell features; oxyphilic changes and secretory changes; and spindle cell patterns with hyalinization and even

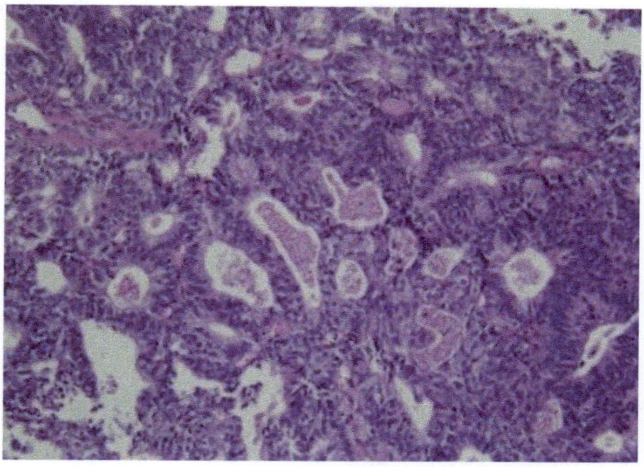

Fig. 15.1 EOC grade 1

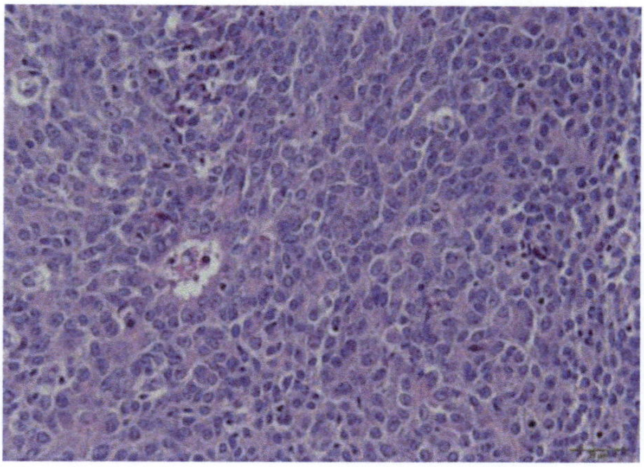

Fig. 15.2 EOC grade 3

heterologous elements. Unusual appearances can cause major problems in differential diagnosis. The most common of such variants are EOC with sex cord-like patterns that can be confused with sex cord-stromal tumors like adult granulosa cell tumors or sertoli cell tumors. Immunohistochemistry of inhibin and EMA is helpful in this setting, as EC is inhibin negative and EMA positive, whereas granulosa and sertoli cell tumors are EMA negative and inhibin positive [25, 26].

Clear-cell change in secretory EOC or EOC with squamous differentiation may be confused with clear-cell carcinoma. Recently, a panel of immunohistochemical markers containing HNF1β, napsin A, ER, and PR showed a very good specificity of napsin A in differentiating EC from CCC. In addition, ER and PR are diffusely and strongly expressed in EC, but absent or only focally positive in CCC [25, 27, 28].

EOC with spindle cell features, hyalinization, and corded aspects with heterologous elements may be confused with carcinosarcoma. In contrast to spindle cell

Table 15.1 Immunohistochemistry of ovarian carcinomas [27, 32, 33]

	PAX8	WT1	p16	p53	ER	PR	Napsin A
EOC	84 %	4 %	±	wt	86 %	72 %	3–5.3 %
LGSC	100 %	100 %	±	wt	96 %	50 %	1 %
HGSC	98 %	92 %	+++	93 %[a]	80 %	30 %	1 %
MC	50–60 %	4 %	∓	50 %[b]	6 %	0 %	0 %
CCC	99 %	0 %	±	12 %[a]	13 %	6 %	88 %

LGSC low-grade serous carcinoma, *HGSC* high-grade serous carcinoma, *MC* mucinous carcinoma, *CCC* clear-cell carcinoma, *wt* wild-type p53 expression (not associated with p53 mutation)
[a]Aberrant expression >60 % of strong nuclear or totally absent or <5 % of stained nuclei
[b]Loss of nuclear staining

EOC, heterologous sarcomatous components of carcinosarcoma have high-grade cytological features, and the border between carcinomatous and sarcomatous components is clear-cut showing no merging of epithelial and spindle cell areas as encountered in spindle cell EOC.

Endometrioid yolk sac tumors (YSTs) may be distinguished from endometrioid carcinoma by the absence of EMA and cytokeratin 7 expression. On the other hand, YSTs express SALL4, a marker of germ cell neoplasia, negative in EOC.

Papillary low-grade endometrioid carcinomas may challenge differential diagnosis with serous carcinoma. In this setting, the morphological clue to diagnosis is the discordance between architectural and cytological features.

Among high-grade tumors, grade 3 EOC may be confused with serous carcinoma with a prominent glandular pattern. Immunohistochemistry is helpful as serous carcinomas most often harbor p53 mutations, show diffuse and intense p16 and nuclear WT1 expression, and are vimentine negatives. However, as some grade 3 EOC may be p53 mutated (11–33 %), overlapping features can render distinction of the two types difficult [28]. Some of the high-grade endometrioid carcinomas represent probably glandular forms of serous carcinoma [29, 30]. As serous carcinomas behave more aggressively than grade 3 EOC, immunohistochemistry should be employed in order to correctly classify the tumor [31] – see Table 15.1.

EOC should further be distinguished from metastasis of extraovarian adenocarcinomas as colorectal adenocarcinoma (cytokeratin 20 and CDX2 positive and cytokeratin 7 negative) or endocervical adenocarcinoma (mostly showing diffuse expression of p16 and negative staining for vimentine, RE, RP, as well as positive cytoplasmic staining for CEA).

In cases of concomitant uterine and ovarian EC, a low-grade uterine EC with minimal or no myometrial invasion favors two independent primaries [33].

Prognosis of Endometrioid Ovarian Carcinoma

Given the differences in carcinogenesis, supporting that type I and II carcinomas are separate entities, plus the fact that most endometrioid carcinomas of the ovary belong to the type I class, one may speculate that patient outcomes are different as well. In an analysis of 929 patients (270 with pure endometrioid carcinoma and 659 with high-grade serous tumors), Storey et al. showed that endometrioid carcinoma patients did better in terms of progression-free and overall survival [4]. Not surprisingly, although the majority of patients had high-grade tumors, less patients harbored this subtype in the endometrioid carcinoma group, and more endometrioid carcinoma patients were at earlier FIGO stages. The authors reported that more endometrioid patients were "debulked" to less than 2 cm residual lesions, but fewer had chemotherapy. Despite the limitations of this study, the median progression-free survival favored the endometrioid patients (24 vs. 13 months, $p<0.001$). However, when the authors compared the outcomes of the subgroup stage III/"optimally" debulked, the difference was not significant (21 vs. 16 months, $p=0.219$), however favoring endometrioid patients. Overall survival again favored the endometrioid carcinoma patients (48 vs. 22 months, $p<0.001$) and remained significantly better in stage II and III patients (81 vs. 46 months, $p=0.0219$, and 33 vs. 22 months, $p=0.002$, respectively). This difference in overall survival was also found in another study, despite having as well the disadvantages of being retrospective and having recruited patients over decades [34]. Conversely, in a small study recruiting 42 patients, no survival difference was found [35]. Wang et al. investigated patients' outcome according to the presence of concomitant endometriosis. Not surprisingly, those patients were younger and had earlier FIGO stage and more low-grade tumors. The presence of concomitant endometriosis was linked to a better survival in univariate, but not multivariate analysis [36].

Interestingly, response to platinum-based chemotherapy was similar in both groups in the study by Storey et al. that is consistent with the fact that most patients had high-grade tumors that are more likely to be chemosensitive than low-grade tumors [4].

Treatment

The treatment guidelines for ovarian cancer (irrespectively to pathologic subtypes) include several cornerstones, among which are adequate staging, carcinologic surgery, and chemotherapy [37]. Among the past years, a number of phase III trials have established the standards of medical care for advanced ovarian cancer, again, not specifically focusing on a particular subtype, excepted perhaps for clear-cell carcinoma. Platinum-based combination with paclitaxel combined with bevacizumab in advanced ovarian cancers is considered as the frontline treatment standard and applies to all epithelial ovarian cancer subtypes. Of note, the recent phase III trials focusing onto advanced ovarian cancer have enrolled an overwhelming majority of high-grade serous tumors, as compared to endometrioid carcinomas. For example, the GOG 218 trial that investigated upfront/maintenance bevacizumab recruited a mean of 84 % of high-grade serous tumors versus 3 % of endometrioid carcinomas [38]. In the ICON-7 trial that also investigated bevacizumab, 69 % of enrolled patient had serous carcinoma, but the number of endometrioid carcinoma patients enrolled was not reported [39]. It is therefore extremely difficult (and probably impossible) to speculate on potential differences of treatment efficacy that may arise from pathologic subtypes.

Future Directions

As in a number of other malignancies such as lung, breast, colorectal cancer, and others, recent advances have focused on the dismemberment of cancers according to their molecular profile. More than providing evidences regarding carcinogenesis, this effort undoubtedly drives advances in tumor management especially toward the identification of "druggable" targets. Of note, a recent translational study in endometrial cancer (the TransPORTEC-3 initiative) identified four different prognosis groups according to molecular profiles that are (in part) close to those encountered in ovarian endometrioid cancer [40]. However, low-grade endometrioid carcinomas of the endometrium and the ovary do have distinct molecular profiles as PTEN mutations are far more frequent in endometrial tumors (67 vs. 17 %, $p<0.0001$), whereas CTNNB1 mutations are in turn more frequent in ovarian tumors (57 vs. 28 %, $p<0.0057$), possibly due to distinct microenvironments [32, 41]. These data reinforce the need for designing innovative translational approaches to ovarian cancer, particularly at the scale of cooperative groups (such as the GINEGEPS within the French GINECO group).

References

1. Soslow RA. Histologic subtypes of ovarian carcinoma: an overview. Int J Gynecol Pathol. 2008;27(2):161–74.
2. Seidman JD, Horkayne-Szakaly I, Haiba M, Boice CR, Kurman RJ, Ronnett BM. The histologic type and stage distribution of ovarian carcinomas of surface epithelial origin. Int J Gynecol Pathol. 2004;23(1):41–4.
3. Prat J. New insights into ovarian cancer pathology. Ann Oncol. 2012;23 Suppl 10:x111–7.
4. Storey DJ, Rush R, Stewart M, Rye T, Al-Nafussi A, Williams AR, et al. Endometrioid epithelial ovarian cancer : 20 years of prospectively collected data from a single center. Cancer. 2008;112(10):2211–20.
5. Quirk JT, Natarajan N. Ovarian cancer incidence in the United States, 1992-1999. Gynecol Oncol. 2005;97(2):519–23.
6. Kline RC, Wharton JT, Atkinson EN, Burke TW, Gershenson DM, Edwards CL. Endometrioid carcinoma of the ovary: retrospective review of 145 cases. Gynecol Oncol. 1990;39(3):337–46.
7. Kurman RJ, Shih IM. The origin and pathogenesis of epithelial ovarian cancer: a proposed unifying theory. Am J Surg Pathol. 2010;34(3):433–43.
8. Suchy J, Kurzawski G, Jakubowska A, Lubinski J. Ovarian cancer of endometrioid type as part of the MSH6gene mutation phenotype. J Hum Genet. 2002;47(10):529–31.
9. Irving JA, Catasus L, Gallardo A, Bussaglia E, Romero M, Matias-Guiu X, et al. Synchronous endometrioid carcinomas of the uterine corpus and ovary: alterations in the beta-catenin (CTNNB1) pathway are associated with independent primary tumors and favorable prognosis. Hum Pathol. 2005;36(6):605–19.

10. Nagle CM, Olsen CM, Webb PM, Jordan SJ, Whiteman DC, Green AC, et al. Endometrioid and clear cell ovarian cancers: a comparative analysis of risk factors. Eur J Cancer. 2008;44(16):2477–84.
11. Prat J. Ovarian carcinomas: five distinct diseases with different origins, genetic alterations, and clinicopathological features. Virchows Arch. 2012;460(3):237–49.
12. Tothill RW, Tinker AV, George J, Brown R, Fox SB, Lade S, et al. Novel molecular subtypes of serous and endometrioid ovarian cancer linked to clinical outcome. Clin Cancer Res. 2008;14(16):5198–208.
13. Ayhan A, Mao TL, Seckin T, Wu CH, Guan B, Ogawa H, et al. Loss of ARID1A expression is an early molecular event in tumor progression from ovarian endometriotic cyst to clear cell and endometrioid carcinoma. Int J Gynecol Cancer. 2012;22(8):1310–5.
14. Lowery WJ, Schildkraut JM, Akushevich L, Bentley R, Marks JR, Huntsman D, et al. Loss of ARID1A-associated protein expression is a frequent event in clear cell and endometrioid ovarian cancers. Int J Gynecol Cancer. 2012;22(1):9–14.
15. Wiegand KC, Shah SP, Al-Agha OM, Zhao Y, Tse K, Zeng T, et al. ARID1A mutations in endometriosis-associated ovarian carcinomas. N Engl J Med. 2010;363(16):1532–43.
16. Sato N, Tsunoda H, Nishida M, Morishita Y, Takimoto Y, Kubo T, et al. Loss of heterozygosity on 10q23.3 and mutation of the tumor suppressor gene PTEN in benign endometrial cyst of the ovary: possible sequence progression from benign endometrial cyst to endometrioid carcinoma and clear cell carcinoma of the ovary. Cancer Res. 2000;60(24):7052–6.
17. Chen CA, Chiang YC, Chang MC, Hu YH, You SL, Cheng YY, et al. Gene methylation profiles as prognostic markers in ovarian clear cell and endometrioid adenocarcinomas. Am J Transl Res. 2015;7(1):139–52.
18. Fukunaga M, Nomura K, Ishikawa E, Ushigome S. Ovarian atypical endometriosis: its close association with malignant epithelial tumours. Histopathology. 1997;30(3):249–55.
19. Stewart CJ, Leung Y, Walsh MD, Walters RJ, Young JP, Buchanan DD. KRAS mutations in ovarian low-grade endometrioid adenocarcinoma: association with concurrent endometriosis. Hum Pathol. 2012;43(8):1177–83.
20. Geyer JT, Lopez-Garcia MA, Sanchez-Estevez C, Sarrio D, Moreno-Bueno G, Franceschetti I, et al. Pathogenetic pathways in ovarian endometrioid adenocarcinoma: a molecular study of 29 cases. Am J Surg Pathol. 2009;33(8):1157–63.
21. Okuda T, Otsuka J, Sekizawa A, Saito H, Makino R, Kushima M, et al. p53 mutations and overexpression affect prognosis of ovarian endometrioid cancer but not clear cell cancer. Gynecol Oncol. 2003;88(3):318–25.
22. Sainz de la Cuesta R, Eichhorn JH, Rice LW, Fuller Jr AF, Nikrui N, Goff BA. Histologic transformation of benign endometriosis to early epithelial ovarian cancer. Gynecol Oncol. 1996;60(2):238–44.
23. Czernobilsky B, Morris WJ. A histologic study of ovarian endometriosis with emphasis on hyperplastic and atypical changes. Obstet Gynecol. 1979;53(3):318–23.
24. Van Gorp T, Amant F, Neven P, Vergote I, Moerman P. Endometriosis and the development of malignant tumours of the pelvis. A review of literature. Best Pract Res Clin Obstet Gynaecol. 2004;18(2):349–71.
25. Zhao C, Bratthauer GL, Barner R, Vang R. Comparative analysis of alternative and traditional immunohistochemical markers for the distinction of ovarian sertoli cell tumor from endometrioid tumors and carcinoid tumor: a study of 160 cases. Am J Surg Pathol. 2007;31(2): 255–66.
26. Murray SK, Clement PB, Young RH. Endometrioid carcinomas of the uterine corpus with sex cord-like formations, hyalinization, and other unusual morphologic features: a report of 31 cases of a neoplasm that may be confused with carcinosarcoma and other uterine neoplasms. Am J Surg Pathol. 2005;29(2):157–66.
27. Lim D, Ip PP, Cheung AN, Kiyokawa T, Oliva E. Immunohistochemical comparison of ovarian and uterine endometrioid carcinoma, endometrioid carcinoma with clear cell change, and clear cell carcinoma. Am J Surg Pathol. 2015;39(8):1061–9.

28. Zannoni GF, Vellone VG, Arena V, Prisco MG, Scambia G, Carbone A, et al. Does high-grade endometrioid carcinoma (grade 3 FIGO) belong to type I or type II endometrial cancer? A clinical-pathological and immunohistochemical study. Virchows Arch. 2010;457(1):27–34.
29. Gilks CB, Oliva E, Soslow RA. Poor interobserver reproducibility in the diagnosis of high-grade endometrial carcinoma. Am J Surg Pathol. 2013;37(6):874–81.
30. McCluggage WG. Morphological subtypes of ovarian carcinoma: a review with emphasis on new developments and pathogenesis. Pathology. 2011;43(5):420–32.
31. Bartosch C, Manuel Lopes J, Oliva E. Endometrial carcinomas: a review emphasizing overlapping and distinctive morphological and immunohistochemical features. Adv Anat Pathol. 2011;18(6):415–37.
32. Fadare O, Zhao C, Khabele D, Parkash V, Quick CM, Gwin K, et al. Comparative analysis of Napsin A, alpha-methylacyl-coenzyme A racemase (AMACR, P504S), and hepatocyte nuclear factor 1 beta as diagnostic markers of ovarian clear cell carcinoma: an immunohistochemical study of 279 ovarian tumours. Pathology. 2015;47(2):105–11.
33. Kurman R, Carcangiu M, Herrington C, Young RH. WHO classification of tumors of female reproductive organs. Lyon: IARC; 2014.
34. Grosso G, Raspagliesi F, Baiocchi G, Di Re E, Colavita M, Cobellis L. Endometrioid carcinoma of the ovary: a retrospective analysis of 106 cases. Tumori. 1998;84(5):552–7.
35. Zwart J, Geisler JP, Geisler HE. Five-year survival in patients with endometrioid carcinoma of the ovary versus those with serous carcinoma. Eur J Gynaecol Oncol. 1998;19(3):225–8.
36. Wang S, Qiu L, Lang JH, Shen K, Huang HF, Pan LY, et al. Prognostic analysis of endometrioid epithelial ovarian cancer with or without endometriosis: a 12-year cohort study of Chinese patients. Am J Obstet Gynecol. 2013;209(3):241e1–9.
37. Ledermann JA, Raja FA, Fotopoulou C, Gonzalez-Martin A, Colombo N, Sessa C, et al. Newly diagnosed and relapsed epithelial ovarian carcinoma: ESMO Clinical Practice Guidelines for diagnosis, treatment and follow-up. Ann Oncol. 2013;24 Suppl 6:vi24–32.
38. Burger RA, Brady MF, Bookman MA, Fleming GF, Monk BJ, Huang H, et al. Incorporation of bevacizumab in the primary treatment of ovarian cancer. N Engl J Med. 2011;365(26):2473–83.
39. Perren TJ, Swart AM, Pfisterer J, Ledermann JA, Pujade-Lauraine E, Kristensen G, et al. A phase 3 trial of bevacizumab in ovarian cancer. N Engl J Med. 2011;365(26):2484–96.
40. Stelloo E, Bosse T, Nout RA, MacKay HJ, Church DN, Nijman HW, et al. Refining prognosis and identifying targetable pathways for high-risk endometrial cancer; a TransPORTEC initiative. Mod Pathol. 2015;28(6):836–44.
41. McConechy MK, Ding J, Senz J, Yang W, Melnyk N, Tone AA, et al. Ovarian and endometrial endometrioid carcinomas have distinct CTNNB1 and PTEN mutation profiles. Mod Pathol. 2014;27(1):128–34.

Mucinous Carcinoma of the Ovary

16

Jubilee Brown and Michael Frumovitz

Abstract

Mucinous ovarian carcinoma is a rare tumor, but deserves separate attention, as its clinical behavior is quite different from other types of ovarian carcinoma. This has implications for both surgical therapy as well as adjuvant treatment.

Introduction

Mucinous carcinoma of the ovary is a rare ovarian cancer that is distinct from other epithelial subtypes based on specific clinical, histologic, and molecular features. Until recently, all epithelial ovarian cancers have been eligible for the same clinical trials, and treatment recommendations have been generalized to specific subtypes. Clinical decision making and prognostic information have been applied in a similar fashion to all subtypes, despite the difference in clinical behavior and outcomes between mucinous ovarian cancer (MOC) and other more common histologic subtypes. Since 2004, the subtleties of MOC have been investigated, and the clinical presentation, biologic behavior, and outcomes data appear to be specific to this histology [1, 2]. Comparative genomic hybridization (CGH) reveals differences between mutational profiles of mucinous and serous ovarian carcinomas. Mucinous carcinomas have fewer alterations (additions or deletions), while serous carcinomas have multiple alterations throughout the genome (Fig. 16.1).

J. Brown, MD (✉) • M. Frumovitz, MD
Department of Gynecologic Oncology and Reproductive Sciences, The University of Texas M.D. Anderson Cancer Center, 1155 Herman Pressler Blvd., Unit 1362, P.O. Box 301439, Houston, TX 77030, USA
e-mail: jbbrown@mdanderson.org; jubilee.brown@me.com

E. Pujade-Lauraine et al. (eds.), *Ovarian Cancers*,
DOI 10.1007/978-3-319-32110-3_16

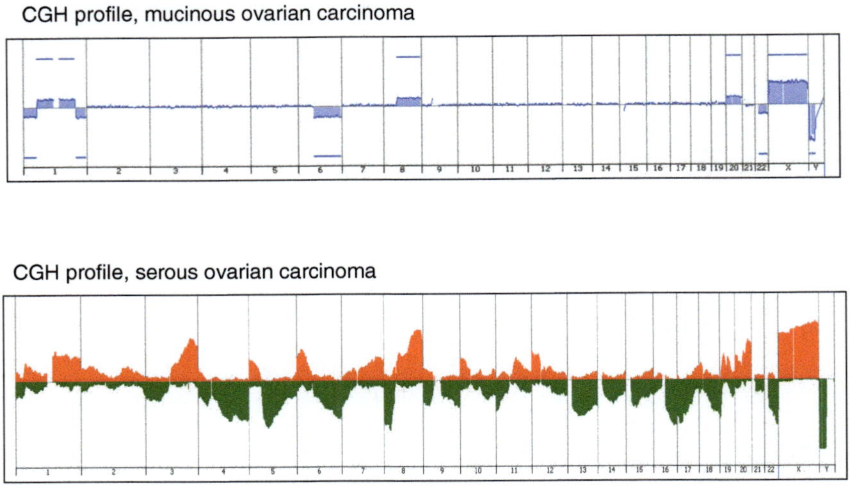

Fig. 16.1 (Courtesy of Drs/Treilleux, D Pissaloux and Pr/Ray-Coquard from centre leon berard, Lyon)

While the low incidence is a barrier to performing effective clinical trials specific to MOC, international involvement has been key to a better understanding of this entity and has resulted in improved diagnostics, assessment, and treatment.

Epidemiology

Mucinous carcinoma of the ovary is a rare subtype of epithelial ovarian cancer. The true incidence has been difficult to determine due to challenges in pathologic diagnosis in differentiating benign, borderline (low malignant potential), and metastatic tumors from primary invasive MOC [3, 4]. Most mucinous tumors are actually benign or borderline neoplasms; benign mucinous tumors account for 10–15 % of all benign ovarian neoplasms [5, 6]. Borderline (low malignant potential) tumors account for 67 % of tumors not considered strictly benign and thus are more common than invasive MOC [7]. Until recently, MOC was thought to account for 5–10 % of epithelial ovarian malignancies, but a systematic review to exclude tumors of low malignant potential and metastatic lesions from gastrointestinal, pancreatic, or other gynecologic primary tumors suggested that MOCs are less common and represent 2.4 % of all epithelial ovarian cancers [4]. Subsequently, Shimada et al. reviewed and reclassified 1400 cases of epithelial ovarian carcinoma. While 16 % were initially diagnosed as primary MOC, upon review only 4.9 % were found to be invasive, with the remainder intraepithelial, borderline, or metastatic in origin [3].

This low incidence is supported by a similar percentage enrollment of mucinous histology in cooperative group trials. In Gynecologic Oncology Group (GOG) trial 111, 14 of 410 patients (3.4 %) had MOC [8]. Intergroup trial IV-10 enrolled 30 of

680 patients (4.4 %) with mucinous histology [9]. Enrollment in GOG trial 132 included 16 of 614 patients (2.6 %) with mucinous histology [10], and enrollment in GOG trial 182 included 71 of 4312 patients (1.6 %) with mucinous histology [11].

The age at diagnosis of MOC is usually described between ages 20–50 years, which is younger than that for epithelial ovarian cancer in general [12]. While family history does not appear to be a risk factor, a history of smoking is associated with a twofold increase in the incidence of both invasive and borderline disease [13].

Pathology

The diagnosis and classification of mucinous tumors has been problematic and controversial. Accurate diagnosis is essential for appropriate treatment, as standard approaches for serous epithelial ovarian cancer are futile, failure to diagnose benign or borderline histology results in overtreatment, and failure to identify ovarian disease as metastatic leads to a missed diagnosis of a gastrointestinal primary and incorrect therapy [2].

Upon gross inspection, these tumors are typically large, unilocular, or multilocular cysts filled with mucoid liquid that becomes gelatinous at room temperature. The mean size at diagnosis is 18 cm, but these tumors can be massive and fill the abdomen and pelvis [1, 14].

The World Health Organization lists specific criteria for the diagnosis of intestinal-type mucinous borderline tumor. These include the following: (1) tumors contain cystic spaces lined by gastrointestinal-type mucinous epithelium with stratification and may form filiform papillae with at least minimal stromal support, (2) nuclei are slightly larger than those seen in cystadenomas, (3) mitotic activity is present, and (4) goblet cells and sometimes Paneth cells are present but stromal invasion is absent [15]. Marked cytologic atypia without stromal invasion represents intraepithelial carcinoma and is a separate entity [2].

The diagnosis of invasive mucinous carcinoma rests on the presence of stromal invasion more than 5 mm in depth or more than 10 mm in area. Invasive MOC is further subdivided into expansile (confluent) and infiltrative types. The expansile (confluent) type consists of a glandular growth pattern without intervening normal ovarian parenchyma, whereas the infiltrative pattern consists of glands, nest, or individual cells which infiltrate the stroma; the latter appears to be more clinically aggressive [16, 17].

The challenge of differentiating among these subtle diagnoses is compounded by the frequent coexistence of benign, borderline, intraepithelial, and/or invasive mucinous carcinoma within one mass. While this may suggest a continuum of malignancy from benign to invasive disease, direct evidence is lacking. These issues make accurate intraoperative diagnosis difficult due to limitations of sampling and time. The tumor size and coexistence of multiple degrees of malignancy may also lead to failure to diagnose a small focus of carcinoma within a large benign or borderline tumor [15].

An additional challenge in mucinous carcinoma is determining whether the source of the tumor is primary in the ovary or metastatic from another site. Primary ovarian tumors tend to be more often unilateral and larger than metastatic tumors (16–20 cm versus 11–12 cm). However, large size is not specific to primary disease, as 32–48 % of metastatic tumors are over 10 cm [1, 14]. Primary ovarian tumors are more likely to have coexistent benign or borderline components, an expansile (confluent) pattern of invasion, and other ovarian pathologies (e.g., mural nodule, Brenner tumor, or teratoma). Metastatic disease is more often associated with a prominent desmoplastic response, nodular or infiltrative pattern of invasion, small clusters of tumor cells within corpora lutea or albicantia, numerous pools of mucin dissecting the ovarian stroma (i.e., pseudomyxoma ovarii) in the absence of a coexistent teratoma, extensive signet-ring cell pattern, ovarian surface involvement, vascular invasion, and hilar involvement [18]. The most common primary sites for disease metastatic to the ovary are gastrointestinal, pancreas, cervix, breast, and uterus, and these sites should be clearly investigated as a source of malignancy when metastatic disease is suspected [4].

Molecular Biology and Genetics

Mucinous and serous epithelial ovarian cancers have distinct molecular characteristics, further supporting the functional separation between these histologic subtypes. In contrast to serous carcinomas, *K-ras* mutations are identified in 43–65 % of MOCs, mucinous borderline tumors, and mucinous cystadenomas [12, 17, 19–21]. Mutations in the p53 tumor suppressor gene occur less frequently than in serous ovarian carcinomas but are present in some cases (16 % versus 60 %) [22]. Gene expression profiling also differs between serous and mucinous histologies [23, 24]. MOC does not appear to be linked to BRCA gene mutations, as only about 2 % of ovarian cancers associated with BRCA mutations are of mucinous histology [25, 26]. One recent study has identified amplification of *Her2* in 19 % of mucinous tumors, which may provide a rationale for directed therapy in these cancers [27, 28].

Other immunohistochemical and molecular alterations characterize mucinous tumors [29–32]. Mucinous tumors are more likely to express E-cadherin and less likely to express N-cadherin than serous tumors [33]. Matrix metalloproteinases and WT-1 have also been characterized [34]. Src kinase has been recently identified as a targetable non-receptor tyrosine kinase expressed in many MOCs and may represent a therapeutic strategy [35].

Clinical Presentation and Diagnosis

The constellation of symptoms at presentation, unilaterality, stage, lack of lymphatic involvement, and serum tumor markers may suggest a mucinous ovarian neoplasm. These tumors are usually quite large, with a median size of 18 cm, but may be extremely large, presenting with a mass effect or ureteral obstruction [36, 37].

Primary tumors are larger than metastatic tumors, and nearly 80 % of primary mucinous ovarian tumors are unilateral, a feature that distinguishes these tumors from serous ovarian carcinomas and from mucinous cancers metastatic to the ovary [16]. Based on these characteristics, Seidman has developed an algorithm to predict primary ovarian versus metastatic origin, in which a unilateral tumor great than 10 cm correctly predicts primary ovarian origin in 82 % of cases. Conversely, bilateral tumors less than 10 cm accurately predict metastatic disease in 95 % of cases [4].

The stage at diagnosis in primary MOCs is more likely to be early stage than in serous ovarian carcinomas. Whereas 83 % of MOCs are stage I at diagnosis, only 4 % of serous ovarian cancers are stage I at diagnosis [38]. Lymphatic dissemination does not occur in mucinous ovarian tumors, a finding which affects not only stage but also the surgical staging procedure [39].

The profile of serum tumor markers elevated in MOC also suggests the histology and the primary disease site. Serum carcinoembryonic antigen (CEA) and CA19-9 are often elevated in primary mucinous ovarian cancer but to a lesser extent than in colorectal tumors. These markers do not help to determine the site of primary origin [40]. The ratio of CA125 to CEA, when greater than 25, suggests primary ovarian origin [17]. In total, CEA, elevated in over 30 % of all ovarian cancers, is the most useful marker in suggesting a preoperative diagnosis of MOC and in following a patient's disease course following initial diagnosis. Other biomarkers that tend to be elevated in MOC include CA72-4, matrix metalloproteinase-9, CD40L, insulin-like growth factor-binding protein-1, myeloperoxidase, and tissue plasminogen activator-1 [41].

Initial Treatment

The cornerstone of treatment is surgery. Any suspected ovarian mass should be removed intact, typically with the involved adnexa being removed and sent for intraoperative pathologic evaluation. Pelvic washings are obtained upon entry into the peritoneal cavity. In a woman who has completed childbearing, surgery should consist of total hysterectomy and bilateral salpingo-oophorectomy. A benign mucinous cystadenomy requires no additional surgery. Upon return of pathology indicating a mucinous tumor of low malignant potential or invasive cancer, the entire abdominopelvic cavity is inspected with careful attention to the gastrointestinal tract to evaluate a possible focus of gastrointestinal primary, and the appendix is removed [42–44]. If there is no evidence of extra ovarian disease, the appendix may be retained, but this is controversial, and others advocate appendectomy even in the setting of a benign mucinous tumor [45]. Any extra ovarian disease is removed entirely with the goal of leaving no macroscopic residual disease. If the extent and distribution of disease precludes complete resection, surgery is directed to alleviate patient symptoms, surgery is stopped, and chemotherapy is initiated. Interval debulking surgery proceeds after 3 cycles of neoadjuvant chemotherapy if the patient responds [42, 46]. If no extra ovarian disease is identified, a staging procedure is performed, consisting of peritoneal biopsies, omentectomy, and biopsy of any suspicious area. The incidence of lymphatic metastases is extremely low in mucinous tumors, so lymphadenectomy is omitted from the staging procedure, but enlarged lymph nodes should be removed [39, 47]. Accurate determination of the presence of an invasive component may be difficult at the time of intraoperative pathology evaluation due to the size of the mass [48]. Therefore, staging is performed any time a mucinous tumor of low malignant potential or invasive cancer is identified.

The route of surgery in the setting of known metastatic disease should be through a vertical midline incision. In the absence of known metastatic disease, minimally invasive surgery may be superior in terms of postoperative recovery and is acceptable when the mass can be removed in a specimen retrieval bag without intentional spill or rupture [49, 50]. Rupture of the mass should be avoided, as this upstages the patient and may increase the risk of recurrence. Morcellation in the abdominal cavity or trocar sites should absolutely be avoided [16]. The correct technique involves placing the detached specimen into the specimen retrieval bag and drawing the edges of the bag out through one trocar site, enlarging it if necessary. Once the circumference of the bag opening is externalized, a large bore spinal needle or suction device is used to aspirate the fluid, decompress the cyst, and the mass is removed without contact with the peritoneum, subcutaneous tissues, or skin [51].

Patients who wish to retain childbearing potential may undergo fertility-sparing surgery, with conservation of the normal-appearing uterus and contralateral ovary in early-stage disease. A recent study reported 7 patients with clinically early-stage MOC who underwent fertility-sparing surgery; all were without evidence of recurrence at a median follow-up of 47.3 months, and one patient had a term pregnancy resulting in a live birth [52]. Another study found no differences in recurrence-free or disease-specific survival among 35 patients who underwent fertility-sparing surgery compared with 55 patients who underwent radical surgery for clinically apparent early-stage MOC [53]. Fertility-sparing surgery does not imply ovarian cystectomy, as the involved adnexa should be removed, nor does it obviate the need for staging.

Adjuvant Therapy

Patients with stage IA or IB grade 1 tumors do not require adjuvant therapy. According to the NCCN guidelines, patients with stage IB grade 2 tumors may undergo observation or 3–6 cycles of adjuvant chemotherapy. Patients with stage IC grade 3 disease or greater should receive 3–6 cycles of adjuvant chemotherapy [42]. However, adjuvant chemotherapy in the setting of early disease is not clearly of benefit. The two largest trials of adjuvant chemotherapy in this setting, ICON 1 and ACTION, enrolled a total of 180 patients with a mucinous-type tumor. While 18 % of patients overall relapsed, there were no differences in relapse rate or outcome of the treated patients compared with patients undergoing observation [54].

Definitive recommendations for effective chemotherapy are lacking based on poor results with paclitaxel and carboplatin, chemotherapy that is usually effective in this setting in serous ovarian carcinoma. The results of several retrospective analyses demonstrate resistance to this regimen. The Hellenic Cooperative Group reported a lower response rate (38.5 versus 70 %, $p=0.001$) in 47 patients with advanced MOC when compared to 94 matched controls with serous ovarian cancers. Time to progression and overall survival were not significantly different [55]. A similar study from the Royal Marsden Hospital found a similar response rate but lower PFS (5.7 versus 14.1 months) and OS (12.0 versus 36.7 months) among 27 patients with MOC compared with 54 controls with serous ovarian carcinoma [1]. Additionally, a Dutch Cancer Registry showed that patients with advanced-stage MOC have a worse prognosis than patients with advanced-stage serous ovarian carcinoma (11 versus 26 % 5-year survival, $p<0.01$) [56].

Although the percentage enrollment of primary MOC is small, pooled data from multiple cooperative group trials have demonstrated the limited efficacy of paclitaxel and carboplatin in patients with MOC (see Prognosis). A pooled analysis of 7 Gynecologic Cancer InterGroup trials including 8704 patients, 264 (3 %) of whom had mucinous tumors, reveals that despite a higher resection rate at primary surgery, the hazard ratio for progression was 2.1 and for death was 2.7 when compared to serous ovarian carcinomas [57]. Additionally, a pooled analysis of GINECO (French cooperative group) found that 5 % of enrolled patients had MOC, and these patients were less likely to have advanced disease and more likely to achieve complete cytoreduction, but had a worse prognosis with a greater proportion of visceral metastases, a lower response rate to paclitaxel and carboplatin, and a shorter progression-free (PFS) and overall survival (OS) when compared with serous ovarian carcinoma [58]. A pooled analysis of 7 Gynecologic Oncology Group (GOG) trials including 1896 patients, 34 (1.8 %) of whom had MOC and received 6 cycles of paclitaxel and carboplatin, revealed that these patients had a worse PFS (10.5 versus 16.9 months) and OS (14.8 versus 45.1 months) when compared with serous carcinoma [59].

The search for alternative, more effective chemotherapy has included regimens utilized for gastrointestinal cancer based on the histologic appearance and biologic similarities. The combination of oxaliplatin and a fluoropyrimidine using either 5-fluorouracil or capecitabine has been used, but there are no published data clearly supporting their use in this setting. An international combined cooperative group trial including the GCIG, GOG, NCRI, and NCT compared oxaliplatin and capecitabine with carboplatin and paclitaxel ± bevacizumab in each arm. This trial had slow accrual so was closed prior to completion [51]. Review of the preliminary results indicates difficulty in accurate diagnosis of primary disease, as many enrolled patients were in fact extraovarian primary malignancies metastatic to the ovary [personal communication, David Gershenson, January 19, 2016]. This highlights the need for prospective pathology evaluation in any trial involving primary MOC.

Recurrent Disease

A paucity of information exists on the treatment of recurrent mucinous ovarian cancer. Patients with platinum-sensitive disease (platinum-free interval greater than 6 months) also appear to do worse than their counterparts with recurrent serous ovarian cancer.

In the only study to evaluate outcomes in the recurrent setting, the response rate to second-line treatment with platinum-based chemotherapy was lower in patients with mucinous histology (36 % versus 62 %, $p=0.04$), PFS was worse (4.5 versus 8 months, $p=0.03$), and OS was worse (17.9 versus 28.8 months, $p=0.003$) [60].

Prognosis

The prognosis of MOC varies by stage. Compared to patients with serous ovarian cancer, a greater proportion of patients with MOC are diagnosed at an early stage, and these patients have a 5-year survival of 90.8 % [36]. This is significantly better than the 5-year survival for serous carcinoma of the ovary, reported at 75.9 % [5]. A large analysis of the Dutch Cancer Registry confirmed these findings, demonstrating an improved prognosis for MOCs compared with serous ovarian carcinomas in early-stage disease (79 % versus 73 % 5-year survival, $p<0.01$) [56]. Risk of recurrence is also lower than for other histologic subtypes, with a hazard ratio of 0.37, and 5-year survival independent of stage is better for mucinous than for serous when all patients are considered (58 % versus 40 % 5-years survival, $p<0.01$) [56, 61]. Similarly, the median OS for over 6000 patients with ovarian cancer in the Swedish family study was also significantly better for mucinous than serous histology (970 versus 34 months) [62]. This is likely due to the preponderance of early-stage disease and its excellent prognosis.

Women with advanced-stage mucinous carcinoma of the ovary, however, do poorly and have a worse outcome than women with other histologic subtypes of ovarian cancer. This was demonstrated in a matched cohort study of patients with stage III and IV disease, in which 27 patients with mucinous ovarian cancer and 54 patients with other histologic subtypes were evaluated. The only factors that differed between groups were PFS (5.7 versus 14.1 months, $p<0.001$) and OS (12.0 versus 36.7 months, $p<0.001$) [1].

Future Research

Future research centers on finding active agents against MOC. Cell line studies have shown resistance to single-agent platinum and taxane agents, but some activity was demonstrated with oxaliplatin, etoposide, and 5-fluorouracil (5-FU). The most active combination was oxaliplatin and 5-FU. A mouse xenograft model confirmed these findings [63]. This has lead to a clinical trial currently enrolling women in Japan with advanced or recurrent MOC in a single-arm phase II trial of oxaliplatin in combination with S-1, a drug comprised of tegafur, gimeracil, and oteracil [2].

Other investigators have previously evaluated CPT-11 and mitomycin-C [64]. As noted, the GCIG initiated a 4-arm, phase III trial which randomized carboplatin and paclitaxel ± bevacizumab with oxaliplatin and capecitabine ± bevacizumab. The trial closed early due to low accrual [51].

Other areas of interest include the role of Src kinase, a non-receptor tyrosine kinase which regulated tumor progression. This is a mutation targetable with a novel agent which inhibits both Src signaling and pre-tubulin [35]. Additionally, therapeutics targeting the ras pathway may be useful to investigate in the recurrent setting.

Conclusions

Primary mucinous ovarian cancer is a distinct entity which differs from other histologic subtypes. Surgical management, including fertility-sparing surgery, is key in the management of these tumors. Early-stage tumors do not require chemotherapy and have an excellent prognosis. Late-stage and recurrent tumors, however, do not have a defined therapy at this time, as paclitaxel and carboplatin are not useful in this setting. Current research focuses on identifying active combination regimens and targeted therapy potentially useful in managing this difficult disease.

References

1. Hess V, A'Hern R, Nasiri N, et al. Mucinous epithelial ovarian cancer: a separate entity requiring specific treatment. J Clin Oncol. 2004;22:1040–4.
2. Frumovitz M, Schmeler KM, Malpica A, et al. Unmasking the complexities of mucinous ovarian carcinoma. Gynecol Oncol. 2010;117:491–6.
3. Shimada M, Kigawa J, Ohishi Y, et al. Clinicopathological characteristics of mucinous adenocarcinoma of the ovary. Gynecol Oncol. 2009;113:331–4.
4. Seidman JD, Kurman RJ, Ronnett BM. Primary and metastatic mucinous adenocarcinomas in the ovaries: incidence in routine practice with a new approach to improve intraoperative diagnosis. Am J Surg Pathol. 2003;27:985–93.
5. Mondal SK, Banyopadhyay R, Nag DR, et al. Histologic pattern, bilaterality and clinical evaluation of 957 ovarian neoplasms: a 10-year study in a tertiary hospital in eastern India. J Cancer Res Ther. 2011;4:433–7.
6. Koonings PP. Relative frequencies of primary ovarian neoplasms: a 10-year review. Obstet Gynecol. 1989;74:921–6.
7. Shappell HW, Riopel MA, Smith Sehdev AE, et al. Diagnostic criteria and behavior of ovarian seromucinous (endocervical-type mucinous and mixed cell-type) tumors: atypical proliferative (borderline) tumors, intraepithelial, microinvasive, and invasive carcinomas. Am J Surg Pathol. 2002;26:1529–41.
8. McGuire WP, Hoskins WJ, Brady MF, et al. Cyclophosphamide and cisplatin compared with paclitaxel and cisplatin in patients with stage III and stage IV ovarian cancer. N Engl J Med. 1996;334:1–6.
9. Piccart MJ, Bertelsen K, James K, et al. Randomized intergroup trial of cisplatin–paclitaxel versus cisplatin–cyclophos-phamide in women with advanced epithelial ovarian cancer: three-year results. J Natl Cancer Inst. 2000;92:699–708.
10. Muggia FM, Braly PS, Brady MF, et al. Phase III randomized study of cisplatin versus paclitaxel versus cisplatin and paclitaxel in patients with suboptimal stage III or IV ovarian cancer: a gynecologic oncology group study. J Clin Oncol. 2000;18:106–15.
11. Bookman MA, Brady MF, McGuire WP, et al. Evaluation of new platinum-based treatment regimens in advanced-stage ovarian cancer: a Phase III Trial of the Gynecologic Cancer Intergroup. J Clin Oncol. 2009;27:1419–25.

12. Kelemen LE, Kobel M. Mucinous carcinomas of the ovary and colorectum: different organ, same dilemma. Lancet Oncol. 2011;12:1071–80.
13. Collaborative Group on Epidemiological Studies of Ovarian C; Beral V, Gaitskell K, et al. Ovarian cancer and smoking: individual participant meta-analysis including 28,114 women with ovarian cancer from 51 epidemiological studies. Lancet Oncol. 2012;13:946–56.
14. Siegel R, Naishadham D, Jemal A. Cancer statistics, 2013. CA Cancer J Clin. 2013;63:11–30.
15. Chiesa AG, Deavers MT, Veras E, et al. Ovarian intestinal type mucinous borderline tumors: are we ready for a nomenclature change? Int J Gynecol Pathol. 2010;29:108–12.
16. Lee KR, Scully RE. Mucinous tumors of the ovary: a clinicopathologic study of 196 borderline tumors (of intestinal type) and carcinomas, including an evaluation of 11 cases with 'pseudomyxoma peritonei'. Am J Surg Pathol. 2000;24:1447–64.
17. Rodriguez IM, Prat J. Mucinous tumors of the ovary: a clinicopathologic analysis of 75 borderline tumors (of intestinal type) and carcinomas. Am J Surg Pathol. 2002;26:139–52.
18. Lee KR, Young RH. The distinction between primary and metastatic mucinous carcinomas of the ovary: gross and histologic findings in 50 cases. Am J Surg Pathol. 2003;27:281–92.
19. Gemignani ML, Schlaerth AC, Bogomolniy F, et al. Role of KRAS and BRAF gene mutations in mucinous ovarian carcinoma. Gynecol Oncol. 2003;90:378–81.
20. Mok SC, Bell DA, Knapp RC, et al. Mutation of K-ras protooncogene in human ovarian epithelial tumors of borderline malignancy. Cancer Res. 1993;53:1489–92.
21. Mackenzie R, Kommoss S, Winterhoff BJ, et al. Targeted deep sequencing of mucinous ovarian tumors reveals multiple overlapping RAS-pathway activating mutations in borderline and cancerous neoplasms. BMC Cancer. 2015;15:415. doi:10.1186/s12885-015-1421-8.
22. Schuijer M, Berns EM. TP53 and ovarian cancer. Hum Mutat. 2003;21:285–91.
23. Marchini S, Mariani P, Chiorino G, et al. Analysis of gene expression in early-stage ovarian cancer. Clin Cancer Res. 2008;14:7850–60.
24. Heinzelmann-Schwarz VA, Gardiner-Garden M, Henshall SM, et al. A distinct molecular profile associated with mucinous epithelial ovarian cancer. Br J Cancer. 2006;94:904–13.
25. Risch HA, McLaughlin JR, Cole DE, et al. Prevalence and penetrance of germline BRCA1 and BRCA2 mutations in a population series of 649 women with ovarian cancer. Am J Hum Genet. 2001;68:700–10.
26. Evans DG, Young K, Bulman M, et al. Probability of BRCA1/2 mutation varies with ovarian histology: results from screening 442 ovarian cancer families. Clin Genet. 2008; 73:338–45.
27. Anglesio MS, Kommoss S, Tolcher MC, et al. Molecular characterization of mucinous ovarian tumours supports a stratified treatment approach with HER2 targeting in 19% of carcinomas. J Pathol. 2013;229:111–20.
28. McAlpine JN, Wiegand KC, Vang R, et al. HER2 overexpression and amplification is present in a subset of ovarian mucinous carcinomas and can be targeted with trastuzumab therapy. BMC Cancer. 2009;9:433.
29. Vang R, Gown AM, Barry TS, et al. Cytokeratins 7 and 20 in primary and secondary mucinous tumors of the ovary: analysis of coordinate immunohistochemical expression profiles and staining distribution in 179 cases. Am J Surg Pathol. 2006;30:1130–9.
30. Moh M, Krings G, Ates D, Aysal A, Kim GE, Rabban JT. SATB2 expression distinguishes ovarian metastases of colorectal and appendiceal origin from primary ovarian tumors of mucinous or endometrioid type. Am J Surg Pathol. 2016;40:419–32.
31. Cao D, Ji H, Ronnett BM. Expression of mesothelin, fascin, and prostate stem cell antigen in primary ovarian mucinous tumors and their utility in differentiating primary ovarian mucinous tumors from metastatic pancreatic mucinous carcinomas in the ovary. Int J Gynecol Pathol. 2005;24:67–72.
32. Oien KA. Pathologic evaluation of unknown primary cancer. Semin Oncol. 2009;36:8–37.
33. Sarrio D, Moreno-Bueno G, Sanchez-Estevez C, et al. Expression of cadherins and catenins correlates with distinct histologic types of ovarian carcinomas. Hum Pathol. 2006;37:1042–9.

34. Brun JL, Cortez A, Commo F, Uzan S, Rouzier R, Darai E. Serous and mucinous ovarian tumors express different profiles of MMP-2, -7, -9, MT1-MMP, and TIMP-1 and -2. Int J Oncol. 2008;33:1239–46.
35. Matsuo K, Masato M, Nishimura M, et al. Targeting Src in mucinous ovarian carcinoma. Clin Cancer Res. 2011;17:5367–78.
36. Riopel MA, Ronnett BM, Kurman RJ. Evaluation of diagnostic criteria and behavior of ovarian intestinal-type mucinous tumors: atypical proliferative (borderline) tumors and intraepithelial, microinvasive, invasive, and metastatic carcinomas. Am J Surg Pathol. 1999;23:617–35.
37. Tait DL, Miller DS. Multicystic ovarian tumor weighing 156 lbs: the second largest tumor in Texas. Tex Med. 1997;93:89.
38. Seidman JD, Horkayne-Szakaly I, Haiba M, et al. The histologic type and stage distribution of ovarian carcinomas of surface epithelial origin. Int J Gynecol Pathol. 2004;23:41–4.
39. Schmeler KM, Tao X, Frumovitz M, et al. Prevalence of lymph node metastasis in primary mucinous carcinoma of the ovary. Obstet Gynecol. 2010;116:269–73.
40. Kelly PJ, Archbold P, Price JH, et al. Serum CA19.9 levels are commonly elevated in primary ovarian mucinous tumours but cannot be used to predict the histological subtype. J Clin Pathol. 2010;63:169–73.
41. Nolen B, Marrangoni A, Velikokhatnaya L, et al. A serum based analysis of ovarian epithelial tumorigenesis. Gynecol Oncol. 2009;112:47–54.
42. NCCN guidelines – ovarian cancer. Version 2.2013. Accessed on 20 Jan 2016.
43. Schilder JM, Thompson AM, DePriest PD, et al. Outcome of reproductive age women with stage IA or IC invasive epithelial ovarian cancer treated with fertility-sparing therapy. Gynecol Oncol. 2002;87:1–7.
44. Wright JD, Shah M, Mathew L, et al. Fertility preservation in young women with epithelial ovarian cancer. Cancer. 2009;115:4118–26.
45. Lin JE, Seo S, Kushner DM, Rose SL. The role of appendectomy for mucinous ovarian neoplasms. Am J Obstet Gynecol. 2013;208:46e41–4.
46. Bristow RE, Tomacruz RS, Armstrong DK, et al. Survival effect of maximal cytoreductive surgery for advanced ovarian carcinoma during the platinum era: a meta-analysis. J Clin Oncol. 2002;20:1248–59.
47. Cho YH, Kim DY, Kim JH, et al. Is complete surgical staging necessary in patients with stage I mucinous epithelial ovarian tumours? Gynecol Oncol. 2006;103:878–82.
48. Naik JD, Seligmann J, Perren TJ. Mucinous tumours of the ovary. J Clin Pathol. 2012;65:580–4.
49. Leys CM, Gasior AC, Hornberger LH, St. Peter SD. Laparoscopic resection of massive ovarian mucinous cystadenoma. J Laparoendosc Adv Surg Tech. 2012;22:307–10.
50. Eltabbakh GH, Charbonneau AM, Eltabbakh NG. Laparoscopic surgery for large benign ovarian cysts. Gynecol Oncol. 2008;108:72–6.
51. Ledermann JA, Luvero D, Shafer A, O'Connor D, Mangili G, Friedlander M, Pfisterer J, Mirza MR, Kim JW, Alexandre J, Oza A, Brown J. Gynecologic Cancer InterGroup (GCIG) consensus review for mucinous ovarian carcinoma. Int J Gynecol Cancer. 2014;24(9 Suppl 3): S14–9.
52. Park JY, Heo EJ, Lee JW, Lee YY, Kim TJ, Kim BG, Bae DS. Outcomes of laparoscopic fertility-sparing surgery in clinically early-stage epithelial ovarian cancer. J Gynecol Oncol. 2016;27(2):e20.
53. Lee JY, Kim TH, Kim HS, Kim MA, Kim JW, Parek NH, Song YS. Safety of fertility-soaring surgery in primary mucinous carcinoma. Cancer Res Treat. 2015;47(2):290–7.
54. Trimbos JB, Parmar M, Vergote I, et al. International Collaborative Ovarian Neoplasm trial 1 and Adjuvant ChemoTherapy In Ovarian Neoplasm trial: two parallel randomized phase III trials of adjuvant chemotherapy in patients with early- stage ovarian carcinoma. J Natl Cancer Inst. 2003;95:105–12.
55. Pectasides D, Fountzilas G, Aravantinos G, et al. Advanced stage mucinous epithelial ovarian cancer: the Hellenic Cooperative Oncology Group experience. Gynecol Oncol. 2005;97:436–41.

56. Simons M, Ezendam N, Bulten J, Nagtegall I, Massuger L. Survival of patients with mucinous ovarian carcinoma and ovarian metastases: a population-based cancer registry study. Int J Gynecol Cancer. 2015;25(7):1208–15.
57. Mackay HJ, Brady MF, Oza AM, et al. Prognostic relevance of uncommon ovarian histology in women with stage III/IV epithelial ovarian cancer. Int J Gynecol Cancer. 2010;20: 945–52.
58. Alexandre J, Ray-Coquard I, Selle F, et al. Mucinous advanced epithelial ovarian carcinoma: clinical presentation and sensitivity to platinum-paclitaxel-based chemotherapy, the GINECO experience. Ann Oncol. 2010;21:2377–81.
59. Winter WE, Maxwell GL, Tian C, et al. Prognostic factors for stage III epithelial ovarian cancer: a gynecologic oncology group study. J Clin Oncol. 2007;25:3621–7.
60. Pignata S, Ferrandina G, Scarfone G, et al. Activity of chemotherapy in mucinous ovarian cancer with a recurrence free interval of more than 6 months: results from the SOCRATES retrospective study. BMC Cancer. 2008;8:252.
61. Vergote I, De Brabanter J, Fyles A, et al. Prognostic importance of degree of differentiation and cyst rupture in stage I invasive epithelial ovarian carcinoma. Lancet. 2001;357: 176–82.
62. Ji J, Forsti A, Sundquist J, Lenner P, Hemminki K. Survival in ovarian cancer patients by histology and family history. Acta Oncol. 2008;47:1133–9.
63. Sato S, Itamochi H, Kigawa J, et al. Combination chemotherapy of oxaliplatin and 5-fluorouracil may be an effective regimen for mucinous adenocarcinoma of the ovary: a potential treatment strategy. Cancer Sci. 2009;100:546–51.
64. Shimizu Y, Umezawa S, Hasumi K. A phase II study of combined CPT-11 and mitomycin-C in platinum refractory clear cell and mucinous ovarian carcinoma. Ann Acad Med Singapore. 1998;27:650–6.

Gynecological Carcinosarcomas

17

D. Berton-Rigaud, J.S. Frenel,
M. Devouassoux-Shisheboran, and I. Ray-Coquard

Abstract

- Carcinosarcomas (also known as malignant mixed müllerian tumors) are rare and highly aggressive epithelial malignancies that contain both malignant sarcomatous and carcinomatous elements.
- Uterine carcinosarcomas (UCs) are uncommon with more than 35 % presenting with extrauterine disease at diagnosis. Up to 90 % of ovarian carcinosarcomas (OCs) will have spread beyond the ovary.
- Prognosis for localized stage disease is poor with a high risk of recurrences, both local and distant, occurring within 1 year. The survival of women with advanced uterine or ovarian carcinosarcoma is worse than in endometrioid or high-grade serous histologies. No improvement in survival rates has been observed in recent decades with an overall median survival of less than 2 years.
- Currently, there is no clear evidence to establish consensus guidelines for the therapeutic management of carcinosarcomas.
- Until recently, gynecological carcinosarcomas were considered as a subtype of sarcoma and treated as such. However, carcinosarcomas are now thought to be related to metaplastic carcinomas and so should be treated as endometrial or ovarian high-risk carcinomas, despite the lack of specific data.

D. Berton-Rigaud (✉) • J.S. Frenel
ICO Centre René Gauducheau, Saint Herblain, France
e-mail: Dominique.Berton-Rigaud@ico.unicancer.fr; Jean-Sebastien.Frenel@ico.unicancer.fr

M. Devouassoux-Shisheboran
Centre Hospitalier Universitaire Lyon Sud, Lyon, France
e-mail: mojgan.devouassoux@chu-lyon.fr

I. Ray-Coquard
Centre Leon Bérard, Lyon, France
e-mail: isabelle.ray-coquard@lyon.unicancer.fr

E. Pujade-Lauraine et al. (eds.), *Ovarian Cancers*,
DOI 10.1007/978-3-319-32110-3_17

- For uterine carcinosarcomas (UCs), a comprehensive management approach is recommended with complete surgical staging followed by systemic chemotherapy in patients with both early- and advanced-stage disease. Active agents include Paraplatin, cisplatin, ifosfamide, and paclitaxel. The carboplatin-paclitaxel combination is the most widely used regimen in the adjuvant and advanced setting. Adjuvant radiotherapy (external beam radiation and/or vaginal brachytherapy) has not shown any overall survival benefit but could reduce local recurrences.
- For ovarian carcinosarcomas (OCs) as for other ovarian epithelial cancers, the mainstay of treatment remains cytoreductive surgery followed by platinum-based chemotherapy, usually carboplatin-paclitaxel, even in early stages.

Epidemiology

Carcinosarcoma is a rare gynecological neoplasm that belongs to the category of mixed müllerian tumors, with both components (epithelial and mesenchymal) being malignant. These tumors can occur in any part of the gynecological tract but are most often seen in the uterine cavity where they accounts for less than 5 % of malignancies, followed by the ovary (1–3 % of ovarian tumors). According to an analysis of the Surveillance, Epidemiology, and End Results (SEER) program, the adjusted rate of uterine and ovarian carcinosarcomas is 0.6 per 100,000 and 0.19 per 100,000 women, respectively.

Although a higher incidence has been reported in African-Americans, the risk factors associated with the development of uterine carcinosarcomas are identical to other endometrial carcinomas, such as obesity, nulliparity, exogenous estrogen use, or tamoxifen therapy (RR = 2–7) with a median time to occurrence of 9 years. Prior pelvic radiotherapy has been implicated as a risk factor in 5–30 % of patients [1]. The risk factors are not well established for ovarian carcinosarcomas.

Clinical Features

Carcinosarcoma is a highly aggressive tumor. Up to two thirds of patients present with advanced-stage disease, with tumor extending outside the uterus or ovary and involving the peritoneum. 40–60 % of women with uterine carcinosarcoma present with stage I or II disease; at diagnosis, the majority of ovarian carcinosarcomas (>90 %) have spread beyond the ovary.

Uterine and ovarian carcinosarcomas typically occur in postmenopausal women at a median age of 65 years, later than other epithelial tumors. Clinical symptoms are those typically found in standard uterine endometrial carcinomas, with vaginal bleeding, pelvic mass, lower abdominal pain, or abnormal pap smears. In the ovary, the tumor is often diagnosed at the time of peritoneal spread and presents as a pelvic mass with peritoneal carcinomatosis.

Clinical and radiological staging tend to underestimate the extent of the disease, as up to 60 % of clinical stage I uterine tumors are found to have lymph node metastases.

Table 17.1 FIGO ovarian cancer staging 2014

Stage I: tumor confined to ovaries	*IA*	Tumor limited to 1 ovary, capsule intact, no tumor on surface, negative washings
	IB	Tumor involves both ovaries otherwise like IA
	IC	IC1: surgical spill
		IC2: capsule rupture before surgery or tumor on ovarian surface
		IC3: malignant cells in ascites or peritoneal washings
Stage II: tumor involves 1 or both ovaries with pelvic extension (below the pelvic brim) or primary peritoneal cancer	*IIA*	Extension and/or implant on the uterus and/or fallopian tubes
	IIB	Extension to other pelvic intraperitoneal tissues
Stage III: tumor involves 1 or both ovaries with cytologically or histologically confirmed spread to the peritoneum outside the pelvis and/or metastasis to the retroperitoneal lymph nodes	*IIIA*	Positive retroperitoneal lymph nodes and/or microscopic metastasis beyond the pelvis
	IIIA1	Positive retroperitoneal lymph nodes only
	IIIA1(i)	Metastasis ≤10 mm
	IIIA1(ii)	Metastasis >10 mm
	IIIA2	Microscopic, extrapelvic (above the brim) peritoneal involvement ± positive retroperitoneal lymph nodes
	IIIB	Macroscopic, extrapelvic, peritoneal metastasis ≤2 cm ± positive retroperitoneal lymph nodes. Includes extension to capsule of the liver/spleen
	IIIC	Macroscopic, extrapelvic, peritoneal metastasis >2 cm ± positive retroperitoneal lymph nodes. Includes extension to capsule of the liver/spleen
Stage IV: distant metastasis excluding peritoneal metastasis	*IVA*	Pleural effusion with positive cytology
	IVB	Hepatic and/or splenic parenchymal metastasis, metastasis to extra-abdominal organs (including inguinal lymph nodes and lymph nodes outside of the abdominal cavity)

Table 17.2 FIGO endometrial cancer staging 2014

IA	Tumor confined to the uterus, no or <½ myometrial invasion
IB	Tumor confined to the uterus, >½ myometrial invasion
II	Cervical stromal invasion, but not beyond uterus
IIIA	Tumor invades the serosa or adnexa
IIIB	Vaginal and/or parametrial involvement
IIIC1	Pelvic node involvement
IIIC2	Para-aortic involvement
IVA	Tumor invasion bladder and/or bowel mucosa
IVB	Distant metastases including abdominal metastases and/or inguinal lymph nodes

The staging system for carcinosarcomas is the same as that applied to endometrial and ovarian carcinomas (FIGO 2014) [2] (Tables 17.1 and 17.2).

Morphological Features

Uterine carcinosarcoma is typically a polypoid, bulky mass filling the entire uterine cavity, with a hemorrhagic and necrotic component. Myometrial invasion is frequent as well as extension beyond the uterus. Ovarian carcinosarcoma is also typically a very large tumor with massive areas of hemorrhage and necrosis. The morphological features and biology of this tumor appear identical irrespective of its site of origin in the female genital tract [3].

Histologically (Fig. 17.1), the tumor is biphasic, with both malignant epithelial and mesenchymal elements. The carcinomatous component comprises an admixture of high-grade carcinomas of endometrioid grade 3, serous, clear cell, or undifferentiated features. The sarcomatous component is either homologous or heterologous. Homologous sarcoma comprises high-grade undifferentiated round cell or spindle cell sarcomatous proliferation, with some features similar to an endometrial stromal sarcoma or fibrosarcoma. Heterologous elements, which are seen in approximately 50% of cases, may show cartilaginous, osteosarcomatous, rhabdomyosarcomatous, or liposarcomatous differentiation. Neural or angiomatoid differentiation may also be seen. Myxoid change with hyaline globules is a prominent feature. The proportion of each carcinoma or sarcoma component may vary from one tumor to another [3].

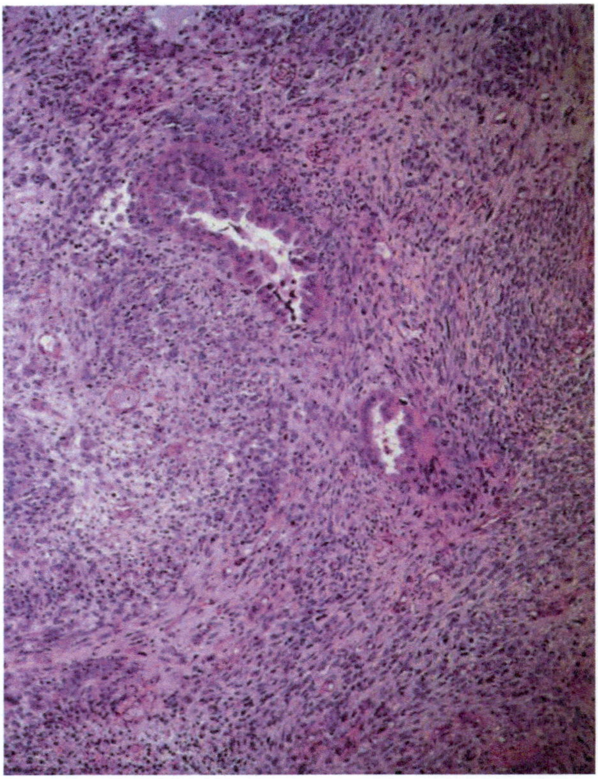

Fig. 17.1 Uterine carcinosarcoma

The histology of the metastatic component is more in keeping with an epithelial origin, since myometrial and lymphovascular invasion often display an epithelial morphology. The metastatic tumors show an epithelial component, in approximately 70 % of cases, while both carcinomatous and sarcomatous elements are found in 25 % of cases and sarcoma in only 6 % of metastatic tumors [4]

Molecular Genetics

The histogenesis of female genital tract carcinosarcomas has been debated and several theories have been proposed, including the collision between a carcinoma and an adenosarcoma, and the combination theory, in which both components arise from a single stem cell clone. However, the conversion theory postulating that sarcoma derives from carcinoma is currently favored [4]. Recent immunohistochemical and molecular findings support the hypothesis that gynecological carcinosarcomas are metaplastic carcinomas. Cell lines established from carcinosarcomas are able to differentiate into either epithelial components, mesenchymal components, or both [5]. Immunohistochemistry demonstrates the expression of epithelial markers in the sarcomatous component of carcinosarcoma. Moreover, clonality study patterns, genomic analysis, and loss of heterozygosity (LOH) studies have shown that the carcinomatous and sarcomatous components of these tumors share common genetic alterations and are monoclonal [6]. The transformation of a carcinoma to a sarcoma in these tumors may represent transdifferentiation as seen in epithelial to mesenchymal transition phenomena [7]. Several studies have demonstrated the expression of EMT-related genes in these tumors. A loss of epithelial characteristics, including an E-cadherin to N-cadherin switch, and an acquisition of mesenchymal phenotype were seen along with changes in the miRNA expression profile and the upregulation of all the E-cadherin repressors analyzed. Specifically, the miR-200 family appears to be a key regulator of EMT, through the downregulation of the *E-cadherin* repressors Zeb1 and Zeb2, thereby maintaining the epithelial phenotype. In addition, phospho-Akt (which plays a key role in EMT) is increased in the mesenchymal component and correlated negatively with E-cadherin expression, and this was associated with significant upregulation of an EMT transcription factor, Slug [8].

The molecular alterations seen in uterine carcinosarcomas are more akin to type II non-endometrioid than type I endometrioid uterine carcinomas. Data concerning molecular alterations in ovarian and uterine carcinosarcomas are scarce and based on analysis of a relatively small number of samples [9]. TP53 mutations and/or protein overexpression is considered to be the most frequent events with p53 positivity observed in up to 60 % of tumors and TP53 mutations in 23 % of cases [10]. *PI3KCA* mutations have also been reported in 19 % of uterine carcinosarcomas and *KRAS* mutations in 24 % [11]. Contradictory results have been found with *PTEN* mutations: 0–14 %. In rare cases, mutations affecting β-*catenin* (7 %) and *NRAS* (2 %) have been identified. Studies have demonstrated that up to 45 % of uterine carcinosarcomas express Abl, 19 % HER-2/neu, 100 % PDGF-R β, 32 % ER-β, and 23 % EP-B. Overexpression of Cox-2 (33 %), EGFR (30 %), Trop-2 (35–57 %), c-KIT (16–25 %), TGF-β, and PARP has also been reported. VEGF is strongly expressed in uterine carcinosarcomas [12]. Consistent with the high frequency of P53 alterations, most uterine carcinosarcomas exhibit high chromosomal instability. Cytogenetic studies of uterine carcinosarcomas have revealed extremely complex karyotypes with gross chromosomal anomalies, such as polysomy 8. Comparative genomic hybridization studies have demonstrated gains and losses at multiple chromosomal loci [6]. Gains (85 %) were observed more frequently than losses (30 %). The most frequently occurring CGH changes were gains on chromosomes 1q, 2p, 8q, 12p, 19q, and 20q and losses on 4q, 9q, and 13q.

Prognosis

Female genital tract carcinosarcomas have a very poor prognosis with overall 5-year survival of less than 30 %.

Uterine Carcinosarcoma

Although stage I uterine carcinosarcoma has a better prognosis (50 % of 5-year overall survival), it is still significantly worse than in stage I high-grade endometrial carcinoma (80 % 5-year overall survival) [1]. Median overall survival varies from 8 to 26 months [13]. Most patients experience a relapse within 1 year after completion of treatment. The FIGO stage, patient's age (over 55), depth of myometrial invasion, and patient's race are the most frequently reported prognostic factors in uterine carcinosarcoma. Lymph node dissection, tumor size, lymphovascular space invasion, parity, and grade of the sarcomatous compound have a less certain prognostic value, while data on the presence of heterologous elements or previous pelvic radiotherapy are contradictory [12–15].

Ovarian Carcinosarcoma

Overall, the prognosis for ovarian carcinosarcomas appears worse than in uterine carcinosarcomas [13] even if controversial [14] and surely worse than in high-grade ovarian carcinomas of a similar FIGO stage [16]. Most (90 %) present with an advanced disease (>stage I), and the median overall survival ranges from 7 to 27 months. Five-year overall survival is only 7–20%for patients with advanced-stage (III or IV) disease.

For ovarian carcinosarcomas, the FIGO stage is the strongest prognostic factor. Some reports indicate that complete cytoreduction, advanced age, sarcomatous component grade, and the use of adjuvant chemotherapy are prognostic factors [16]. It should be noted that the limited number of patients, with various regimens used over an extended period, and the lack of central pathological review in such retrospective studies make it impossible to draw definitive conclusions.

Initial Treatment

Optimal treatment remains uncertain. Ovarian and uterine carcinosarcomas are routinely excluded from upfront clinical trials. Treatment recommendations are mainly based upon retrospective studies with small patient populations especially for ovarian carcinosarcomas.

Surgery

Uterine Carcinosarcoma

Primary treatment includes peritoneal lavage for cytology, total abdominal hysterectomy, bilateral salpingo-oophorectomy with dissection of the pelvic and para-aortic lymph nodes, and maximal tumor debulking. Surgical staging for these tumors should follow the procedures performed for ovarian carcinoma, including detailed examination of the entire abdominal cavity and retroperitoneal spaces and appropriate biopsies. Although the role of omentectomy is unclear, it is recommended in women with early-stage disease. The role of lymphadenectomy is a subject of current debate. However, given the relatively high incidence of lymph node involvement (14–38 % in early stage), regarding impact on survival, the majority of the retrospective studies suggest a significant survival benefit of the lymph node dissection in uterine carcinosarcomas [17, 18]. Nemani et al. [17] reported a significant OS benefit associated with lymph node dissection, with a 5-year OS of 49 % versus 35 % for patients who had not undergone lymph node dissection. Therefore, adequate lymphadenectomy appears necessary for both staging and therapeutic reasons. In advanced disease, primary cytoreductive surgery is generally performed, despite the lack of clear evidence. In a recent series, cytoreductive surgery was found to improve overall survival in patients with advanced carcinosarcomas [19].

Ovarian Carcinosarcoma

Cumulative retrospective data support the benefit of an optimal surgical cytoreduction with total abdominal hysterectomy, bilateral salpingo-oophorectomy, omentectomy, abdominal fluid aspiration, pelvic and para-aortic lymph node dissection, and tumor debulking. Given the rarity of ovarian carcinosarcomas, the role of cytoreductive surgery has not been prospectively evaluated. Several small retrospective studies with fewer than 50 patients have reported an improved outcome for patients undergoing an optimal debulking surgery, without residual disease. One of the largest studies, including 50 patients, reported DFS of 19 months for patients with only microscopic disease, compared to 10 months for those with less than 1 cm residual disease and 5 months for those with more than 1 cm ($p=0.01$). Overall survival is 47, 18, and 8 months, respectively ($p=0.02$) [16]. From the SEER database, Garg reported improved survival for patients with lymphadenectomy suggesting the benefit of lymph node dissection, although this may reflect stage migration. The risk of death was reduced by 34 % after lymphadenectomy (HR = 0.66, 95 % CI = 0.56–0.78) [13]. Conservative surgery is never indicated for ovarian carcinosarcoma even in adequately staged stage IA disease.

Adjuvant Treatment for Early Stage

Due to the high rate of local and distant recurrences, even for early-stage disease, adjuvant systemic treatment is generally considered. There is still no clear consensus on the best adjuvant therapy for patients with carcinosarcoma as most studies are retrospective and describe the outcome in a small number of patients who were given a variety of treatment regimens.

Uterine Carcinosarcomas

Adjuvant Radiotherapy

Pelvic recurrence is common, even for patients with early-stage disease; therefore, pelvic radiotherapy (with or without brachytherapy) has been commonly used and reduces the incidence of local pelvic recurrence [20]. However, its impact on patient survival is not proven and remains controversial. The only phase III study comparing pelvic radiotherapy and observation is Reed's EORTC study.

Two hundred and twenty-four (224) FIGO stage I–II uterine sarcomas, including 91 carcinosarcomas, were randomized between observation and RT. Analysis of all patients revealed a reduction in local relapse ($p=0.004$) but no effect on either overall or disease-free survival. The local recurrences rate was 18.8 % for patients treated with radiotherapy and 35.9 % in the observation arm. The same results were observed among patients with carcinosarcomas. However, most patients relapsed simultaneously at distant sites, and therefore radiotherapy appears to be of limited value [20].

The SEER database from Wright recorded 1819 patients with stage I–II uterine carcinosarcomas and reported, in a multivariate model, a 21 % reduction of death for women who underwent radiotherapy. The benefit was only observed for women who did not undergo lymph node dissection [21]. In the second study using also SEER data ($n=2461$), Clayton Smith reported an improvement in overall survival for women with uterine carcinosarcomas treated with postoperative radiotherapy compared to surveillance. The overall 5-year survival was 41.5 %, using adjuvant radiotherapy compared to 33.2 % ($p<0{,}001$) [22]. However, a third SEER analysis ($n=1855$) did not show any impact of radiotherapy on further prognosis (also in the group of patients without lymphadenectomy) [17]. Large database reviews present limitations because of the lack of standardization in surgery, radiotherapy, and chemotherapy, the absence of centralized pathological review, and the potential impact of patients and physicians preference on adjuvant treatment.

The Gynecologic Oncology Group (GOG) has performed one of the few prospective randomized trials in uterine carcinosarcomas. Whole abdominal radiotherapy (WART) was compared to 3 cycles of ifosfamide-cisplatin in 206 patients with stage I–IV patients after complete resection. The local and distant recurrence rates were 44.7 % and 25.7 %, respectively, with WART and 42.5 % and 23.3 % with chemotherapy. Although there was no statistically significant survival benefit, an improved recurrence and survival rate was noted in the chemotherapy group (21 % lower recurrence and 29 % lower death, but this was not statistically significant).

Table 17.3 Phase III adjuvant study in uterine sarcomas including carcinosarcomas

Study and year of publication	No patients	Treatment regimen	RO	Overall survival	PFS
Omura et al. [24] 1983	156 93 CS Stages I–II	Doxorubicin 60 mg/m² D1–D21 8 cycles	41 %	73.7 months	NA
		No adjuvant treatment	53 %	55 months NS	40.2 months NS
Pautier et al. [25] 2013	81 uterine sarcomas (19 CS) Stages I–III	Doxorubicin (50), cisplatin (75) Ifosfamide(3 g/m² D1–D2) D1–D21+ Pelvic radiotherapy	38.4 %		72 %
		Pelvic radiotherapy	26 %		55 % NS
Wolfson et al. [23] 2007	206 CS Stages I–IV	Ifosfamide(1,5 g/m² D1 to D4) Cisplatin (20 mg/m² D1 to D4) D1–D21 3 cycles	51.4 %		45 %
		Abdominal radiotherapy	57.2 % $P=0.24$		35 % NS

Toxicity was lower with chemotherapy compared to whole abdominal radiotherapy (WART), but this is no longer performed, due to its toxicity [23].

In conclusion, external pelvic radiotherapy does not improve overall survival, but decreases local recurrence rates, which could in theory impact favorably on quality of life.

Adjuvant Chemotherapy (Table 17.3)

Only one trial has prospectively addressed the question of adjuvant chemotherapy (3 cycles of ifosfamide-cisplatin) for completely resected uterine carcinosarcomas in comparison with radiotherapy (WART). This study was not able to demonstrate a significant difference in relapse rate or OS, but a slight advantage favors the use of chemotherapy: The recurrence rate was 21 % lower and death rate 29 % lower in the chemotherapy arm [23]. Another trial, also including gynecologic sarcomas, failed to show a significant advantage with adjuvant chemotherapy on PFS and OS [24]. In a small study of 81 patients with a variety of uterine sarcoma histologies and FIGO stages, chemotherapy, using Adriamycin, ifosfamide, and cisplatin, followed by radiation therapy, was superior to radiation therapy alone in terms of 3-year disease-free survival (55 % versus 41 %) but not overall survival. These data cannot be used to support a recommendation for adjuvant chemotherapy as standard treatment, given the heterogeneity of the tumor types and stages, the very small sample size, and the lack of overall survival benefit [25]. In the prospective phase II GOG 232B study, 65 stage I–II completely resected uterine carcinosarcomas received 3 cycles of ifosfamide-cisplatin chemotherapy; PFS and OS at 7 years were 54 and

52 % [26]. Due to its activity and favorable toxicity profile shown in advanced carcinosarcomas, the carboplatin-paclitaxel combination is commonly used in the adjuvant setting [27].

Multimodal Therapy

Several retrospective studies have shown a favorable survival outcome with sequential multimodality therapy including pelvic radiotherapy and chemotherapy with cisplatin-ifosfamide, paclitaxel-ifosfamide, or paclitaxel-carboplatin. Some studies suggest a better outcome with combined treatment versus radiotherapy alone. A retrospective study reported by Makker included 49 stage I–IV patients receiving platinum-based chemotherapy after surgery (mainly carboplatin-paclitaxel), with or without radiation therapy or radiotherapy alone; the 3-year DFS in the chemotherapy group was 35 % compared to 9 % in the radiotherapy group, and 3-year OS rates were 66 % and 34 %, respectively (NS) [28]. In contrast, other publications do not report the benefit of combination therapy (CT + RT) versus chemotherapy alone in patients with uterine carcinosarcomas.

The 2012 National Comprehensive Cancer Network (NCCN) guidelines recommend adjuvant treatment for all stage of uterine carcinosarcoma, except stage IA without myometrial invasion, similar to type II carcinomas [29].

Ovarian Carcinosarcomas

Adjuvant Radiotherapy

There is little rationale for using radiotherapy in ovarian carcinosarcomas as most are advanced at presentation. In patients with early OCs, the role of radiotherapy remains unknown.

Adjuvant Chemotherapy

The recommendations, based on retrospective data, are to use platinum-based chemotherapy, either carboplatin-paclitaxel or ifosfamide-cisplatin [30]. The optimal combination regimen is still to be determined. The largest study of patients treated postoperatively with carboplatin-paclitaxel involved only 50 patients [16]. A recent Cochrane review found no evidence to inform decisions on adjuvant or neoadjuvant chemotherapy [31].

Advanced/Metastatic Disease and Relapse

Uterine Carcinosarcomas (Table 17.4)

The main cytotoxic agents studied in uterine carcinosarcomas are ifosfamide (32 % response rate (RR)), cisplatin (RR, 19 %), and paclitaxel (RR, 18 % as first- or second-line therapy) [33]. Responses are usually partial and short in duration with a PFS of 8 months.

In contrast to other gynecological sarcomas, doxorubicin is only minimally active (10 % RR) [34], but the data are limited. Some responses have been reported with pegylated liposomal doxorubicin [35].

Table 17.4 Phase III study in the first-line treatment for advanced uterine carcinosarcomas

Study and year of publication	No pat	Chemotherapy regimen	RO (%)	RC	RP	Overall survival	Median PFS
Homesley et al. [32] 2007	179	Ifosfamide 2 g/m² D1–D2–D3/D1–D21	29			8.4 months	3.6 months
		Ifosfamide 1 g6/m² D1–D2–D3 + Paclitaxel 135 mg/m² D1/D1–D21	45			13.5 months *P = 0.03*	5.8 months *P = 0.03*
Sutton et al. [33] 2000	194	Ifosfamide 1 g5/m² D1 to D5/D1–D21	36	24 %	12 %	7.6 months	4 months
		Ifosfamide 1 g5/m² D1 to D5 + CCDP 20 mg/m² D1 to D5/D1–D21	54	31 %	23 %	9.4 months *P = 0.07*	6 months *P < 0.02*

Two prospective randomized trials compared mono- and polychemotherapy with ifosfamide. Sutton et al reported on 194 patients who received ifosfamide with or without cisplatin. Although response rates were higher with the combination (54 % versus 36 %) and PFS significantly higher (6 versus 4 months), no improvement in overall survival was observed, and the toxicity of the combination was notably increased [33]. The GOG 161 study included 179 patients treated with ifosfamide with or without paclitaxel and reported a significant difference in the objective response rate (45 % versus 29 %), PFS (5.8 versus 3.6 months), and overall survival (13.5 versus 8.4 months) in favor of combination [32]. Finally, the Cochrane database, including 579 women, concluded that in advanced-stage uterine carcinosarcoma as well as in recurrent disease, combination chemotherapy with ifosfamide and paclitaxel is associated with a lower risk of death compared with ifosfamide alone (HR = 0.75, 95 % CI, 0.60–0.94, and HR = 0.72, 95 % CI, 0.58–0.90, for OS and PFS, respectively) [36]. Thus, the ifosfamide-paclitaxel combination is currently considered as standard arm treatment in most countries.

The paclitaxel-carboplatin combination is another option as it is a well-tolerated outpatient regimen. Several phase II trials have reported high response rates (ranging from 54 to 69 %), with a number of patients achieving a complete response. The median PFS was 7.6 months and the OS 14.7 months [27, 37]. The GOG 261 study is testing this regimen in an ongoing phase III non-inferiority trial comparing ifosfamide-paclitaxel and carboplatin-paclitaxel.

As a result, paclitaxel-carboplatin is commonly used as routine therapy.

Due to the very poor prognosis of patients with gynecological carcinosarcomas, palliative treatments are a major issue.

Many biological anticancer treatments have been evaluated (sorafenib, imatinib, thalidomide, VEGF-Trap, pazopanib, and iniparib plus paclitaxel and carboplatin). Response rates to targeted agents are poor in unselected populations (0–5 %) [38].

Ovarian Carcinosarcomas

Some data have led to the conclusion that the chemosensitivity of ovarian carcinosarcomas is similar to that of uterine carcinosarcomas, but less than that of serous epithelial ovarian cancer. As a consequence, the conclusions drawn from the effects of chemotherapy in uterine carcinosarcomas are applied to the less common ovarian carcinosarcomas [12].

Published data evaluating benefit of chemotherapy are based on a few nonrandomized prospective studies and some retrospective analysis. Common treatment combinations include platinum-paclitaxel and platinum-ifosfamide. In the phase II ROSIA trial evaluating the feasibility of paclitaxel-carboplatin plus bevacizumab in the neoadjuvant setting, ovarian carcinosarcomas could be included.

Perspectives

The poor survival for gynecological carcinosarcoma highlights the need to improve treatment strategies.

Further research on genetic and molecular signaling pathways should be considered to improve understanding of these tumor subtypes, including descriptive and functional analyses. Further prospective trials are clearly warranted in a larger group of patients. Ideally, these should be randomized trials or well-designed nonrandomized studies that use multivariate analysis to adjust for baseline imbalances.

Studies should incorporate molecular-targeted therapies alone or in combination with cytotoxic drugs, e.g., Paraplatin-paclitaxel. Although both uterine and ovarian carcinosarcomas are rare, care should be taken to stratify patients based on a molecular profile. Such studies can only be conducted with international cooperation.

References

1. Amant F, Cadron I, Fuso L, Berteloot P, de Jonge E, Jacomen G, et al. Endometrial carcinosarcomas have a different prognosis and pattern of spread compared to high-risk epithelial endometrial cancer. Gynecol Oncol. 2005;98:274–80.
2. FIGO Committee on Gynecologic Oncology. FIGO staging for carcinoma of the vulva, cervix, and corpus uteri. Int J Gynaecol Obstet. 2014;125(2):97–8.
3. D'Angelo E, Prat J. Pathology of mixed Müllerian tumours. Best Pract Res Clin Obstet Gynaecol. 2011;25(6):705–18.
4. Sreenan JJ, Hart WR. Carcinosarcomas of the female tract. A pathological study of 29 metastatic tumors: further evidence for the dominant role of the epithelial component and the conversion theory of histogenesis. Am J Surg Pathol. 1995;19:666–74.
5. Gorai I, Yanagibashi T, Taki A, Udagawa K, Miyagi E, Nakazawa T, Hirahara F, Nagashima Y, Minaguchi H. Uterine carcinosarcoma is derived from a single stem cell: an in vitro study. Int J Cancer. 1997;72:821–7.
6. Fujii H, Yoshida M, Gong ZX, Matsumoto T, Hamano Y, Fukunaga M, Hruban RH, Gabrielson E, Shirai T. Frequent genetic heterogeneity in the clonal evolution of gynecological carcinosarcoma and its influence on phenotic diversity. Cancer Res. 2000;60:114–20.

7. Amant F, Vloeberghs V, Woestenborghs H, Moerman P, Vergote I. Transition of epithelial toward mesenchymal differentiation during ovarian carcinosarcoma tumorigenesis. Gynecol Oncol. 2003;90:372–7.
8. Tanaka Y, Terai Y, Kawaguchi H, Fujiwara S, Yoo S, Tsunetoh S, Takai M, Kanemura M, Tanabe A, Ohmichi M. Prognostic impact of EMT(epithelial-mesenchymal-transition)-related protein expression in endometrial cancer. Cancer Biol Ther. 2013;14(1):13–9.
9. Murray S, Linardou H, Mountzios G, Manokoulos M, Markaki S, Eleutherakis-Papaiakovou E, Dimopoulos MA, Papadimitriou CA. Low frequency of somatic mutations in uterine sarcomas: a molecular analysis and review of the literature. Mutat Res. 2010;686:68–73.
10. De Jong RA, Nijman HW, Wilbrandi TF, Reyners AK, Boezen HM, Hollema H. Molecular markers and clinical behavior of uterine carcinosarcomas: focus on the epithelial component. Mol Pathol. 2011;24(10):1368–79.
11. Growdon W, Roussel B, Scialabba V, Foster R, Dias-Santagata D, Iafrate A, Ellisen L, Tambouret R, Rueda B, Borger D. Tissue-specific signatures of activating PI3CA and RAS mutations in carcinosarcomas of gynecologic origin. Gynecol Oncol. 2011;121:212–7.
12. Cimbaluk D, Rotmensch J, Scudiere J, Gown A, Bitterman P. Uterine carcinosarcoma: Immunohistochemical studies on tissue microarrays with focus on potential therapeutic targets. Gynecol Oncol. 2007;105:138–44.
13. Garg G, Shah J, Kumar S, Bryant C, Munkarah A, Morris R. Ovarian and uterine carcinosarcomas: a comparative analysis of prognostic variables and survival outcomes. Int J Gynecol Cancer. 2010;20:888–94.
14. Rauh-Hain JA, Shoni M, Shorge JO, Goodman A, Horowitz N, Del Carmen M. Prognostic determinants in patients with uterine and ovarian carcinosarcomas. J Reprod Med. 2013;58: 297–304.
15. Ferguson SE, Tornos C, Hummer A, Barakat RR, Soslow RA. Prognostic features of surgical stage I uterine carcinosarcoma. Am J Surg Pathol. 2007;31(11):1653–61.
16. Rauh-Hain JA, Growdon WB, Rodriguez N, Goodman AK, Boruta II DM, Schorge JO, Horowitz NS, Del Carmen MG. Carcinosarcoma of the ovary: a case control study. Gynecol Oncol. 2011;121:477–81.
17. Nemani D, Mitra N, Guo M, et al. Assessing the effects of lymphadenectomy and radiation therapy in patients with uterine carcinosarcoma: a SEER analysis. Gynecol Oncol. 2008;III:82–8.
18. Vorgias G, Fotiou S. The role of lymphadenectomy in uterine carcinomas: a critical literature review Arch. Gynecol Obstet. 2010;282:659–64.
19. Tanner EJ, Leitao Jr MM, Garg K. The role of cytoreductive surgery for newly diagnosed-stage uterine carcinosarcoma. Gynecol Oncol. 2011;25:751–60.
20. Reed NS, Mangioni C, Malmstrom H, et al. Phase III randomised study to evaluate the role of adjuvant pelvic radiotherapy III the treatment of uterine sarcomas stages I and II: an European Organisation for Research and Treatment of Cancer Gynaecological Cancer Group Study (protocol 55874). Eur J Cancer. 2008;44:808–18 [Erratum appears in Eur J Cancer. 2008;44:1612].
21. Wright JD, Seshan VE, Shah M, Schiff PB, Burke WM, Cohen CJ, Herzog TJ. The role of radiation in improving survival for early-stage carcinosarcoma and leiomyosarcoma. Am J Obstet Gynecol. 2008;199(5):531–8.
22. Clayton Smith D, Kenneth Macdonald O, Gaffney DK, et al. The impact of adjuvant radiation therapy on survival in women with uterine carcinosarcoma. Radiother Oncol. 2008;88:227–32.
23. Wolfson AH, Brady MF, Rocereto T, Mannel RS, Lee YC, Futoran RJ, et al. A gynecologic oncology group randomized phase III trial of whole abdominal irradiation (WAI) vs. cisplatin-ifosfamide and mesna (CIM) as post-surgical therapy in stage I–IV carcinosarcoma (CS) of the uterus. Gynecol Oncol. 2007;107:177–85.
24. Omura GA, Major FJ, Blessing JA, Sedlacek TV, Thigpen JT, Creasman WT, et al. A randomized study of adriamycin with and without dimethyl triazenoimidazolecarboxamide in advanced uterine sarcomas. Cancer. 1983;52:626–32.
25. Pautier P, Floquet A, Gladieff L, et al. A randomized clinical trial of adjuvant chemotherapy with doxorubicin, ifosfamide and cisplatin followed by radiotherapy versus radiotherapy alone in patients with localized uterine sarcomas (SARCGYN study). Ann Oncol. 2013;24(4):1099–104.

26. Sutton G, Kauderer J, Carson LF, Lentz SS, Whitney CW, Gallion H. Adjuvant ifosfamide and cisplatin in patients with completely resected stage I or II carcinosarcomas (mixed mesodermal tumors) of the uterus: a Gynecologic Oncology Group study. Gynecol Oncol. 2005;96: 630–4.
27. Powell MA, Filiaci VL, Rose PG, Mannel RS, Hanjani P, DeGeest K, et al. Phase II evaluation of paclitaxel and carboplatin in the treatment of carcinosarcoma of the uterus: a Gynecologic Oncology Group Study. J Clin Oncol. 2010;28:2727–31.
28. Makker V, Abu-Rustum NR, Alektiar KM, et al. A retrospective assessment of outcomes of chemotherapy-based versus radiation-only adjuvant treatment for completely resected stage I-IV uterine carcinosarcoma. Gynecol Oncol. 2008;3:249–54.
29. NCCN Guidelines Version 3.2012 Endometrial carcinoma. http://www.nccn.org/professionals/physician_gls/pdf/uterine.pdf. Accessed on 19 Sept 2012.
30. Duska LR, Garett A, Eltabbakh MD, Oliva E, Penson R, Fuller A. Paclitaxel and Platinum Chemotherapy for malignant mixed mullerian tumors of the ovary. Gynecol Oncol. 2002;85: 459–63.
31. Shylasree TS, Bryant A, Athavale R. Chemotherapy and/or radiotherapy in combination with surgery for ovarian carcinosarcoma. Cochrane Database Syst Rev. 2013;2:CD006246.
32. Homesley HD, Filiaci V, Markman M, Bitterman P, Eaton L, Kilgore LC, et al. Phase III trial of ifosfamide with or without paclitaxel in advanced uterine carcinosarcoma: a Gynecologic Oncology Group Study. J Clin Oncol. 2007;25:526–31.
33. Sutton G, Brunetto VL, Kilgore L, Soper JT, McGehee R, Olt G, et al. Trial of ifosfamide with or without cisplatin in carcinosarcoma of the uterus: a gynecologic oncology group study. Gynecol Oncol. 2000;79:147–53.
34. Morrow CP, Bundy BN, Hoffman J, Sutton G, Homesley H. Adriamycin chemotherapy for malignant mixed mesodermal tumor of the ovary. A Gynecologic Oncology Group Study. Am J Clin Oncol. 1986;9(1):24–6.
35. Pectasides D, Pectasides E, Papaxoinis G, Xiros N, Sykiotis C, Papachristodoulou A, Tountas N, Panayiotides J, Economopoulos T, et al. Combination chemotherapy with carboplatin, paclitaxel and pegylated liposomal doxorubicin for advanced or recurrent carcinosarcoma of the uterus: clinical experience of a single institution. Gynecol Oncol. 2008;110:299–303.
36. Galaal K, van der Heijden E, Godfrey K, et al. Adjuvant radiotherapy and/or chemotherapy after surgery for uterine carcinosarcoma. Cochrane Database Syst Rev. 2013;2:CD006812.
37. Hoskins PI, Le N, Ellard S, et al. Carboplatin plus paclitaxel for advanced or recurrent uterine malignant mixed mullerian tumors. The British Columbia Cancer Agency experience. Gynecol Oncol. 2008;108:58–62.
38. Huh WK, Sill MW, Darcy KM, et al. Efficacy and safety of imatinib mesylate (Gleevec®) and immunohistochemical expression of c-Kit and PDGFR-β in a Gynecologic Oncology Group Phase II Trial in women with recurrent or persistent carcinosarcomas of the uterus. Gynecol Oncol. 2010;117:248–54.

Malignant Ovarian Germ Cell Tumours: An Overview of Management and Controversies

18

Constantine Alifrangis and Michael J. Seck

Abstract

Non-epithelial malignancies of the ovary account for around 10 % of all ovarian malignancies, but display a striking disparity in epidemiology and outcomes. Over the previous decades, epidemiological trends have suggested that malignant ovarian germ cell tumours (MOGCTs) are presenting earlier and that overall survival in this category as a whole is excellent, even in the setting of advanced disease. Indeed since the advent of cisplatin-based multimodality treatment, this is a tumour type which one can argue has been understudied in comparison to the other more prevalent gynaecological malignancies.

As such many questions remain unanswered. MOGCT is a disease that is poorly understood at the molecular level despite the serendipitous finding of high response rates to cytotoxic chemotherapy. Much of our evidence base stems from small single-centre retrospective case series, and as such true randomised prospective trial data is lacking in this field. Subsequently questions such as the optimal treatment of relapsed disease are currently not well defined. This overview will present the state of our knowledge to date on the management of MOGCT and seek to outline areas of controversy.

C. Alifrangis, PhD, MRCP • M.J. Seck, PhD, FRCP (✉)
Department of Medical Oncology, Charing Cross Hospital Campus of Imperial College London, London W68RF, UK
e-mail: costi@doctors.org.uk; m.seckl@imperial.ac.uk

E. Pujade-Lauraine et al. (eds.), *Ovarian Cancers*,
DOI 10.1007/978-3-319-32110-3_18

Epidemiology

Non-epithelial malignancies of the ovary account for between 5 and 10 % of all ovarian cancers. The two major groups of these cancers include germ cell tumours (GCTs) and sex cord-stromal tumours (SCSTs) which will not be discussed in this article. Unlike epithelial ovarian cancer which peaks in postmenopausal women, the peak incidence of MOGCT is in the second decade of life affecting adolescent girls and young women. MOGCTs have a yearly adjusted incidence rate of 3.7/1,000,000 in the USA [1], although higher incidences have been reported in some ethnic subgroups: with an increased incidence of MOGCTs among paediatric black females and Hispanic girls aged 10–19, as compared to non-Hispanics [2]. Dysgerminomas occur less frequently in black females, and immature teratomas occur less frequently in white females compared with other racial and ethnic groups. A family history of cancer appears to be inversely correlated with the risk of developing germ cell tumours [4], and no genetic susceptibility has been identified related to the development of MOGCT. However, there have been several case reports of germ cell tumours noted to cluster within families, which may suggest a rare familial gonadal tumour syndrome that has not yet been fully characterised. These cancers account for 58 % of all ovarian tumours diagnosed in patients younger than 20 years old [2]. One recent cohort has demonstrated the association between syndromes of gonadal dysgenesis and a predisposition to MOGCT. In a cohort of 50 patients, 7 were found to have a karyotype of XY, and these patients were more likely to present with dysgerminoma [3]. Interestingly concurrent benign gonadoblastoma was found in five.

Clinical Presentation and Staging

MOGCT usually presents with pelvic pain (the presenting feature in 50–80 % of patients at diagnosis) or symptoms resulting from a rapidly enlarging pelvic mass and occasionally menstrual irregularities [4]. The duration of symptoms is usually noted to be fairly short at presentation (2–4 weeks) indicating rapid growth of the tumour, once again sharply contrasting with the more protracted presentation associated with epithelial ovarian cancer in older women. This speed of onset is reflected in the distribution of staging of MOGCT seen at presentation. This is classified according to the modified International Federation of Gynaecologic Oncology (FIGO) staging criteria initially applied to epithelial ovarian cancer [5, 6]. The majority of MOGCTs are diagnosed at an early stage – FIGO stage IA–II (60–70 %), and 20–30 % are stage III with the minority presenting with stage IV disease [5].

Histopathological Subtypes and Tumour Markers

Histopathological identification of subtypes of ovarian GCTs is well established (Table 18.1) and is usually performed according to the WHO classification [5, 6]. The different histological subtypes reflect the continuum of developmental stages in the oocyte from primordial undifferentiated germ cells to adult tissues, an

Table 18.1 Histological subtypes of MOGCT

Histological subtype	AFP	HCG
Primitive germ cell tumours		
Dysgerminoma	–	±
Yolk sac tumour	++	–
Embryonal carcinoma	±	±
Polyembryona	±	+
Non-gestational choriocarcinoma	–	++
Mixed germ cell tumour	±	±
Biphasic or triphasic teratoma		
Immature teratoma	+	–
Mature teratoma	–	–
Monodermal teratoma and somatic-type tumours		

observation initially characterised by Kleinsmith and Pierce in the 1960s [7]. The three major categories are (1) primitive GCTs, including dysgerminoma, yolk sac tumours (otherwise referred to as endodermal sinus tumours), embryonal carcinoma and tumours with overlapping features of the above known as mixed germ cell tumours. The other main histologic category is that of (2) biphasic or triphasic teratoma, which includes the entities mature-differentiated teratoma and undifferentiated immature teratoma. This can be graded according to the number and characteristics of neural tissues present in the tumour [8], as this has important therapeutic and prognostic implications. The third and least common category is that of monodermal-type tumours and somatic-type tumours. MOGCTs share many histologic features with their male testicular germ cell tumour counterparts, and this link also extends to the frequent observation of 12p karyotypic abnormalities [9, 10]. However, biologically/clinically the tumours as we will see below can behave differently between the sexes.

In most large case series, dysgerminoma represents approximately 15–25 % of cases, teratoma 12–20 %, yolk sac tumours 25–30 % and mixed germ cell tumours 30–35 %. The importance of correct histological diagnosis is underpinned by the therapeutic implications for the patient.

Some authorities have recommended a two-tier grading system for immature teratomas because of inter- and intraobserver inconsistency with a three-grade system. Additionally, the criteria to establish malignant behaviour in immature teratomas vary among reports and institutions based on the amounts of immature neural and/or nonneural elements and yolk sac elements.

As these tumours are chemosensitive and fertility-preserving surgery is utilised, the recent ESMO guidelines [6] stipulate that all such tumours should be considered for second review by an expert histopathologist. Indeed in some centres, this central review of pathology is mandatory. In the UK there has now been a move to centralise the care of MOGCT to mirror the successful approach used used in Gestational Trophoblastic Disease (GTD) [11].

Tumour markers play an important role in the diagnosis and management of germ cell tumours. The serum alpha-fetoprotein (AFP), lactate dehydrogenase

(LDH) and serum human chorionic gonadotropin (hCG) should be measured at baseline in all patients. AFP is secreted by yolk sac tumour elements and may be secreted by embryonal carcinoma and immature teratomas. The pregnancy hormone, hCG, is secreted by choriocarcinoma elements and can be produced in a small subset of dysgerminomas at lower levels [8]. Mixed germ cell tumours may secrete a combination of AFP and hCG, and approximately 16 % may be negative for all tumour markers. Dysgerminoma never secretes AFP, and about 10–20 % produces hCG [12, 13]. All MOGCT may be associated with an elevated lactate dehydrogenase level and CA125 both of which are non-specific for the disease but may nevertheless give an indication of response and relapse. In practical terms, the ability to regularly monitor tumour markers following any intervention, such as either surgery or chemotherapy, allows the clinician to have an early readout of response, resistance and relapse. For example, failure to normalise tumour markers after curative surgery in stage 1 disease would be an indicator for further treatment (stage 1 M disease). Furthermore, knowledge of the normal half-life of these tumour markers is helpful in this regard. If all the tumour has been removed, then for patients with normal renal and liver function, the half-life of hCG is 1–2 days and for AFP is about 6–7 days. If the markers are falling slower than this, then suspicion about residual disease should be high. If gonadal dysgenesis is suspected based on history and physical examination, a karyotype should be performed before surgery, if possible, to ensure both ovaries are removed if clinically indicated.

Prognostic Factors

FIGO stage at presentation is the most critical indicator of prognosis. Evidence from many centres indicates that stage I (including 1a, 1c and 1 m) has an excellent prognosis of approaching 100 % survival rates. This cure rate progressively declines to approximately 80–90 % in stage II and stage III disease and around 60 % cure rates in stage IV disease (see Fig. 18.1) [14–16]. Other factors have been identified that can be independent prognostic indicators in univariate and multivariate analyses. Indeed, in those patients receiving chemotherapy (stages 1c/1 m through stage IV at diagnosis), the presence of elevated AFP and hCG at diagnosis was associated

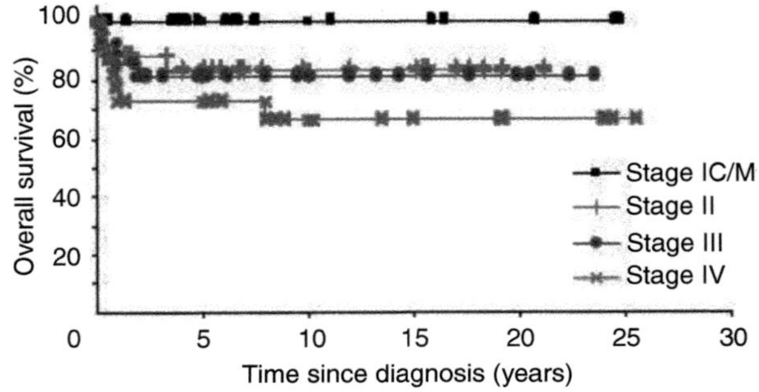

Fig. 18.1 Survival of MOGCT by stage (Adapted from Zanetta et al. [14], Murugaesu et al. [16])

with a much poorer outcome when compared to those patients with both tumour markers being normal at baseline [16]. The role of age as an independent prognostic factor is more controversial with some studies suggesting this and others not [15, 17]. It is clear however that paediatric MOGCT may represent biologically different group diseases as recent studies have indicated significant differences in transcriptional signatures more suggestive of pluripotency compared to adult tumours [18]. Indeed outcomes in the paediatric population differ with seemingly higher survival when matched stage for stage with adults [19]. Residual disease after surgery and histological subtype (dysgerminoma vs non-dysgerminoma) have also been implicated as prognostic factors in retrospective case series [20].

Management of Early Disease

Surgery is the mainstay of management of early MOGCT. In other gynaecologic malignancies, the principles of cancer surgery dictate maximal clearance with a bilateral salpingo-oophorectomy (BSO), total abdominal hysterectomy (TAH) and peritoneal exploration. However, in MOGCT, fertility-preserving surgery should be utilised [21]. For most patients with early stage disease (stage 1A/1B), a unilateral salpingo-oophorectomy (USO), peritoneal washings and careful exploration of the abdomen are appropriate. Routine biopsy of the remaining ovary should be avoided unless there is clinical suspicion of bilateral disease. This last point is important as most MOGCTs are unilateral, with dysgerminomas having the greatest propensity for contralateral disease in the other ovary, and this is said to be seen in up to 15 % of these tumours although in our experience, it seems less than this [22]. Avoiding the contralateral ovarian biopsy potentially helps future fertility by preventing scar formation over the ovary surface.

The management of early MOGCTs that have been pathologically staged as 1A/1B (and as such are confined to the ovary with no capsular rupture) has been controversial with some centres advocating the use of adjuvant chemotherapy in addition to fertility-preserving surgery, particularly in non-dysgerminomatous histologies (grade II–III immature teratoma, mixed GCT and yolk sac tumours) [23]. Studies by Williams et al. [24], Gershenson [25] and Dimopoulous et al. [26] have demonstrated excellent survival outcomes in completely resected MOGCT treated with adjuvant bleomycin, etoposide and cisplatin (BEP), but these studies have to be interpreted with caution as they also include stage II and III diseases. There is consensus that stage 1A dysgerminoma should be managed with surgery alone with many studies showing survival of close to 100 % with a policy of surveillance after fertility-sparing surgery [27]. A policy of careful surveillance after surgery for stage 1A/1B disease of all histological subtypes has been adopted by Charing Cross and Mount Vernon hospitals with long-term survival in excess of 95 % in these patients, reserving chemotherapy only for those patients that relapse [27]. This approach has subsequently been adopted, and its efficacy validated in other centres [23] as well as in a prospective study in the paediatric and adolescent population [28]. In keeping with this, the recent ESMO guidelines assert that chemotherapy is not mandated in the adjuvant setting in non-dysgerminomatous early stage MOGCT and can be reserved for documented relapse after a policy of close surveillance.

The Management of Advanced Disease

Cytotoxic chemotherapy has altered the landscape of MOGCT prognosis. In the pre-chemotherapy era, even patients with early stage disease would be at significant risk of relapse and death, and all patients with advanced disease would die from their disease. Early studies demonstrated some efficacy of VAC (vincristine, dactinomycin and cyclophosphamide) combination chemotherapy in patients with MOGCT [29], but most lessons have been learnt from the randomised studies undertaken in testicular germ cell tumours. As a result of this work, the regimes used in MOGCT have been optimised to allow maximal preservation of fertility, whilst decreasing risk of long-term complications from agents such as cyclophosphamide (in its propensity to cause acute leukaemia). Cisplatin-based regimens with PVB (cisplatin, vinblastine, bleomycin) [30] then most recently BEP chemotherapy (bleomycin, etoposide, cisplatin) have become the gold standard therapy for advanced or relapsed MOGCT. Studies using platinum-based combination regimens have demonstrated overall survival in all MOGCT patients requiring chemotherapy (both those with relapsed early stage disease following surveillance and advanced disease) of between 62 and 85 % (Table 18.2) [20, 29, 31–33]. Although BEP is the most commonly utilised regimen in this setting, with evidence demonstrating efficacy and overall survival of 82–90 % [14, 20, 31, 34] across all stages, the optimum regimen is still unclear due to the lack of a randomised evidence base in this cohort of patients with MOGCT. Studies in germ cell tumours have examined the efficacy of substituting carboplatin with cisplatin due its markedly different toxicity profile including less nausea, ototoxicity and renal toxicity. However, the data available does not demonstrate that two platinum agents are comparable, and there is a suggestion (in testicular GCT) that carboplatin outcomes may be inferior [35]. Most centres would therefore recommend using cisplatin-containing regimens in MOGCT unless there are specific contraindications that make safe delivery of cisplatin impossible.

Table 18.2 Studies of platinum-based chemotherapy in advanced MOGCT

Study	Patients (*n*)	Regimen	Overall survival	Includes stage 1A
Williams et al.	93	BEP	96 %	Yes
Murugaescu et al.	113	BEP/POMB-ACE	82 %	No
Gershenson et al.	26	BEP	96 %	Yes
Dimopoulous et al.	16	BEP	88 %	Yes
Lai et al.	93	BEP	97 %	Yes
Billmire et al.	131	BEP	97 %	Yes
Zanetta et al.	105	BEP/PVB	95 %	Yes

The POMB-ACE regimen was introduced by Charing Cross Hospital to manage patients with high-risk-advanced testicular germ cell tumours. It was found to be a well-tolerated and effective method of introducing seven cytotoxic agents in a two-weekly alternating regimen to try and overcome drug resistance and maximise cure rates [36]. Indeed, in poor prognosis testicular GCTs, the cure rate with POMB/ACE is around 70 % which from nonrandomised data appears better than four cycles of BEP. In stage IV MOGCT, cure rates appear to be around 65 % with this regimen, but data are still limited, and there is a clear need to improve outcomes for this group of patients [16].

A current consensus would indicate that for relapsed stage I disease or for stage 1c and 1 m and completely resected stage II–III disease, three cycles of BEP chemotherapy would be standard treatment. In incompletely resected stage III or IV disease with a higher burden of tumour, including patients with very high tumour markers, a longer course of platinum-based chemotherapy is utilised, commonly four cycles of BEP over 12 weeks or 5–7 treatments with POMB-ACE chemotherapy over 10–14 weeks [6, 16]. However, there is a clear need to improve management for these advanced cases to improve overall survival results.

The value of aggressive surgery prior to chemotherapy in advanced disease is debatable. This is because residual microscopic disease grows back so fast that by the time chemotherapy is commenced post-operatively, much of the cytoreduction advantage of the surgery is lost. Moreover, with so much disease in the pelvis, fertility-preserving surgery becomes very difficult. Consequently, many centres now practise neoadjuvant chemotherapy for advanced MOGCT and reserve surgery for once the chemotherapy is completed. In some instances this will mean that only the affected ovary is left to remove, but in others, the disease will become more cystic and large residual masses will need to be excised. Leaving these masses is not sensible as one cannot be certain that there is no active cancer left, and over time they may continue to grow in up to 30 % of patients and in a small proportion may dedifferentiate back in to active cancer.

With chemotherapy, once the tumour markers have normalised, it may help to continue treatment for a further 4–6 weeks to help minimise the possibility of relapse. Re-imaging after treatment with an MRI pelvis, CT chest and abdomen all with contrast will help define what needs surgical resection. Various features of the clinical course may cause concern for the managing clinicians. Thus, in some patients the AFP will fail to return to normal or might start rising towards the end of chemotherapy which can reflect liver repair and production of AFP rather than progressing disease. In addition, some patients with cystic differentiation may develop mature teratoma-growing syndrome, so post-chemotherapy imaging may show enlarging masses that make the clinicians feel their treatment has failed. However, once this is resected, this will nearly always turn out to be mature teratoma which requires no further chemotherapy. It is essential that residual masses are removed. Small lesions of 1 cm or less that appear non-cystic can be observed with repeat imaging 2–3 months post-completion of chemotherapy. Figure 18.2 illustrates an example of residual cystic pelvic mass post-POMB-ACE chemotherapy and marker normalisation. This mass was resected and

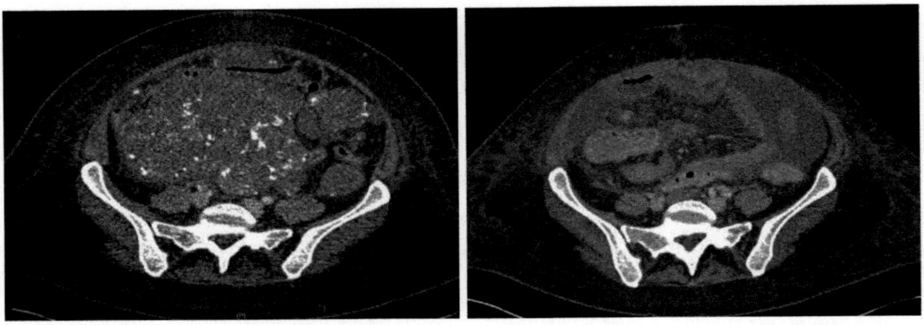

Post chemotherapy residual pelvic mass.

1 month post surgical resection

Fig. 18.2 Resection of residual disease post-chemotherapy

showed mature-differentiated cystic teratoma. The CT images show the appearances before and after surgery [6].

Relapse of MOGCT After Platinum-Based Multimodality Therapy

The frequency of relapse after platinum-containing therapies for advanced MOGCT varies from approximately 14–20 % of patients [16, 37]. The dominant pathology at relapse post-platinum appears to be yolk sac [38, 39], but the data are limited. In contrast to male patients with testicular germ cell tumours who can expect a cure rate of up to 50 % in response to salvage chemotherapy, women with MOGCT who relapse following initial chemotherapy appear to do exceptionally badly. Indeed, in one series the salvage rate was only 10 % [15]. This suggests that testicular and ovarian GCTs are in some way biologically different. Conventional relapse regimens investigated in germ cell tumours include re-challenging with platinum, ifosfamide-containing regimens [40], taxane [41] or gemcitabine-based regimens [42]. These therapies can provoke excellent responses in relapsed disease; however, drug resistance is extremely difficult to overcome in this setting, and patients usually die of their disease. Given its utility in relapsed advanced testicular germ cell tumours, high-dose chemotherapy with stem cell rescue (HD) has been investigated in MOGCT patients. In one series the relapse rate was 10 %, and only one of the four patients who underwent HD achieved long-term disease control [16]; in another series [20] two patients with relapsed disease were salvaged with HD. The largest series reported includes 13 patients of which 4 achieved long-term responses [39] following upfront tandem HD autografts. In very carefully selected patients re-look surgery or indeed multiple rounds of surgery to maximally remove macroscopic disease in combination with relapse regimens can deliver long-term remission [43].

It follows from the above discussion that we need improved stratification biomarkers to help identify which MOGCT will do badly from the outset so that these individuals can be treated differently to prevent relapse. Moreover, in those that do relapse, new agents and approaches are needed to increase the salvage rates. If, for example, tandem transplants are better than single transplants, will triple transplants improve matters further? Given the success of the UK GTD service, it would appear that a very good way to achieve these much needed improvements in MOGCT outcomes would be through centralised care of this rare disease.

Radiotherapy

Radiotherapy had a critical role in the management of MOGCT prior to the advent of effective cytotoxic chemotherapy. Within MOGCT, dysgerminoma is particularly radiosensitive, and radiotherapy has been used with good effect in long-term control. However radiotherapy increases the risk of second cancers and induces infertility with a very high rate of ovarian failure observed in young women treated with pelvic radiotherapy (>50 % in some series [44]). Consequently, it is no longer included routinely in modern management algorithms.

Complications of Therapy and Survivorship Issues

Most women with MOGCT will be cured of their disease with modern multimodality therapy as described above. However as in other tissue types where the application of cytotoxic chemotherapy has resulted in high cure rates such as Hodgkin lymphoma and acute lymphoid leukaemias, as a community we have to be aware of the impact of treatment on long-term survivorship and quality of life. Acute complications with regimens used in MOGCT include life-threatening infections and neutropaenia, acute renal injury from cisplatin, but also the small but significant risk of fatal pulmonary fibrosis from bleomycin [45]. The risk of bleomycin pulmonary toxicity might be due not only to the total dose but also to peak dose effects seen when the drug is given as a rapid infusion. Consequently, it seems reasonable to try and reduce this risk by using a slow IV infusion over several hours and to avoid giving bleomycin with the fourth cycle of BEP to limit the total dose. Even so physicians prescribing bleomycin need to be extremely aware of any cough or dyspnoea on treatment to minimise the risk of this rare but devastating complication, and we would advocate regular physical examination of the thorax with baseline pulmonary function tests to include transfer factor. Should the patient develop cough or shortness of breath, then a high-resolution CT chest and/or repeat pulmonary function tests should be requested.

Long-term complications of treatment with cytotoxic chemotherapy have been well studied in diseases such as Hodgkin disease and GCT [46]. A primary goal of the modification of curative treatment algorithms in recent decades has been the identification of secondary malignancies, particularly myeloid leukaemias in patients treated with curative intent with prolonged courses of alkylating agents [47] or with cumulative doses of etoposide >2000 mg/m^2 following the cure of the primary cancer [48]. Fortunately, cumulative doses of etoposide in conventional BEP and POMB-ACE regimens, and in etoposide mobilisation for HD, fall below this threshold.

Two recent studies to address long-term toxicity issues have compared survivors of MOGCT having had platinum-based chemotherapy with healthy matched controls [49, 50]. Indeed in one such study [50], no increased rate of malignancy was observed in 123 MOGCT survivors. This matches our experience in young women treated with combination agent chemotherapy for gestational trophoblastic neoplasia where we now have over 30,000 patient years of follow-up [51]. However, platinum-based chemotherapy is associated with an increased incidence of hypertension and chronic functional problems such as tinnitus and Raynaud's phenomenon, and these issues have been observed in MOGCT patients. Moreover, and of significant importance for these patients, 15.9 % of MOGCT survivors vs 4.5 % of healthy controls were denied health insurance because of their perceived additional health risks.

Fertility is also one area of concern for patients undergoing combined modality treatment. Many studies have now demonstrated that following fertility-preserving surgery and standard chemotherapy with platinum-containing regimens, fertility is preserved for the vast majority of patients [52–54]. However some studies have suggested that there may be a relationship between duration of therapy and the risk of subsequent ovarian failure – 0 % for those having three cycles of BEP in one study versus 33 % of those having >4 cycles of platinum-containing therapy [15]. However, the data are still rather limited. Interestingly, research in women with GTD has failed to show a significant impact of multiagent chemotherapy on fertility other than bringing forwards the date of the menopause by a few years [51, 55, 56]. In contrast, women undergoing high-dose chemotherapy are at very high risk of ovarian failure. There has been interest in hormonal suppression of ovarian function to preserve long-term fertility during standard chemotherapy; however previous studies analysing the effect LHRH analogue therapy in premenopausal women undergoing intensive chemotherapy regimens (in breast cancer) did not show a benefit in long-term ovarian function [57]. This is also our experience in GTD and in MOGCT. What we observe is that the ovaries naturally shut down with chemotherapy and restart within 7 months (range 1–12 months) of completing treatment.

Conclusions

Overall the outlook for MOGCT is vastly superior to that of epithelial ovarian cancer. The application of clinical research and international collaborations has enabled significant progress in optimising and refining therapy to allow many young women to be cured of this disease, with a minimal burden of treatment-related morbidity and mortality. However as physicians we are still challenged by many issues in MOGCT management as a result of its rarity and the lack of randomised evidence base for many decisions we have to make in the care of our patients. This is particularly so in the context of relapsed disease post-platinum therapy where prognosis is bleak despite the advent of high-dose chemotherapy with stem cell rescue. The only way we will secure progress in these areas is to further strengthen collaborations on basic and clinic science research to understand the molecular drivers of this group of diseases and to ensure young women with these rare illnesses are managed in large centres with the greatest accumulated experience in treating MOGCT. The development of national reference centres is an important step in this process.

References

1. Smith HO, et al. Incidence and survival rates for female malignant germ cell tumors. Obstet Gynecol. 2006;107(5):1075–85.
2. Quirk JT, Natarajan N, Mettlin CJ. Age-specific ovarian cancer incidence rate patterns in the United States. Gynecol Oncol. 2005;99(1):248–50.
3. Lin KY, et al. Malignant ovarian germ cell tumor – role of surgical staging and gonadal dysgenesis. Gynecol Oncol. 2014;134(1):84–9.
4. Norris HJ, Zirkin HJ, Benson WL. Immature (malignant) teratoma of the ovary: a clinical and pathologic study of 58 cases. Cancer. 1976;37(5):2359–72.
5. Brown J, et al. Gynecologic Cancer Intergroup (GCIG) consensus review for ovarian germ cell tumors. Int J Gynecol Cancer. 2014;24(9 Suppl 3):S48–54.
6. Colombo N, et al. Non-epithelial ovarian cancer: ESMO clinical practice guidelines for diagnosis, treatment and follow-up. Ann Oncol. 2012;23 Suppl 7:vii20–6.
7. Kleinsmith LJ, Pierce Jr GB. Multipotentiality of single embryonal carcinoma cells. Cancer Res. 1964;24:1544–51.
8. Nogales FF, Dulcey I, Preda O. Germ cell tumors of the ovary: an update. Arch Pathol Lab Med. 2014;138(3):351–62.
9. Cossu-Rocca P, et al. Chromosome 12p abnormalities in dysgerminoma of the ovary: a FISH analysis. Mod Pathol. 2006;19(4):611–5.
10. Sheikine Y, et al. Molecular genetics of testicular germ cell tumors. Am J Cancer Res. 2012;2(2):153–67.
11. Seckl MJ, Sebire NJ, Berkowitz RS. Gestational trophoblastic disease. Lancet. 2010; 376(9742):717–29.
12. Gershenson DM. Management of ovarian germ cell tumors. J Clin Oncol. 2007;25(20): 2938–43.
13. Lu KH, Gershenson DM. Update on the management of ovarian germ cell tumors. J Reprod Med. 2005;50(6):417–25.
14. Zanetta G, et al. Survival and reproductive function after treatment of malignant germ cell ovarian tumors. J Clin Oncol. 2001;19(4):1015–20.
15. Solheim O, et al. Prognostic factors in malignant ovarian germ cell tumours (the surveillance, epidemiology and end results experience 1978–2010). Eur J Cancer. 2014;50(11):1942–50.
16. Murugaesu N, et al. Malignant ovarian germ cell tumors: identification of novel prognostic markers and long-term outcome after multimodality treatment. J Clin Oncol. 2006;24(30):4862–6.
17. Solheim O, et al. Malignant ovarian germ cell tumors: presentation, survival and second cancer in a population based Norwegian cohort (1953–2009). Gynecol Oncol. 2013;131(2):330–5.
18. Palmer RD, et al. Pediatric malignant germ cell tumors show characteristic transcriptome profiles. Cancer Res. 2008;68(11):4239–47.
19. Frazier AL, et al. Revised risk classification for pediatric extracranial germ cell tumors based on 25 years of clinical trial data from the United Kingdom and United States. J Clin Oncol. 2015;33(2):195–201.
20. Lai CH, et al. Outcome and prognostic factors in ovarian germ cell malignancies. Gynecol Oncol. 2005;96(3):784–91.

21. Peccatori F, et al. Surgical management of malignant ovarian germ-cell tumors: 10 years' experience of 129 patients. Obstet Gynecol. 1995;86(3):367–72.
22. Gordon A, Lipton D, Woodruff JD. Dysgerminoma: a review of 158 cases from the Emil Novak Ovarian Tumor Registry. Obstet Gynecol. 1981;58(4):497–504.
23. Mangili G, et al. Is adjuvant chemotherapy indicated in stage I pure immature ovarian teratoma (IT)? A multicentre Italian trial in ovarian cancer (MITO-9). Gynecol Oncol. 2010;119(1): 48–52.
24. Williams S, et al. Adjuvant therapy of ovarian germ cell tumors with cisplatin, etoposide, and bleomycin: a trial of the Gynecologic Oncology Group. J Clin Oncol. 1994;12(4):701–6.
25. Gershenson DM. Management of early ovarian cancer: germ cell and sex cord-stromal tumors. Gynecol Oncol. 1994;55(3 Pt 2):S62–72.
26. Dimopoulos MA, et al. Treatment of ovarian germ cell tumors with a 3-day bleomycin, etoposide, and cisplatin regimen: a prospective multicenter study. Gynecol Oncol. 2004;95(3):695–700.
27. Dark GG, et al. Surveillance policy for stage I ovarian germ cell tumors. J Clin Oncol. 1997;15(2):620–4.
28. Billmire DF, et al. Surveillance after initial surgery for pediatric and adolescent girls with stage I ovarian germ cell tumors: report from the Children's Oncology Group. J Clin Oncol. 2014;32(5):465–70.
29. Gershenson DM, et al. Treatment of malignant nondysgerminomatous germ cell tumors of the ovary with vincristine, dactinomycin, and cyclophosphamide. Cancer. 1985;56(12):2756–61.
30. Gershenson DM, et al. Treatment of malignant nondysgerminomatous germ cell tumors of the ovary with vinblastine, bleomycin, and cisplatin. Cancer. 1986;57(9):1731–7.
31. Zanagnolo V, et al. Clinical review of 55 cases of malignant ovarian germ cell tumors. Eur J Gynaecol Oncol. 2004;25(3):315–20.
32. Gershenson DM. Update on malignant ovarian germ cell tumors. Cancer. 1993;71(4 Suppl):1581–90.
33. Gershenson DM. Chemotherapy of ovarian germ cell tumors and sex cord stromal tumors. Semin Surg Oncol. 1994;10(4):290–8.
34. Gershenson DM, et al. Treatment of malignant germ cell tumors of the ovary with bleomycin, etoposide, and cisplatin. J Clin Oncol. 1990;8(4):715–20.
35. Horwich A, et al. Randomized trial of bleomycin, etoposide, and cisplatin compared with bleomycin, etoposide, and carboplatin in good-prognosis metastatic nonseminomatous germ cell cancer: a Multiinstitutional Medical Research Council/European Organization for Research and Treatment of Cancer Trial. J Clin Oncol. 1997;15(5):1844–52.
36. Bower M, et al. Treatment of men with metastatic non-seminomatous germ cell tumours with cyclical POMB/ACE chemotherapy. Ann Oncol. 1997;8(5):477–83.
37. Messing MJ, et al. Primary treatment failure in patients with malignant ovarian germ cell neoplasms. Int J Gynecol Cancer. 1992;2(6):295–300.
38. Nawa A, et al. Prognostic factors of patients with yolk sac tumors of the ovary. Am J Obstet Gynecol. 2001;184(6):1182–8.
39. Reddy Ammakkanavar N, et al. High-dose chemotherapy for recurrent ovarian germ cell tumors. J Clin Oncol. 2015;33(2):226–7.
40. Loehrer Sr PJ, et al. Vinblastine plus ifosfamide plus cisplatin as initial salvage therapy in recurrent germ cell tumor. J Clin Oncol. 1998;16(7):2500–4.
41. Kondagunta GV, et al. Combination of paclitaxel, ifosfamide, and cisplatin is an effective second-line therapy for patients with relapsed testicular germ cell tumors. J Clin Oncol. 2005;23(27):6549–55.
42. Bokemeyer C, et al. Combination chemotherapy with gemcitabine, oxaliplatin, and paclitaxel in patients with cisplatin-refractory or multiply relapsed germ-cell tumors: a study of the German Testicular Cancer Study Group. Ann Oncol. 2008;19(3):448–53.
43. Munkarah A, et al. Salvage surgery for chemorefractory ovarian germ cell tumors. Gynecol Oncol. 1994;55(2):217–23.
44. Mitchell MF, et al. The long-term effects of radiation therapy on patients with ovarian dysgerminoma. Cancer. 1991;67(4):1084–90.

45. Azambuja E, et al. Bleomycin lung toxicity: who are the patients with increased risk? Pulm Pharmacol Ther. 2005;18(5):363–6.
46. Aleman BM, et al. Long-term cause-specific mortality of patients treated for Hodgkin's disease. J Clin Oncol. 2003;21(18):3431–9.
47. Canellos GP. Can MOPP be replaced in the treatment of advanced Hodgkin's disease? Semin Oncol. 1990;17(1 Suppl 2):2–6.
48. Boshoff C, et al. Secondary tumours following etoposide containing therapy for germ cell cancer. Ann Oncol. 1995;6(1):35–40.
49. Matei D, et al. Chronic physical effects and health care utilization in long-term ovarian germ cell tumor survivors: a Gynecologic Oncology Group study. J Clin Oncol. 2009;27(25):4142–9.
50. Solheim O, et al. Fertility and gonadal function after adjuvant therapy in women diagnosed with a malignant ovarian germ cell tumor (MOGCT) during the "cisplatin era". Gynecol Oncol. 2015;136(2):224–9.
51. Savage P, et al. Effects of single-agent and combination chemotherapy for gestational trophoblastic tumors on risks of second malignancy and early menopause. J Clin Oncol. 2015; 33(5):472–8.
52. Gershenson DM. Menstrual and reproductive function after treatment with combination chemotherapy for malignant ovarian germ cell tumors. J Clin Oncol. 1988;6(2):270–5.
53. Pektasides D, et al. Fertility after chemotherapy for ovarian germ cell tumours. Br J Obstet Gynaecol. 1987;94(5):477–9.
54. Gaffan J, et al. Infertility rates following POMB/ACE chemotherapy for male and female germ cell tumours – a retrospective long-term follow-up study. Br J Cancer. 2003;89(10):1849–54.
55. Woolas RP, et al. Influence of chemotherapy for gestational trophoblastic disease on subsequent pregnancy outcome. Br J Obstet Gynaecol. 1998;105(9):1032–5.
56. Bower M, et al. Chemotherapy for gestational trophoblastic tumours hastens menopause by 3 years. Eur J Cancer. 1998;34(8):1204–7.
57. Gerber B, et al. Effect of luteinizing hormone-releasing hormone agonist on ovarian function after modern adjuvant breast cancer chemotherapy: the GBG 37 ZORO study. J Clin Oncol. 2011;29(17):2334–41.

Ovarian Sex Cord Tumors

19

Annalisa Garbi, Maria Teresa Achilarre, and Nicoletta Colombo

Abstract

Sex cord–stromal tumors (SCSTs) account for approximately 10% of all malignant ovarian neoplasms. The low incidence, the histological heterogeneity, and the variable biologic behavior, makes their optimal management difficult. SCSTs constitute a heterogeneous group of tumors and according to the World Health Organization, they are classified into these categories: pure stromal tumors, pure sex cord tumors (i.e. granulosa cell tumor) and mixed sex cord-stromal tumors (Sertoli-Leydig cell tumors).

Histologically, these tumors are considered malignant neoplasms; their natural history, however, is indolent with a very favorable long-term prognosis. Treatment principles have generally based on small series and borrowed from clinical management of epithelial tumors. Adequate knowledge of these neoplasms is imperative to the appropriate diagnosis, choice of surgical treatment and adjuvant therapy.

Epidemiology

Non-epithelial ovarian malignancies, mainly comprising germ cell tumors and sex cord-stromal tumors, account for approximately 10 % of all primary ovarian cancers. In particular, sex cord-stromal tumors (SCSTs) are rare neoplasms, and they account for only 7 % of all ovarian malignancies [1].

A. Garbi • M.T. Achilarre • N. Colombo (✉)
Division of Gynecologic Oncology, European Institute of Oncology, Milan, Italy
e-mail: annalisa.garbi@ieo.it; maria.achilarre@ieo.it; nicoletta.colombo@ieo.it

E. Pujade-Lauraine et al. (eds.), *Ovarian Cancers*,
DOI 10.1007/978-3-319-32110-3_19

Table 19.1 Classification of sex cord-stromal tumors and steroid cell tumors – WHO 2014

Pure stromal tumors
Fibroma
Cellular fibroma
Thecoma
Luteinized thecoma associated with sclerosing peritonitis
Fibrosarcoma
Sclerosing stromal tumor
Signet-ring stromal tumor
Microcystic stromal tumor
Leydig cell tumor
Steroid cell tumor
Steroid cell tumor, malignant
Pure sex cord tumors
Adult granulosa cell tumor
Juvenile granulosa cell tumor
Sertoli cell tumor
Sex cord tumor with annular tubules
Mixed sex cord-stromal tumors
Sertoli–Leydig cell tumors Well differentiated
Moderately differentiated with heterologous elements
Poorly differentiated with heterologous elements
Retiform with heterologous elements
Sex cord-stromal tumors, not otherwise specified

The yearly adjusted incidence rate for SCSTs is 2.1 per 1,000,000 women [1], and they are more common in adult women (perimenopausal and postmenopausal); familial forms have been described [2].

SCSTs constitute a heterogeneous group of tumors, and according to the World Health Organization (WHO), they are classified into the categories shown in Table 19.1.

Granulosa cell tumors (GCTs) account for approximately 70 % of malignant SCSTs; adult granulosa cell tumors (AGCTs) are the most frequent (95 % of GCTs), and they occur more often in postmenopausal than premenopausal women, with a peak incidence between 50 and 55 years.

Juvenile granulosa cell tumors (JGCTs) were described the first time by Young in 1984, and they account for approximately 5 % of all GCTs. They have a natural history and histologic characteristics very different from the typical GCTs; approximately 90 % of JGCTs occur in prepubertal girls. In Young et al. series of 125 cases, 44 % of the tumors occurred before age of 10 years and only 3 % after the third decade of life [3, 4].

Sertoli–Leydig cell tumors or androblastomas (SLCTs) occur most frequently in the second and third decades, with 75 % of the lesions seen in women younger than 40 years. These neoplasms are extremely rare, accounting for less than 0.2 % of ovarian cancers [5].

Etiopathogenesis

Granulosa and Sertoli cells arise from the sex cords of the developing gonads, which originate from celomic epithelium. Granulosa cells derive from the cortical sex cord, while the Sertoli cells originate from medullary cords of mesonephric origin.

Very little is known about the etiology of SCSTs; one theory is that the degeneration of follicular granulosa cells after oocyte loss and the consequent compensatory rise in pituitary gonadotropins may induce an irregular proliferation. This hypothesis could be applied with the oocyte depletion and high levels of gonadotropins observed in menopausal patients; however, this explanation is not applicable to those tumors developing in young women.

A more recent hypothesis points toward the involvement of granulosa stem cells supported by the evidence of their ability to express telomerase [6].

However the most relevant discovery related to the etiopathogenesis of AGCTs is the finding of a somatic 402C>G missense point mutation in the gene encoding the FOXL2 (forkhead box L2). This finding is frequent, and more than 95 % of ovarian AGCTs harbor this type of mutation. FOXL2 somatic mutations may be involved in the tumorigenesis of these tumors due to a partial loss of function in its ability to induce apoptosis [7]. Moreover, Cheng et al. showed that the mutated form of FOXL2 may lead to the development of AGCT by reducing the expression of GnRH receptors, conferring resistance to GnRH-induced apoptotic effect [8].

These insights could have a clinical impact in developing targeted therapeutic strategies for AGCT patients.

FOXL2 shows a molecular interaction with others genes involved in the etiopathogenesis of AGCT such as SMAD3, CCND2, and GATA4 [9]. The clinical implications of these knowledges include the use of FOXL2 in the differential diagnosis of AGCT with an excellent specificity, considering that up to now there are no reports of any other tumor types being positive for this mutation [10].

FOXL2 has also clinical implication in the prognosis of AGCTs: patients with higher FOXL2 protein expression had worse overall survival and disease-free survival than those with negative or weak expression [11].

Chang et al. demonstrated that another molecule involved in the tumorigenesis of AGCT is activin A [12].

The other major recent finding regarding SCSTs is the mutation of DICER1; Schultz et al. reported that children with both pleuropulmonary blastoma (PPB) and SLCTs had germ line DICER1 mutations. They found these germinal mutations among family members of these patients [13]. Somatic DICER1 mutations are also described in SLCTs [14].

Peutz–Jeghers syndrome (PJS) is a rare autosomal dominant disorder characterized by mucocutaneous pigmentation, hamartomatous polyposis, and predisposition to benign and malignant tumors of the gastrointestinal tract, breast, ovary, uterine cervix, and testis. Germ line-inactivating mutations in 1 allele of the STK11/LKB1 gene at chromosome 19p13.3 have been found in most PJS patients. Although ovarian sex cord tumors with annular tubules (SCTATs) are very rare in the general population, they occur with increased frequency in women with PJS. Germ line mutations in the STK11 gene, accompanied by loss of heterozygosity were found in PJS-associated SCTATs [15].

Histopathology

SCSTs develop from the dividing cell population surrounding the oocytes, including the cells that produce ovarian hormones (the non-germ cell and non-epithelial components of the gonads), and therefore they vary in their capacity to produce clinically significant amounts of steroid hormones.

They are usually expressed at least one of the following markers (inhibin, calretinin, and FOXL2), but in 15 % of them, FOXL2 is the unique marker of sex cord differentiation.

AGCTs

Gross Findings

AGCTs vary from tiny lesions to huge masses with a mean diameter of about 13 cm. AGCTs are bilateral in only 2 % of cases. The external surface may be smooth or bosselated. The cut surface is often solid and sometimes partly solid and partly cystic. Hemorrhage and necrosis are common [16].

Microscopic Findings

The tumor cells grow in a variety of patterns, including microfollicular, macrofollicular, trabecular, insular, tubular, diffuse, moiré silk, and gyriform. The microfollicular variant, the most easily recognized, is characterized by multiple small rounded spaces formed by cystic degeneration in small aggregates of granulosa cells, containing eosinophilic PAS-positive material and often fragments of nuclear debris or pyknotic nuclei. These spaces, known as Call–Exner bodies, are found in only 30–50 % of tumors [17].

JGCTs

Gross Findings

JGCTs' appearance is similar to the adult variant.

Microscopic Findings

JGCT is typically a solid cellular neoplasm, with focal follicle formation. The follicles are of variable sizes and shapes but generally don't reach the large size of the follicles in the macrofollicular variant of adult granulosa cell tumor. Their lumens contain basophilic or eosinophilic fluid. Variable layers of granulosa cells line the follicles and occasionally surrounded by mantle of theca cells. The neoplastic granulosa cells have abundant eosinophilic and/or vacuolated cytoplasm and rounded hyperchromatic nuclei. Nuclear grooves are rare. Nuclear atypia in JGCTs varies from minimal to marked. The mitotic rate is also variable but is generally higher than adult granulosa cell tumor.

SLCT

Gross Findings

SLCTs are variable in dimension but frequently are smaller than 10 cm. They mostly are solid, firm, encapsulated, and lobulated masses, typically yellow or tan in color. They are typically unilateral.

Microscopic Findings

SLCTs are derived from mesenchyme and sex cords, which regroup histologically all the embryonic phases of testicular development, from an undifferentiated cord to well-differentiated Sertoli tubes. These tumors contain variable proportions of sertolian and leydigian elements. Tumors with only a sertolian component (Sertoli tumors) belong to the benign group. Tumors containing both types are classified into three groups: (1) benign differentiated forms (androgenic, secretory in 60 % of the cases), (2) intermediate differentiation (immature Sertoli cells), and (3) poorly differentiated forms (sarcomatoid or retiform).

In the forms with poor or intermediate differentiation (primarily epithelial or mesenchymatous), it is possible to see heterogeneous elements. In the largest series of SLCTs with greater than 200 tumors, 18 % contains glands and cysts lined by well-differentiated intestinal-type or gastric-type epithelium, 16 % has microscopic foci of carcinoid tumor, and 5 % has stromal heterologous elements, including islands of cartilage and/or areas of embryonal rhabdomyosarcoma [18]. Other heterologous elements that have been associated with SLCTs include hepatocyte-like cells, retinal tissue, neuroblastoma, and mucinous adenocarcinoma [19, 20]. Interestingly, tumors that contain heterologous or the retiform type are more frequently cystic.

SCTAT

Gross Findings

SCTAT is a tumor composed of sex cord (Sertoli) cells arranged in simple and complex annular tubules. SCTATs which occur in conjunction with the PJS are usually multifocal, bilateral, and almost always very small tumorlets found incidentally in ovaries. In patients without the PJS, SCTAT is usually unilateral and presents as a solitary, large solid mass up to 33 cm in diameter.

SCTAT typically exhibits well-circumscribed, rounded or oval, epithelial islands made up of ring-shaped, lumenless tubules encircling glassy, acidophilic, PAS-positive, basement membrane-like material.

Others

Gynandroblastomas are probably derived from undifferentiated mesenchyme. This origin would explain their “bisexual” potential; in fact, they could contain a variable amount of granulosa cells and Sertoli–Leydig cells.

In the majority of cases, these tumors are benign; however, certain malignant tumors have been described in the literature, and they are usually large tumors (7–10 cm in diameter).

Also pure Leydig cell tumors are usually benign. In some cases, no evidence of ovarian or testicular differentiation is seen. These tumors belong either to the undifferentiated SCST or to the steroid cell tumors according to cell morphology. Rarely they are malignant but evolution remains unpredictable today [21].

Neoplasms of pure ovarian stroma are mostly benign more than 50 % of them being fibromas. In morphologically ambiguous cases, the reticulin stain, together with mutational analysis of FOXL2, is useful to distinguish adult granulosa cell tumor from fibrothecoma.

Clinical Presentation

The most common symptoms related to SCSTs are pelvic pain, feeling of pelvic pressure due to pelvic mass and menstrual disorders.

GCTs typically occur as an abdominal mass with symptoms suggestive of functioning ovarian tumor. In approximately 5–15 % of patients, hemoperitoneum developed secondary to tumor rupture, and acute pelvic pain due to ovarian torsion could be the first sign [3]. Ascites occurs in about 10 % of cases, and they are asymptomatic in another 10 %.

AGCTs are clinically the most common estrogenic ovarian tumors. Functional symptoms are related to the age and reproductive state of the patient. In prepubertal girls, granulosa cell tumor often induces isosexual pseudoprecocious puberty. In women of reproductive age, the tumor may be associated with menstrual irregularities. In postmenopausal women, irregular uterine bleeding is the most common manifestation due to endometrial alteration such as endometrial hyperplasia that exhibits some degree of atypia (24–80 %) and well-differentiated adenocarcinoma (5 %). In addition, GCTs are associated with an increased incidence of breast cancer [5].

About 80 % of JGCT occurs in children, who typically present with isosexual pseudoprecocity. When JGCT occurs after puberty, patients usually present with abdominal pain or swelling, menstrual irregularities, or amenorrhea.

SLCTs are in 95 % of cases confined to the ovaries, tumor rupture is present in 10 % of cases, and 4 % of patients develop ascites. They are usually associated with hyperandrogenic symptoms (30 %), like hirsutism, acne and seborrhea, oligo- or amenorrhea, and in the most severe cases with clitoris hypertrophy, lower tone of voice, and may have laryngeal protuberance and reduction in breast volume. In some cases they have estrogenic functions and in 50 % of the cases are asymptomatic [22–24].

In gynandroblastomas signs of virilescence generally are more frequent than the estrogenic ones.

Tumor Markers and Diagnostics

Diagnostic work-up should include pelvic ultrasound, abdominopelvic computed tomography (CT scan), and chest X-ray. In young patients, serum human chorionic gonadotropin (hCG), α-fetoprotein (AFP) titers, and lactate dehydrogenase (LDH) can be assessed in order to differentiate germ cell ovarian tumors.

Estradiol is secreted by GCTs, but it is not a reliable marker of disease proliferation. Absence of estradiol secretion is observed in approximately 30 % of patients, and it may be due to a relative lack of theca cells in the tumor stroma. In the rare case of an androgen-secreting GCT, testosterone or its precursors could be used as tumor markers [5].

Inhibin is secreted by granulosa cell tumors and could be a useful marker [25]. Inhibins are mainly formed in granulosa cells and are made of two subunits (subunit bA or bB).

The first report of elevated serum inhibin levels associated with these tumors was published in 1989 by Lappohn et al. Several other studies seem to suggest that inhibin could be a useful marker of GCTs in both pre- and postmenopausal patients [26]. They demonstrated the efficacy of inhibin as a marker for both primary and recurrent disease and showed that a rise in inhibin levels preceded clinical recurrence as early as 20 months. However, elevated inhibin levels are not specific for GCT, as may be observed in epithelial ovarian cancer, especially of the mucinous variety (82 %) [5].

Newer studies using subunit-specific ELISA showed inhibin B to be the major form secreted in GCT and that inhibin B was more accurate than inhibin A to predict primary or recurrent disease. Inhibins act as autocrine and paracrine granulosa cell growth factors, and levels of inhibin reflect the amount of tumor burden.

Another hormone that recently has been evaluated is the anti-Mullerian hormone (AMH); this hormone, in fact, is secreted by granulosa cells only in postnatal females and both prenatally and postnatally by Sertoli cells in the male testis.

AMH is a marker of ovarian reserve, and it disappears in menopausal age or after a bilateral oophorectomy. This marker is highly specific for GCT in postmenopausal women and is related to the extent of disease [27].

AMH and inhibin B level parallel changes predict clinical recurrence as early as 11 months. Several studies show AMH to be a reliable tumor marker with sensitivity between 76 and 100 %. Further studies are required before deciding which tumor marker could be most reliable in detection and management of GCT. One retrospective study suggests AMH to be more sensitive and reliable than inhibin [28].

Regarding instrumental diagnostic work-up, new specific pattern recognition was validated with ultrasound. Van Holsbeke et al. described two typical patterns. The first was a solid mass with heterogeneous echogenicity of the solid tissue as, for example, in necrotic tissue. The second pattern was a multilocular-solid mass containing a considerable amount of solid tissue around relatively small locules, but with no papillary projections. It typically had a 'Swiss cheese' appearance owing to the large number of small locules with a variable thickness of solid tissue around the cystic areas [29].

On the contrary 18F-FDG PET/CT is not useful in the staging and follow-up of the great majority of GCTs which are known to cause false-negative results due to very low FDG avidity [30]. There are two possible explanations of this low sensitivity: one is related to the low metabolic and proliferative activity of GCTs as evidenced by weaker MIB-1 (a monoclonal antibody developed against the Ki-67 antigen proliferation index marker); the other explanation could be related to their tendency to recur as cystic lesions [31].

Treatment

Surgery

Early Stage Disease

Surgery represents the most important therapeutic tool for patients with suspected SCSTs at early stage [32].

The staging system for SCSTs is generally adopted from that for epithelial ovarian cancer as originally defined by the International Federation of Gynecology and Obstetrics staging system (FIGO staging). However, the prognostic significance of certain features within the FIGO classification (such as positive cytology or ovarian surface involvement) has not been well defined for patients with SCSTs [33].

Surgical approach can be carried out through an open route that allows adequate visualization of the upper abdomen or, in selected cases, by laparoscopy or robotics. Minimally invasive surgery could be considered feasible and safe either for primary surgery or restaging procedures in selected patients [34].

The staging procedure includes infracolic omentectomy, biopsy of the diaphragmatic peritoneum, paracolic gutters, pelvic peritoneum, and peritoneal washings [33].

Many reports indicate that more than 90 % of these neoplasms are unilateral and confined to the ovary. Thus, a fertility-sparing surgery with unilateral salpingo-oophorectomy and staging seems to be reasonable in patients wishing to preserve their fertility, in the absence of extra-ovarian spread. For young women who can be offered conservative therapy, uterine curettage should be performed before surgery, because of the frequent association of GCT with endometrial hyperplasia (55 %) or endometrial adenocarcinoma (4–20 %).

Removal of the other ovary and total abdominal hysterectomy are recommended in postmenopausal women, and it is advisable at the conclusion of childbearing, though this issue is still controversial. Some authors reported a worse survival for patients undergoing fertility-sparing surgery, but this was related mostly to a higher stage of disease in the group analyzed [35].

Zanagnolo and Zhang published the two largest series about conservative treatment.

In the series of 63 cases published by Zanagnolo et al., a conservative surgical treatment was performed in 23 % of early stage tumors; none of them recurred, and five of 11 patients became pregnant after treatment [36].

Zhang et al., in a series of 110 patients, showed no statistical difference on survival between the conservative vs demolitive treatment (94.8 % and 94.9 %, $p=0.38$) [37].

SLCTs are frequently low-grade malignancies, although occasionally a poorly differentiated variety may behave more aggressively. Unilateral salpingo-oophorectomy with preservation of the contralateral ovary and the uterus is now considered the adequate surgical treatment for patients in childbearing age.

There is no consensus about the role of systematic lymphadenectomy in SCSTs because of the very low incidence of retroperitoneal metastases in early stages [38, 39].

Thrall et al. confirmed previous reports and strengthened the principle that routine lymphadenectomy is unnecessary in the primary surgical management of SCSTs; they reviewed 47/87 patients, who had some nodal tissue examined as part of the initial or restaging procedure, and all examined nodes were negative [39–41].

In a more recent study of Shim et al., 578 patients were analyzed, and lymph node metastases were not detected in the 86 patients who underwent lymph node removal. This study confirms that the incidence of lymph node metastases in patients with clinical stage I and II SCSTs is low [34].

Node dissection should be carried out only in those cases with evidence of nodal abnormality.

Advanced Stage and Recurrent Disease

In advanced stage SCSTs, surgery is necessary to establish a definitive pathological diagnosis, to perform staging, and to achieve optimal debulking. In patients with advanced stage disease or with bilateral ovarian involvement, abdominal hysterectomy and bilateral salpingo-oophorectomy should be performed with a careful surgical staging/cytoreduction. This includes a thorough exploration of abdominal cavity, washing for cytological analysis, multiple peritoneal biopsies, omentectomy, and pelvic and para-aortic lymph node sampling/dissection. Although no scientific evidence exists on the role of cytoreduction in these tumors, an effort should be made to remove all metastatic disease.

Adjuvant Treatment

Early Stage Disease

The majority of SCSTs are diagnosed at early stage (60–95 %). Given the indolent nature and the overall good prognosis, there are no data to support any kind of postoperative adjuvant treatment for patients with stage I who underwent an adequate staging procedure. Some authors suggest adjuvant therapy for stage IC with high mitotic index with preoperative tumor rupture [5, 35]. For SLCTs, postoperative adjuvant chemotherapy should be considered for those patients with stage I poorly differentiated tumors or with heterologous elements. Platinum-based chemotherapy is the treatment of choice. The most commonly used regimen is the BEP combination (bleomycin, etoposide, cisplatin) for three courses [42–44].

Alternative chemotherapy options include etoposide plus cisplatin, cyclophosphamide, doxorubicin and cisplatin, paclitaxel and carboplatin, or platinum agent alone.

Advanced Stage and Recurrent Disease

In metastatic and recurrent GCTs, debulking surgery continues to be the most effective treatment.

The rarity of GCTs has made it impossible to conduct a well-designed randomized study assessing the value of postoperative therapy after debulking surgery.

Postoperative treatment should be considered in case of residual tumor after surgery [45–49].

Different approaches such as surgery followed by either chemotherapy or hormonal therapy and radiation have been associated with prolonged disease-free survival in some series [17, 35, 36, 42].

Chemotherapy

The rarity of this disease, the different regimens utilized, and the tendency for late relapses make it difficult to draw definitive guidelines. Platinum-based chemotherapy has been the treatment of choice for the past decade with an overall response rate of 63–80 % for advanced and relapsed disease [50].

In the early 1980s, the first promising regimens reported in the literature were the combination of cisplatin with doxorubicin (AP) and the three drugs regimen cisplatin, doxorubicin, and cyclophosphamide (CAP). The response rate was 100 % and 63 %, respectively [47, 51].

Later, PVB (cisplatin-vinblastine-bleomycin) was reported as an effective regimen in two Italian studies and in one EORTC (European Organization for Research and Treatment of Cancer) series, with response rates ranging from 57 to 82 % [46, 48, 52]. Despite these promising results, severe hematologic and non-hematologic toxicities were reported, making this regimen unfeasible in most patients.

The combination of platinum with bleomycin and etoposide (BEP) was subsequently tested.

Gershenson et al. observed an overall response rate of 83 % in a series of nine patients with poor-prognosis SCSTs treated with BEP. Median progression-free survival was 14 months, and median overall survival was 28 months [49].

In 1999, Homesley reported the results of a Gynecologic Oncology Group (GOG) study on the use of BEP in a series of 56 patients. In this trial, with a median follow-up of 3 years, 11 (69 %) of 16 patients in the primary advanced disease category and 21 (51 %) of 41 of recurrent patients were progression-free. However, this active regimen was associated with a severe toxicity, in particular, Grade 4 myelotoxicity occurred in 61 % of patients [43].

In 1995 Tresukosol reported the first case report on paclitaxel response of recurrent GCTs [53].

In a more recent retrospective study from Brown et al., the efficacy and side effects of taxanes, with or without platinum, were historically compared to BEP in the recurrent and advanced setting (222 patients). For newly diagnosed patients treated with BEP versus taxane, no significant differences in response rate (82 % for both regimens), median overall survival (97.2 months for BEP and more than 52 months for taxane), and median progression-free survival (46.1 months for BEP and more than 52 months for taxane) were observed. Median OS and PFS for taxane were not reached.

Among patients treated for recurrent measurable disease, the response rate was higher, but not statistically significant, with BEP (71 %) compared to taxane (37 %); the median progression-free survival was 11.2 and 7.2 months, respectively. The presence of platinum in the taxane-based combination correlated with response in patients with recurrent disease: 60 % with taxane–platinum comparing with 18 % with taxane alone. Many of the latter patients, however, had received platinum before. Toxicity profile was better with taxane regimens [54].

Currently, BEP regimen for three to six cycles (last three without bleomycin) or carboplatin/paclitaxel is recommended for advanced and recurrent SCSTs. A Gynecologic Oncology Group phase II trial is currently ongoing, to compare BEP versus the combination of paclitaxel and carboplatin for patients with newly diagnosed and chemo-naïve recurrent metastatic SCSTs of the ovary (GOG0264) [55].

New perspectives in the systemic treatment of SCSTs are represented by antiangiogenic agents, due to the overexpression of vascular endothelial growth factor and vascularity of these tumors.

In a recent retrospective study conducted at MD Anderson Cancer Center, the potential activity of bevacizumab was tested in eight patients. The median progression-free survival was 7.2 months, and overall survival was not reached at a median follow-up of 23.6 months. VEGF overexpression and microvessel density were associated with poor outcome, but sample size was too small to calculate statistical significance [56].

The Gynecologic Oncology Group conducted a phase II prospective multi-institutional trial (GOG 251) on the use of bevacizumab for women with recurrent SCSTs. In this trial, patients received bevacizumab 15 mg/kg intravenously on day 1 of every 21-day cycle until progression or unacceptable adverse effects. The median progression-free survival was 9.3 months, and the median overall survival was not reached. Inhibin A and B values were lower in patients who responded to treatment, but the difference was not statistically significant ($p = 0.100$) [57].

Another ongoing study (ALIENOR–ENGOT-ov7/GINECO) aims to explore the clinical benefit of adding bevacizumab to weekly paclitaxel followed by bevacizumab as maintenance versus weekly paclitaxel followed by observation in patients with relapsed SCSTs.

Radiation Therapy

Radiation treatment could be considered in selected cases with isolated liver, bone, and mediastinal recurrences, although data on large series are not available.

Wolf et al. reported on 14 advanced or recurrent patients with clinically measurable disease. Six of 14 patients achieved a clinical complete response with an overall response rate of 43 %; three of them remained alive and without evidence of disease 10–21 years after treatment, whereas the other three patients experienced relapse between 4 and 5 years after radiation. The eight nonresponders had a median survival time of 12.3 months [58].

Hormonal Therapy

The use of hormone-based approach is a promising therapeutic strategy in GCTs.

Given the functional hormonal nature of GCTs, it has been suggested that the suppression of endogenous estrogens may provide antiproliferative benefits [59].

Aromatase inhibitors (AI) are a family of oral nonsteroidal (anastrozole and letrozole) and steroidal (exemestane) medications that bind to aromatase, an enzyme involved in the conversion of androstenedione to estriol (E1) and testosterone to estradiol (E2). AI have been widely utilized in the treatment of advanced breast cancer, and they are the current first-line adjuvant hormonal therapy for estrogen receptor-positive postmenopausal breast cancer [60].

AI have been used in the management of six recurrent GCT cases with promising results.

Freeman et al. described the first two cases in the literature. Both patients received treatment with anastrozole following multiple treatment modalities for recurrent GCT, including surgery, chemotherapy (carboplatin/paclitaxel and paclitaxel alone), radiotherapy, and gonadotropin-releasing hormone (GnRH) agonists. These patients experienced normalization of their inhibin levels, which remained normal for 14 and 18 months.

Korach et al. treated four patients with recurrent GCT with AI (two treated with anastrozole and two with letrozole) and showed clinical complete responses in three patients [59, 61].

Response to progestins, gonadotropin-releasing hormone agonists, and tamoxifen has been reported in several case series [62].

Briasoulis et al. observed activity of oral megestrol acetate, 160 mg daily, in the treatment of lung recurrence after platinum-based chemotherapy [63].

Fisherman et al. reported a partial response rate of 40 % to leuprolide acetate in a small series of six patients with refractory or persistent disease without major adverse effects. Thus, he concluded that hormonal therapy can be used in cases of progressive disease that have failed to respond to chemotherapy and/or radiation [64].

In a recent review, van Meurs reported the results of 31 patients treated with hormonal therapy. In 25.8 % of patients, a complete response, and in 45.2 % a partial response, was described. Four patients had stable disease, while five patients had a progression. Various hormone treatments showed different results, for instance, AI demonstrated response in nine out of nine, tamoxifen in none of three. Median progression-free survival after the start of hormone therapy was 18 months (range 0–60).

Despite the limited available data, hormone therapy appears to be a useful treatment alternative for patients with advanced stage or recurrent GCTs. However, study quality is poor, and prospective studies are needed to confirm clinical benefit [65, 66] (Fig. 19.1).

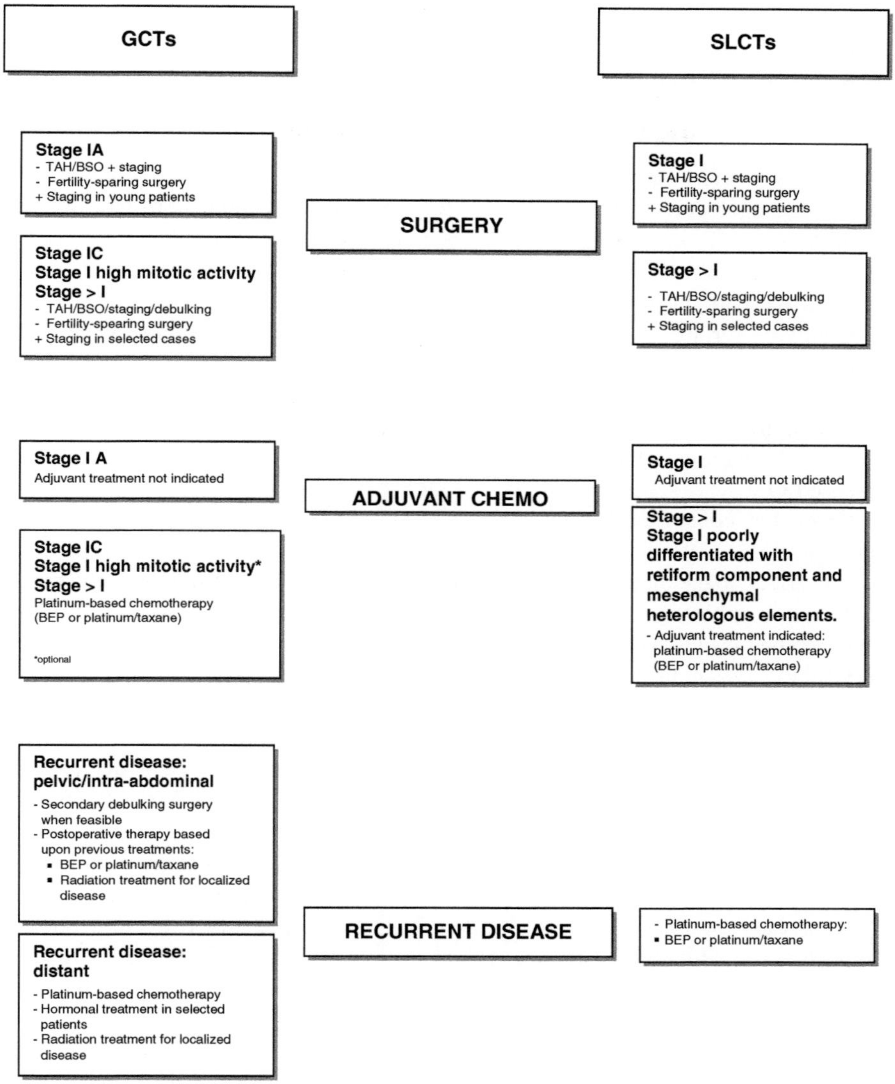

Fig. 19.1 Flow chart on the clinical management of sex cord stromal tumors

Prognosis

AGCTs

Several prognostic factors have been proposed in AGCTs such as stage, grade, residual disease, age, rupture, mitotic activity, nuclear atypia, aneuploidy, p53 overexpression, high Ki-67, and histological pattern [37, 39, 67–69].

However, only stage has been shown as a significant prognostic factor for survival.

In a recent study by Park et al., the 5-year disease-specific survival (DFS) and OS rate in early stage (stages I and II) disease was 89 and 99 %, respectively, while in advanced stages (stages III and IV), it was 72 % and 80 %, respectively. The 10-year DFS and OS rate in early stage disease was 89 % and 90 %, respectively, while in advanced stages, it was 57 and 67 %. Grade I and II tumors had better survival compared to grade III tumors. The disease-specific survival at 5 and 10 years for grade I and II tumors was 96 % and 86 %, respectively, while the disease-specific survival at 5 and 10 years for grade III tumors was 64 % and 59 %, respectively [37].

Complete surgical debulking is associated with better prognosis: the presence of postoperative residual tumor reduces survival from 82 to 22 % [70].

In the study by Ranganathan et al., median survival of patients who underwent optimal cytoreduction was 60 months in contrast to 19 months for those who did not. All the patients who were unable to undergo optimal cytoreduction died of disease [39].

Chan et al. confirmed that absence of residual disease is a predictor for improved survival [71].

The effect of age on prognosis is controversial. Lee et al. have shown a high recurrence rate in patients younger than 40 years. When comparing the survival of patients younger than 40 years to those older than 40 years, the 5- and 10-year disease-free survival rate was reduced from 93 to 82 % and from 84 to 48 %, respectively [68].

However, other studies have shown an improved prognosis in younger patients [71, 72].

A series evaluating the significance of tumor rupture showed a decrease in 25-year survival from 86 % in patients with stage IA disease to 60 % in patients with stage IC [73].

Koukourakis et al. reported a DFS at 80 months of 90 % for tumors with mitotic index <4/10 HPF compared to 25 % for those with a higher mitotic index.

In a study comparing the 25-year survival rate in patients with mild nuclear atypia to those with marked atypia, a fall in survival from 80 to 60 % was noted [73].

Tumors with a follicular pattern seemed to have a better survival compared to tumors with a diffuse or insular histological pattern [73].

GATA4 promotes granulosa cell proliferation; immunohistochemistry studies showed high GATA4 activity in GCTs which positively correlated to the clinical stage (IC and above) and risk of recurrence. This marker can be used as an important tool to predict tumor aggressiveness [9].

Newly diagnosed AGCTs with an intense expression of b-catenin showed a disease-free survival of 16.8 years, as compared with 12.7 years for tumors with a reduced intensity of expression [74].

FOXL2 has also clinical implication in prognosis of GCTs: patients with higher FOXL2 protein expression had worse overall survival and disease-free survival than those with negative or weak expression [11].

JGCTs

In contrast to AGCT, which recurs late, almost all clinically malignant JGCT recurs within 3 years.

Although the JGCTs usually appear less differentiated than the adult form, follow-up data indicate a high cure rate. Young et al. reported on 95 patients with an average follow-up of 5 years and observed that 92 % of patients were alive and free of disease. As in AGCT, the most important prognostic factor for JGCT is stage; the juvenile form is aggressive in advanced stages, and the time to relapse and death is of short duration (<3 years) [75].

SLCTs

In SLCTs prognosis is closely related to their degree of differentiation, the presence of heterologous elements, and stage of disease.

In the report by Young and Scully, none of the well-differentiated tumors, 11 % of those with intermediate differentiation, 59 % of the poorly differentiated tumors, and 19 % of those with heterologous elements, were clinically malignant. In the Zaloudek and Norris series, four of 20 poorly differentiated tumors were malignant, in contrast with one of 44 tumors of intermediate differentiation and none of the seven well-differentiated tumors.

Advanced stages are associated with a poor prognosis, with a mortality rate of 100 %. The collective salvage rates in patients with clinically malignant disease are less than 20 % [2, 76].

Follow-Up

A long-term follow-up is required for GCTs due to their indolent nature and their tendency to late recurrence.

Approximately median time to relapse is 4–6 years, but some authors described relapses at 20 years from diagnosis [35, 77–80].

The upper abdomen (55–70 %) and the pelvis (30–45 %) are the most common sites of recurrence.

Follow-up visit must include history, physical examination with pelvic examination, and tumor markers (inhibin, AMH).

In a cohort of 123 premenopausal and postmenopausal AGCT patients reported by Färkkilä, AMH was highly sensitive (92 %) and specific (81 %) in detecting the presence of a macroscopic AGCT, and the combination of the markers was superior to inhibin B alone [81].

In the absence of strong evidences on follow-up strategy in SCSTs, ESMO guidelines recommend pelvic examination and tumor markers every 3 months for the first 2 years and then every 6 months after the third year until progression; a pelvic ultrasound should be carried out every 6 months in those patients who have undergone fertility-sparing surgery, whereas a CT scan of the abdomen and pelvis is usually carried out according to clinical indication [82].

Because the risk of breast cancer in these patients is not negligible, especially those with the juvenile form, clinical monitoring and regular mammograms should be performed [35, 83].

References

1. Gatta G, van der Zwan JM, et al. Rare cancers are not so rare: the rare cancer burden in Europe. Eur J Cancer. 2011;47:2493–511.
2. Slade I, Bacchelli C, Davies H, et al. DICER1 syndrome: clarifying the diagnosis, clinical features and management implications of a pleiotropic tumour predisposition syndrome. J Med Genet. 2011;48(4):273–8.
3. Young RH, Dickersin GR, Scully RE. Juvenile granulosa cell tumor of the ovary: a clinico-pathological analysis of 125 cases. Am J Surg Pathol. 1984;8:575–96.
4. Zaloudek C, Norris HJ. Granulosa tumors of the ovary in children: a clinical and pathologic study of 32 cases. Am J Surg Pathol. 1982;6:503–12.
5. Colombo N, Parma G, Zanagnolo V, Insinga A. Management of ovarian stromal cell tumors. J Clin Oncol. 2007;25(20):2944–51.
6. Rodgers RJ, Irving-Rodgers HF, Van Wezel IL, et al. Dynamics of the membrana granulosa during expansion of the ovarian follicular antrum. Mol Cell Endocrinol. 2001;171:41–8.
7. Benayoun BA, Anttonen M, te L'Ho D, et al. Adult ovarian granulosa cell tumor transcriptomics: prevalence of FOXL2 target genes misregulation gives insights into the pathogenic mechanism of the p.Cys134Trp somatic mutation. Oncogene. 2013;30:2739–46.
8. Cheng JC, Klausen C, Leung PC. Overexpression of wild-type but not C134W mutant FOXL2 enhances GnRH-induced cell apoptosis by increasing GnRH receptor expression in human granulosa cell tumors. PLoS One. 2013;8(1):e55099.
9. Anttonen M, Pihlajoki M, Andersson N, et al. FOXL2, GATA4, and SMAD3 cooperatively modulate gene expression, cell viability and apoptosis in ovarian granulosa cell tumour cells. PLoS One. 2014;9:e85545.
10. Kommoss S, Gilks CB, Penzel R, et al. A current perspective on the pathological assessment of FOXL2 in adult-type granulosa cell tumours of the ovary. Histopathology. 2014;64:380–8.
11. D'Angelo E, Mozos A, Nakayama D, et al. Prognostic significance of FOXL2 mutation and mRNA expression in adult and juvenile granulosa cell tumors of the ovary. Mod Pathol. 2011;24(10):1360–7.
12. Chang HM, Cheng JC, Taylor E, et al. Oocyte-derived BMP15 but not GDF9 down-regulates connexin43 expression and decreases gap junction intercellular communication activity in immortalized human granulosa cells. Mol Hum Reprod. 2014;20:373–83.
13. Schultz KA, Pacheco MC, Yang J, et al. Ovarian sex cord-stromal tumors, pleuropulmonary blastoma and DICER1 mutations: a report from the International Pleuropulmonary Blastoma Registry. Gynecol Oncol. 2011;122(2):246–50.
14. Heravi-Moussavi A, Anglesio MS, Cheng SW, et al. Recurrent somatic DICER1 mutations in non-epithelial ovarian cancers. N Engl J Med. 2012;366(3):234–42.
15. Connolly DC, Katabuchi H, Cliby WA, et al. Somatic mutations in the STK11/LKB1 gene are uncommon in rare gynecological tumor types associated with Peutz-Jeghers syndrome. Am J Pathol. 2000;156:339–45.
16. Rabban JT, Zaloudek CJ. A practical approach to immunohistochemical diagnosis of ovarian germ cell tumours and sex cord-stromal tumours. Histopathology. 2013;62(1):71–88.

17. Cronje HS, Niemand I, Bam RH, Woodruff JD. Review of the granulosa-theca cell tumors from the emil Novak ovarian tumor registry. Am J Obstet Gynecol. 1999;180(2 Pt 1):323–7.
18. Baker PM, Oliva E. Immunohistochemistry as a tool in the differential diagnosis of ovarian tumors: an update. Int J Gynecol Pathol. 2004;24:39–55.
19. Prat J, Young RH, Scully RE. Ovarian Sertoli-Leydig cell tumor with heterologous elements II, cartilage and skeletal muscles: a clinicopathologic analysis of twelve cases. Cancer. 1982;50:2465–75.
20. Mooney EE, Nogales FF, Tavassoli FA. Hepatocytic differentiation in retiform Sertoli-Leydig cell tumors: distinguishing a heterologous element from leydig cells. Hum Pathol. 1999; 30:611–7.
21. Ray-Coquard I, Brown J, Harter P, et al. Gynecologic Cancer InterGroup (GCIG) consensus review for ovarian sex cord stromal tumors. Int J Gynecol Cancer. 2014;24(9 Suppl 3):S42–7.
22. Oliva E, Alvarez T, Young RH. Sertoli cell tumors of the ovary: a clinicopathologic and immunohistochemical study of 54 cases. Am J Surg Pathol. 2005;29(2):143–56.
23. Litta P, Saccardi C, Conte L, Codroma A, Angioni S, Mioni R. Sertoli-Leydig cell tumors: current status of surgical management: literature review and proposal of treatment. Gynecol Endocrinol. 2013;29(5):412–7.
24. Chen L, Tunnell CD, De Petris G. Sertoli-Leydig cell tumor with heterologous element: a case report and a review of the literature. Int J Clin Exp Pathol. 2014;7(3):1176–81.
25. Hildebrandt RH, Rouse RV, Longacre TA. Value of inhibin in the identification of granulosa cell tumors of the ovary. Hum Pathol. 1997;28:1387–95.
26. Lappöhn RE, Burger HG, Bouma J, Bangah M, Krans M, de Bruijn HW. Inhibin as a marker for granulosa-cell tumors. N Engl J Med. 1989;321:790–3.
27. Lane AH, Lee MM, Fuller Jr AF, et al. Diagnostic utility of mullerian inhibiting substance determination in patients with primary and recurrent granulosa cell tumors. Gynecol Oncol. 1999;73:51–5.
28. Geerts I, Vergote I, Neven P, Billen J. The role of inhibins B and antimullerian hormone for diagnosis and follow-up of granulosa cell tumors. Int J Gynecol Cancer. 2009;19:847–55.
29. Van Holsbeke C, Domali E, Holland TK, et al. Imaging of gynecological disease (3): clinical and ultrasound characteristics of granulosa cell tumors of the ovary. Ultrasound Obstet Gynecol. 2008;31(4):450–6.
30. Caoduro C, Ungureanu CM, Singeorzan CM, et al. Granulosa cell tumor of the ovary with high FDG uptake. Clin Nucl Med. 2013;38(7):553–6.
31. Raj G, Proietto A, Jaaback K. Positron emission tomography and granulosa cell tumor recurrence: a report of 2 cases. Int J Gynecol Cancer. 2009;19(9):1542–4.
32. Garcia AA, Morrow CP. Stromal tumors of the ovary. In: Raghavan D, Brecher M, Johnson DH, et al., editors. Textbook of uncommon cancer. 2nd ed. New York: Wiley; 1999.
33. Schumer ST, Cannistra SA. Granulosa cell tumor of the ovary. J Clin Oncol. 2003;21: 1180–9.
34. Shim SH, Kim DY, Lee SW, et al. Laparoscopic management of early-stage malignant nonepithelial ovarian tumors: surgical and survival outcomes. Int J Gynecol Cancer. 2013;23(2): 249–55.
35. Evans AT, Gaffey TA, Malkasian GDJ, et al. Clinicopathologic review of 118 granulosa and 82 theca cell tumors. Obstet Gynecol. 1980;55:231–8.
36. Zanagnolo V, Pasinetti B, Sartori E. Clinical review of 63 cases of sex cord stromal tumors. Eur J Gynecol Oncol. 2004;25:431–8.
37. Zhang M, Cheung MK, Shin JY, et al. Prognostic factors responsible for survival in sex cord stromal tumors of the ovary: an analysis of 376 women. Gynecol Oncol. 2007;104(2):396–400. Epub 2006 Oct 9.
38. Mahdi H, Swensen RE, Hanna R. Prognostic impact of lymphadenectomy in clinically early stage malignant germ cell tumour of the ovary. Br J Cancer. 2011;105(4):493.
39. Brown J, Sood AK, Deavers MT, et al. Patterns of metastasis in sex cord-stromal tumors of the ovary: can routine staging lymphadenectomy be omitted? Gynecol Oncol. 2009;113(1): 86–90.

40. Abu-Rustum NR, Restivo A, Ivy J, et al. Retroperitoneal nodal metastasis in primary and recurrent granulosa cell tumors of the ovary. Gynecol Oncol. 2006;103:31–4.
41. Ranganath R, Sridevi V, Shirley SS, et al. Clinical and pathologic prognostic factors in adult granulose cell tumors of the ovary. Int J Gynecol Cancer. 2008;18(5):929–33.
42. Schneider DT, Calaminus G, Wessalowski R, et al. Ovarian sex cord-stromal tumors in children and adolescents. J Clin Oncol. 2003;21:2357–63.
43. Homesley HD, Bundy BN, Hurteau JA, et al. Bleomycin, etoposide, and cisplatin combination therapy of ovarian granulosa cell tumors and other stromal malignancies: a Gynecologic Oncology Group study. Gynecol Oncol. 1999;72:131–7.
44. Gershenson DM. Current advances in the management of malignant germ cell and sex cord stromal tumors of the ovary. Gynecol Oncol. 2012;125:515–7.
45. Mangili G, Sigismondi C, Frigerio L, et al. Recurrent granulosa cell tumors (GCTs) of the ovary: a MITO-9 retrospective study. Gynecol Oncol. 2013;130:38–42.
46. Zambetti M, Escobedo A, Pilotti S, et al. Cisplatinum/vinblastine/bleomycin combination chemotherapy in advanced or recurrent granulosa cell tumors of the ovary. Gynecol Oncol. 1990;36:317–20.
47. Jacobs HJ, Deppe G, Cohen CJ. Combination chemotherapy of ovarian granulosa cell tumor with cisplatinum and doxorubicin. Gynecol Oncol. 1982;14:294.
48. Pecorelli S, Wagenaar HC, Vergote IB, et al. Cisplatin, vinblastine, and bleomycin combination chemotherapy in recurrent or advanced granulose cell tumor of the ovary: an EORTC Gynecologic Cancer Cooperative Group study. Eur J Cancer. 1999;35:1331–7.
49. Gershenson DM, Morris M, Burke TW, et al. Treatment of poor-prognosis sex cord-stromal tumors of the ovary with the combination of bleomycin, etoposide and cisplatin. Obstet Gynecol. 1996;87:527–31.
50. Wolf JK, Brown J. Management of stromal tumors of the ovary. ASCO. 2008;2008 Educational Book.
51. Gershenson DM, Copeland LJ, Kavanagh JJ, et al. Treatment of metastatic stromal tumors of the ovary with cisplatin, doxorubicin and cyclophosphamide. Obstet Gynecol. 1987;70: 765–9.
52. Colombo N, Sessa C, Landoni F, et al. Cisplatin, vinblastine, and bleomycin combination chemotherapy in metastatic granulosa cell tumor of the ovary. Obstet Gynecol. 1986;67: 265–8.
53. Tresukosol D, Kudelka AP, Edwards CL, et al. Recurrent ovarian granulosa cell tumor: a case report of a dramatic response to taxol. Int J Gynecol Cancer. 1995;5:156–9.
54. Brown J, Shvartsman HS, Deavers MT, et al. The activity of taxanes compared with bleomycin, etoposide and cisplatin in the treatment of sex cord stromal ovarian tumors. Gynecol Oncol. 2005;97:489–96.
55. Paclitaxel and carboplatin or bleomycin sulfate, etoposide phosphate, and cisplatin in treating patients with advanced or recurrent sex cord-ovarian stromal tumors. Available at: www.clinicaltrials.gov/ct2/show/NCT01042522.
56. Tao X, Sood AK, Deavers MT, et al. Anti-angiogenesis therapy with bevacizumab for patients with ovarian granulosa cell tumors. Gynecol Oncol. 2009;114:431–6.
57. Brown J, Brady WE, Schink J, et al. Efficacy and safety of bevacizumab in recurrent sex cord stromal ovarian tumours. Cancer. 2014;120(3):344–51.
58. Wolf JK, Mullen J, Eifel PJ, et al. Radiation treatment of advanced or recurrent granulosa cell tumor of the ovary. Gynecol Oncol. 1999;73:35–41.
59. Korach J, Perri T, Beiner M, et al. Promising effect of aromatase inhibitors on recurrent granulosa cell tumors. Int J Gynecol Cancer. 2009;19:830–3.
60. Garrett A, Quinn MA. Hormonal therapies and gynecological cancers. Best Pract Res Clin Obstet Gynaecol. 2008;22:407–21.
61. Freeman SA, Modesitt SC. Anastrozole therapy in recurrent ovarian adult granulose cell tumors: a report of 2 cases. Gynecol Oncol. 2006;103:755–8.
62. Hardy RD, Bell JG, Nicely CJ, et al. Hormonal treatment of a recurrent granulosa cell tumor of the ovary: case report and review of the literature. Gynecol Oncol. 2005;96:865–9.

63. Briasoulis E, Karavasilis V, Pavlidis N. Megestrol activity in recurrent adult type granulosa cell tumour of the ovary. Ann Oncol. 1997;8:811–2.
64. Fishman A, Kudelka AP, Tresukosol D, et al. Leuprolide acetate for treating refractory or persistent ovarian granulosa cell tumor. J Reprod Med. 1996;41:393–6.
65. Hs VM, van Lonkhuijzen LR, Limpens J, et al. Hormone therapy in ovarian granulosa cell tumors: a systematic review. Gynecol Oncol. 2014;134(1):196–205.
66. Sommeijer DW, Sjoquist KM, Friedlander M. Hormonal treatment in recurrent and metastatic gynaecological cancers: a review of the current literature. Curr Oncol Rep. 2013;15(6): 541–8.
67. Lee IH, Choi CH, Hong DG, Song JY, Kim YJ, Kim KT. Clinicopathologic characteristics of granulosa cell tumors of the ovary: a multicenter retrospective study. J Gynecol Oncol. 2011;22:188–95.
68. Shah SP, Köbel M, Senz J, et al. Mutation of FOXL2 in granulosa-cell tumors of the ovary. N Engl J Med. 2009;360:2719–29.
69. Sun HD, Lin H, Jao MS, Wang KL, et al. A long-term follow-up study of 176 cases with adult-type ovarian granulosa cell tumors. Gynecol Oncol. 2012;24:244–9.
70. Park JY, Jin KL, Kim DY, et al. Surgical staging and adjuvant chemotherapy in the management of patients with adult granulosa cell tumors of the ovary. Gynecol Oncol. 2012;125:80–6.
71. Chan JK, Zhang M, Kaleb V, et al. Prognostic factors responsible for survival in sex cord stromal tumors of the ovary a multivariate analysis. Gynecol Oncol. 2005;96:204–9.
72. Ayhan A, Salman MC, Velipasaoglu M, et al. Prognostic factors in adult granulosa cell tumors of the ovary: a retrospective analysis of 80 cases. J Gynecol Oncol. 2009;20:158–63.
73. Koukourakis GV, Kouloulias VE, Koukourakis MJ, et al. Granulosa cell tumor of the ovary: tumor review. Integr Cancer Ther. 2008;7:204–15.
74. Stewart CJ, Doherty D, Guppy R, et al. b-Catenin and E-cadherin expression in stage I adult-type granulosa cell tumour of the ovary: correlation with tumour morphology and clinical outcome. Histopathology. 2013;62:257–66.
75. Young RH, Scully RE. Sex cord-stromal, steroid cell, and other ovarian tumor with endocrine, paracrine, and paraneoplastic manifestation. In: Blaustein's pathology of the female genital tract. 5th ed. New York: Springer; 2002.
76. Young RH, Scully RE. Ovarian Sertoli-Leydig cell tumors: a clinicopathological analysis of 207 cases. Am J Surg Pathol. 1985;9:543.
77. Hines JF, Khalifa MA, Moore JL, et al. Recurrent granulosa cell tumor of the ovary 37 years after initial diagnosis: a case report and review of the literature. Gynecol Oncol. 1996; 60:484–8.
78. Fujimoto T, Sakuragi N, Okuyama K, et al. Histopathologic prognostic factors of adult granulose cell tumors of the ovary. Acta Obstet Gynecol Scand. 2001;80:1069–74.
79. Lauszus FF, Peterson AC, Greisen J, et al. Granulosa cell tumor of the ovary: a population based study of 37 women with stage I disease. Gynecol Oncol. 2001;81:456–60.
80. Miller BE, Barron BA, Wan JY, et al. Prognostic factors in adult granulosa cell tumors of the ovary. Cancer. 1997;79:1951–5.
81. Färkkilä A, Koskela S, Bryk S, et al. The clinical utility of serum anti-Müllerian hormone in the follow-up of ovarian adult-type granulosa cell tumors-a comparative study with inhibin B. Int J Cancer. 2015;137(7):1661–71.
82. Colombo N, Peiretti M, Garbi A, et al. ; ESMO Guidelines Working Group. Non-epithelial ovarian cancer: ESMO Clinical Practice Guidelines for diagnosis, treatment and follow-up. Ann Oncol. 2012;23(Suppl 7):vii20–6.
83. Burger HG, Fuller PJ, Chu S, et al. The inhibins and ovarian cancer. Mol Cell Endocrinol. 2001;180:145–8.

Small Cell Carcinoma of the Ovary

20

Patricia Pautier, Aurélie Auguste, and Alexandra Leary

Abstract

Small cell carcinoma of the ovary (SCCO) is a rare tumor in a very young population with a bad prognosis, even when diagnosed as stage 1A. Recent data suggest a possible implication of SMARCA4 gene in SCCOHT oncogenesis and suggest they may simply be an ovarian variant of malignant rhabdoid tumors. Multimodal approach including intensive chemotherapy, radical surgery and possibly radiotherapy is actually often proposed.

Small cell carcinoma of the ovary (SCCO) is a rare tumor that was first described by Dickersin and Scully in the 1980s [1, 2] and which usually affects young women and children. The incidence of these tumors is low, since they account for less than 1 % of ovarian cancers [3]. They grow very aggressively, and the majority of patients present with advanced stage disease and die rapidly (within 6 months); however, even those diagnosed as stage 1A share a poor prognosis with only 30–40 % of long-term survivors with standard treatment [4]. Potential prognostic factors, in addition to disease stage (stage IA versus others), are age >30 years, normal preoperative

P. Pautier, MD (✉)
Département de médecine oncologique, Gustave Roussy, Université Paris-Saclay, F-94805, Villejuif, France
e-mail: Patricia.PAUTIER@gustaveroussy.fr

A. Auguste, PhD
Gynecological Tumor Translational Research Laboratory, INSERM U981, Villejuif, France

A. Leary, MD, PhD
Département de médecine oncologique, Gustave Roussy, Université Paris-Saclay, F-94805, Villejuif, France

Gynecological Tumor Translational Research Laboratory, INSERM U981, Villejuif, France

E. Pujade-Lauraine et al. (eds.), *Ovarian Cancers*,
DOI 10.1007/978-3-319-32110-3_20

calcium level, a tumor size <10 cm, the absence of large cells, surgical resection including bilateral oophorectomy, and postoperative radiotherapy in some cases [5].

Unfortunately, most of the time, these tumors present at advanced stages (>stage IA) with a size exceeding 10 cm and in the second decade of life. SCCO is described as a highly aggressive tumor in a very young patient population (but often with rapid disease progression). In addition, there is no international consensus regarding the optimal treatment of SCCO, and a multimodal approach including chemotherapy, radical surgery, and possibly radiotherapy is often proposed. However, no randomized studies have ever been conducted, and the available published data are composed of case reports or small retrospective series with very heterogeneous management strategies. International guidelines were published in 2015 to help clinicians to offer the best therapeutic options [6].

Pathology

Two types of SCCO are now recognized in the WHO classification and have different clinical patterns. The hypercalcemic is the most common (SCCOHT) and non-small cell neuroendocrine carcinoma (large cell variant) which can be difficult to distinguish from the first one. Well-differentiated neuroendocrine tumors (carcinoids) are not fully discussed in this chapter and include classical primary carcinoid tumors of the ovary, which are equally uncommon [5, 7, 8]. SCCOHTs are the most frequent, tend to arise in younger women, with a mean age 28 years, and often present in nonsmokers.

SCCOHT is suspected when there is an undifferentiated ovarian carcinoma composed of small cells with scanty neoplasm occurring in a young patient and associated with hypercalcemia, which occurs in approximately 70 % of cases, but cannot be diagnostic. The large cell variant may cause some diagnostic confusion as may have a mixture of both large and small cells [6].

As tumors are highly undifferentiated, the histogenesis remained obscure (epithelial, germinal, or mesenchymatous), but most tumors display epithelial markers [5, 8]; interestingly, recent data suggest they may simply be an ovarian variant of malignant rhabdoid tumors [9, 10].

Until recently, literature describing the genomic profile of SCCOHT was scarce. However, recent publications have confirmed that there may be an identifiable molecular pathway in SCCO. Sequencing of cases with available DNA identified recurrent germ line or somatic deleterious *SMARCA4* mutations, suggesting a possible implication of SMARCA4 in SCCOHT oncogenesis. Germ line mutations in *SMARCA4* or *SMARCB1* were already known to predispose to the development of pediatric tumors, namely, atypical teratoid/rhabdoid tumors [11, 12]. Mutations in the SWItch/Sucrose NonFermentable (SWI/SNF) chromatin-remodeling gene, *SMARCA4* encoding BRG1, have now been shown to be a frequent event occurring in 76–100 % of SCCOHT tumors [13–15]. The SWI/SNF complex has been identified as a tumor suppressor that functions primarily by remodeling nucleosome structure and generating sites that are more or less accessible to DNA-binding factors. SWI/SNF acts as a master coordinator of gene activation and repression and appears to be particularly involved in regulating lineage-specific and differentiation gene expression programs [16, 17].

Inactivating germ line and somatic *SMARCA4* mutations have been identified in SCCOHT in three papers published at the same time: the first one identified inactivating biallelic *SMARCA4* mutations in 100 % of the 12 SCCOHT tumors examined [13]. Protein studies confirmed loss of the SWI/SNF chromatin-remodeling complex *SMARCA4* expression, suggesting a key role in SCCOHT; the second one identified germ line and somatic inactivating mutations in the gene *SMARCA4* in 75 % (9/12) of SCCOHT cases in addition to *SMARCA4* protein loss in 82 % (14/17) of SCCOHT tumors, but in only 0.4 % (2/485) of other primary ovarian tumors [14]. In the third article, authors sequenced the exomes of six individuals from three families with SCCOHT [15]. After discovering segregating deleterious germ line mutations in *SMARCA4*, all the familial tumors sequenced harbored either a somatic mutation or loss of the wild-type allele. Immunohistochemical analysis of these cases and additional familial and nonfamilial cases showed loss of *SMARCA4* (BRG1) protein in 38 of 40 tumors overall. Taken together, these data suggest that *SMARCA4* loss of function mutations may have real diagnostic utility; the question is whether these mutations may also have therapeutic implications.

Until, there were no robust immunohistochemical diagnostic markers, SCCOHTs usually stain diffusely for WT1, which is of little diagnostic aid. The "gold standard" for diagnosis remains an evaluation by an expert pathologist. In France, all suspected SCCOHTs are centrally reviewed by a reference pathologist within the National Rare Ovarian Tumor Network [18]. The differential diagnosis included germ cell and granulosa/sex cord tumors, especially if they were more poorly differentiated. Given the diagnostic challenge frequently posed by these rare tumors.

Regarding the rarity and the therapeutic implications in this particularly rare population of women, all suspected cases should benefit from a review by an expert pathologist in a reference center and be discussed in a specialized tumor board.

Surgery

There are no published data on the impact of surgery in SCCO. Most data on epithelial ovarian tumors suggest a statistically significant positive correlation between the percentage of maximum cytoreduction and median survival [19]. Another argument in favor of maximum cytoreduction in SCCOs is that this may facilitate the action of postoperative chemotherapy. On the basis of these two arguments, maximum debulking surgery by a gynecological oncologist is recommended.

Standard primary surgical debulking (hysterectomy, bilateral annexectomy, omentectomy, pelvic and lombo-aortic lymphadenectomy) is the treatment of choice. However, for selected patients with bulky stage III disease or stage IV disease where primary debulking surgery is not considered to be achievable, the use of neoadjuvant chemotherapy may be considered on an individual basis after discussion at the tumor board [6].

Chemotherapy

Similar to small cell carcinomas of the lung, SCCOHTs are particularly chemosensitive at the outset, but can rapidly escape therapy probably as a result of drug resistance. The choice of chemotherapy regimen is generally extrapolated from data in small cell carcinoma of the lung. A combination of a cisplatin and etoposide-based therapy is generally considered most appropriate [6, 20, 21].

To optimize the practical use of anticancer chemotherapy in these young patients with initially good tumor response, some groups have opted for an aggressive strategy with extensive surgery to lower the tumor burden on the one hand and dose intensive chemotherapy to circumvent cell resistance. The only prospective clinical trial reported in SCCOHTs was a prospective trial testing combination intensive therapy for stage I to IV tumors [22]. Patients received multimodality therapy with aggressive debulking surgery, chemotherapy with a platinum etoposide-based regimen (PAVEP, cisplatin, Adriamycin, VP-16, and cyclophosphamide), and one cycle of high-dose consolidation chemotherapy followed by autologous stem cell support in case of complete response. Eighteen patients among 27 achieved a complete remission, and ten proceeded to high-dose chemotherapy with stem cell support. The only long-term survivors had complete surgical resection. This procedure resulted in an encouraging 3-year survival rate for the entire population of 49 %. This study also used neoadjuvant chemotherapy in a small number of cases who went on to undergo delayed primary surgery. As three pelvic relapses have been registered, pelvic radiotherapy has been added to the current protocol to reduce the risk of local relapse.

Prospective collection of data is needed with new protocols to help develop new and more effective treatments; in addition, standardizing management is key. The French National Network proposes decision-making algorithms and treatment recommendations to ensure that all SCCO patients are treated according to a standard protocol [18].

Relapsed Disease

The management of relapsed disease is often very challenging, and prolonged remissions are never achieved with second-line chemotherapy regimens usually used in small cell lung carcinomas. A number of schedules have been reported including the combination of cyclophosphamide, Adriamycin, and vincristine. There are anecdotal reports on carboplatin and paclitaxel including dose-dense regimes, and topotecan has also shown some modest activity as in small cell lung cancers. To date, no targeted therapies have been tested in SCCO. Second-line treatment is likely to achieve short remission rates, and beyond that, patients should be considered for phase I trials if they remain of good performance status [6]. The future probably requires a better understanding of the molecular drivers.

Conclusion

Even with intensive regimens, prognosis remains dismal, and despite frequent initial responses to chemotherapy, relapses are almost inevitable and tend to be refractory to second-line chemotherapy. Every case has to benefit from centralized pathological review and be presented to a tumor board. Efforts should be made to treat patients in a more homogeneous way through national and international networks. More effective therapies are urgently needed.

References

1. Dickersin GR, Kline IW, Scully RE. Small cell carcinoma of the ovary with hypercalcemia: a report of 11 cases. Cancer. 1982;49:188–97.
2. Scully RE. Small cell carcinoma of the hypercalcemic type. Int J Gynecol Pathol. 1993;12:148–52.
3. Gatta G, van der Zwan JM, Casali PG, et al.; RARECARE working group. Rare cancers are not so rare: the rare cancer burden in Europe. Eur J Cancer. 2011;47:2493–511.
4. Young RH, Oliva E, Scully RE. Small cell carcinoma of the ovary, hypercalcemic type. A clinicopathological analysis of 150 cases. Am J Surg Pathol. 1994;18:1102–16.
5. Clement PB. Selected miscellaneous ovarian lesions: small cell carcinomas, mesothelial lesions, mesenchymal and mixed neoplasms, and non-neoplastic lesions. Mod Pathol. 2005;18 Suppl 2:S113–29.
6. Reed NS, Pautier P, Avall-Lundqvist E, et al. Gynecologic Cancer InterGroup (GCIG) consensus review for ovarian small cell cancers. Int J Gynecol Cancer. 2014;24:S30–3.
7. Veras EV, Deavers MT, Silva EG, et al. Ovarian non-small cell neuroendocrine carcinoma. A clinico-pathological and immunohistochemical study of 11 cases. Am J Surg Pathol. 2007;31:774–82.
8. McCluggage WG. Ovarian neoplasms composed of small round cells: a review. Adv Anat Pathol. 2004;11:288–96.
9. Kupryjanczyk J, Dansonka-Mieszkowska A, Moes-Sosnowska J, et al. Ovarian small cell carcinoma of hypercalcemic type – evidence of germline origin and SMARCA4 gene inactivation. A pilot study. Pol J Pathol. 2013;64:238–46.
10. Foulkes WD, Clarke BA, Hasselblatt M, et al. No small surprise – small cell carcinoma of the ovary, hypercalcaemic type, is a malignant rhabdoid tumour. J Pathol. 2014;233:209–14.
11. Hasselblatt M, et al. Nonsense mutation and inactivation of SMARCA4 (BRG1) in an atypical teratoid/rhabdoid tumor showing retained SMARCB1 (INI1) expression. Am J Surg Pathol. 2011;35:933–5.
12. Schneppenheim R, et al. Germline nonsense mutation and somatic inactivation of SMARCA4/BRG1 in a family with rhabdoid tumor predisposition syndrome. Am J Hum Genet. 2010;86:279–84. Young RH, Oliva E, Scully RE. Am J Surg Pathol 18:1102–16 (1994).
13. Jelinic P, Mueller JJ, Olvera N, et al. Recurrent SMARCA4 mutations in small cell carcinoma of the ovary. Nat Genet. 2014;46:424–6.

14. Ramos P, Karnezis AN, Craig DW, et al. Small cell carcinoma of the ovary, hypercalcemic type, displays frequent inactivating germline and somatic mutations in SMARCA4. Nat Genet. 2014;46:427–9.
15. Witkowski L, Carrot-Zhang J, Albrecht S, et al. Germline and somatic SMARCA4 mutations characterize small cell carcinoma of the ovary, hypercalcemic type. Nat Genet. 2014;46:438–43.
16. Wilson BG, Roberts CW. SWI/SNF nucleosome remodellers and cancer. Nat Rev Cancer. 2011;11:481–92.
17. Hoffman GR, Rahal R, Buxton F, et al. Functional epigenetics approach identifies BRM/SMARCA2 as a critical synthetic lethal target in BRG1-deficient cancers. Proc Natl Acad Sci U S A. 2014;111:3128–33.
18. Ray-Coquard I, Weber B, Lotz JP, et al.; GINECO group. Management of rare ovarian cancers: the experience of the French website "Observatory for rare malignant tumours of the ovaries" by the GINECO group: interim analysis of the first 100 patients. Gynecol Oncol. 2010;119:53–9.
19. Bristow RE, Tomacruz RS, Armstrong DK, et al. Survival effect of maximal cytoreductive surgery for advanced ovarian carcinoma during the platinum era: a meta-analysis. J Clin Oncol. 2002;20:1248–59.
20. Senekjian EK, Weiser PA, Talerman A, et al. Vinblastine, cisplatin, cyclophosphamide, bleomycin, doxorubicin and etoposide in the treatment of small cell carcinoma of the ovary. Cancer. 1989;64:1183–7.
21. Harrison ML, Hoskins P, du Bois A, et al. Small cell of the ovary, hypercalcemic type—analysis of combined experience and recommendation for management. A GCIG study. Gynecol Oncol. 2006;100:233–8.
22. Pautier P, Ribrag V, Duvillard P, et al. Results of a prospective dose-intensive regimen in 27 patients with small cell carcinoma of the ovary of the hypercalcemic type. Ann Oncol. 2007;18:1985–9.

CPI Antony Rowe
Chippenham, UK
2017-03-29 21:20